Pediatric Sonography Review

A Q&A REVIEW FOR THE ARDMS PEDIATRIC SONOGRAPHY EXAM

Register Your Book!

It's quick and easy, and it will connect you to study alerts, expert advice, exclusive promotions, and premium content. Register toll-free by phone at 1-877-792-0005 or at DaviesPublishing.com/book-registration. It will be helpful to have the last three digits of your book's ISBN at hand. Need help? Call us toll-free between 9 AM and 5 PM Pacific time. Thank you!

To my husband, Paul
My rock, my best friend, my biggest fan, and my partner in adventure.
Your constant love and encouragement motivate me to be my best.
And to my children, Kyle and Megan.
I hope to inspire you to never stop learning, to believe that
nothing is impossible if you work hard, and to strive to do something good in the world.
You are my greatest accomplishments and I am so proud to be your Mom.

—Julie Plaugher

To my husband Ruben and children Jacniel and Sofia, for their unconditional support.
Thank you for giving me the motivation to achieve what once seemed impossible.

—Marielis Marrero Maldonado

Pediatric Sonography Review
A Q&A REVIEW FOR THE ARDMS PEDIATRIC SONOGRAPHY EXAM

Julie Plaugher, RDMS (AB)(OB/GYN)(PS)
Arnold Palmer Hospital for Children
Winnie Palmer Hospital for Women & Babies
Orlando, Florida

Marielis Marrero Maldonado, RDMS (AB)(OB/GYN)(PS)
Arnold Palmer Hospital for Children
Winnie Palmer Hospital for Women & Babies
Orlando, Florida

Editors in Chief:

Lennard D. Greenbaum, MD
Winnie Palmer Hospital for Women & Babies
Orlando, Florida

John Blake Campbell, MD
Arnold Palmer Hospital for Children & Women
Orlando, Florida

Copyright © 2023, 2020 by Davies Publishing, Inc.

All rights reserved. No part of this work may be reproduced, stored in a retrieval system, or transmitted in any form or by any means, electronic or mechanical, including photocopying, scanning, and recording, without prior written permission from the publisher.

Davies Publishing, Inc.
32 South Raymond Avenue
Pasadena, California 91105-1961
Phone 626-792-3046
Facsimile 626-792-5308
e-mail info@daviespublishing.com
www.daviespublishing.com

Michael P. Davies, Publisher

Christina J. Moose, Editorial Director
Charlene Locke, Production Manager
Janet Heard, Operations Manager
Satori Design Group, Inc., Design
Zara Jump, Illustration

Printed and bound in the United States of America

ISBN 978-0-941022-60-6

Library of Congress Cataloging-in-Publication Data

Names: Plaugher, Julie, author. | Marrero Maldonado, Marielis , author.
Title: Pediatric sonography review : a Q&A review for the ARDMS pediatric sonography exam / Julie Plaugher, Marielis Marrero Maldonado ; editors in chief, Lennard D. Greenbaum, John Blake Campbell.
Description: Pasadena, California : Davies Publishing, Inc., [2020] | Includes bibliographical references.
Identifiers: LCCN 2019019745 | ISBN 9780941022606 (pbk. : alk. paper)
Subjects: | MESH: Ultrasonography | Child | Examination Question
Classification: LCC RC78.7.U4 | NLM WN 18.2 | DDC 616.07/543--dc23
LC record available at https://lccn.loc.gov/2019019745

Reviewers

Catherine Buttermore, RDMS (AB) (OB/GYN)(PS)
Sonographer
Orlando Health
Orlando, Florida

Tara K. Cielma, BS, RDMS, RDCS, RVT, RT(S)
Lead Sonographer, Clinical Education
Department of Diagnostic Imaging and Radiology
Children's National Health System
Washington, DC

Harris L. Cohen, MD, FACR, FSRU, FAIUM, FAAP
Professor and Chair
Department of Radiology, Pediatrics and OBGYN
University of Tennessee Health Science Center
Radiologist-in-Chief
Le Bonheur Children's Hospital
Memphis, Tennessee

Michael DiPietro, MD, FAAP, FAIUM
Former John F. Holt Collegiate Professor of Radiology
Professor Emeritus, Pediatrics and Communicable Diseases
Division of Pediatric Radiology
C. S. Mott Children's Hospital
Ann Arbor, Michigan

Theresa Donovan, RDMS (AB)(OB/GYN)(PS)
Sonographer
Orlando Health
Orlando, Florida

Joanie Grzeszczak, RDMS (AB)(OB/GYN) (NE)
Arnold Palmer Hospital for Children
Winnie Palmer Hospital for Women & Babies
Orlando, Florida

Charlotte Henningsen, MS, RT(R), RDMS, RVT, FSDMS, FAIUM
Associate VP for Faculty Development in Teaching & Learning
Director and Professor – Center for Advanced Ultrasound Education
AdventHealth University
Orlando, Florida

Jason C. Hooper, BS, RDMS, RVT
Sonography Supervisor
Monroe Carell Jr. Children's Hospital
Vanderbilt University Medical Center
Nashville, Tennessee

Sara M. O'Hara, MD, FAAP, FAIUM
Chief, Section of Ultrasound
Radiologist, Department of Radiology and Medical Imaging
Cincinnati Children's Hospital Medical Center
Professor, University of Cincinnati Department of Radiology
Cincinnati, Ohio

Claudia Rumwell, RN, FSVU
Educator and Consultant in Senior Care
Coauthor, *Vascular Technology: An Illustrated Review*

Susan Raatz Stephenson, MS, MA Ed, RDMS, RVT, CIIP
Global Content Manager
Customer Education General Imaging Ultrasound
Siemens Medical Solutions USA, Inc.
Salt Lake City, Utah

Kerry E. Weinberg, PhD, MA, MPA, RT(R), RDMS, RDCS, FSDMS
Associate Professor
Program Director, Diagnostic Medical Sonography Program
School of Health Professions
Long Island University
Brooklyn, New York

Authors' Preface

PEDIATRIC SONOGRAPHY is quickly increasing in popularity as a focused discipline within the imaging spectrum. The American Registry for Diagnostic Medical Sonography (ARDMS) created the Pediatric Sonography (PS) registry exam in response to the evolving pediatric field, and testing began in 2015. While studying for the new PS exam, we realized that we had to rely solely on textbooks and saw the need for a Q&A registry review mock examination.

Combined, we have 37 years of experience in sonography, and we hope that by writing this book, we will have left a little legacy behind in the field we love so much. We knew that working at Arnold Palmer Medical Center, an imaging center accredited by the American College of Radiology, we were in the right environment to create a great teaching tool.

Our intention is to provide a review book that will serve as a comprehensive mock test covering all the clinical tasks outlined by the ARDMS for the PS registry exam—plus supporting diagrams, text to explain the answers and subtleties of the items, and clear ultrasound images. Beyond this, we wanted to provide sonographers with a tool both to introduce them to pediatric sonography and to help them expand their current knowledge.

> ***Important note:*** Although many of our colleagues have remarked on similarities between our questions and those of the actual exam, do not be misled into thinking you should memorize these questions and answers. They are here to give you practice, to teach you things you may not know, and to reveal your strengths and weaknesses so that you know where to put your energy as you prepare for the exam. They also provide a means of assessing your progress as you study.

Writing this book took a great deal of time and commitment. We were fortunate to work with exceptional mentors and would not have been able to realize our project without the help of Dr. Lennard D. Greenbaum and Dr. John B. Campbell. Their time and expertise were critical to our success, and it is an honor to have worked with them on the development of the book.

We are grateful for the pediatric radiologists of Medical Center Radiology Group: Dr. Joseph N. Foss, Dr. Susan Smith, Dr. Michael S. Gurian, Dr. Ruby Lukse, Dr. Allan S. Clayman, and Dr. Kathryn Garrett. Their willingness to help us find images, answer questions along the way, and invest their time and attention in enlightening us on a day-to-day basis is deeply appreciated.

We would also like to thank our manager, Larry C. Simmons, and our supervisor, Olga A. Rasmussen, for their guidance, support, and understanding. We truly appreciate Catherine C. Buttermore, RDMS, and Theresa M. Donovan, RDMS, for dedicating personal time to providing valuable feedback and suggestions as well as notes of encouragement and images for our use. A special expression of gratitude goes out to a host of other colleagues and coworkers for their patience with us during this process and for the quality of the images they helped provide for this book: Brianna Arellano, RDMS, RVT; Jennifer Astor, RDMS; Allison G. Bastian, RDMS; Brittni J. Rivera, RDMS; Edwin Cosme, RDMS; Sandra Dahlstrom, RDMS; Jennifer Deckman, RDMS;

Lexi Furukawa, RDMS, RVT; Stacey L. Garcia, RDMS; Gabrielle Green, RDMS; Joanie Grzeszczak, RDMS; Marie C. Irving, RDMS; Natasha L. Johnson, RDMS; Esta Manso, RDMS; Mindee Mulharan, RDMS; Kiarisel M. Newell Diaz, RDMS, RVT; Cristina Pozdoll, RDMS; Samantha N. Smith, RDMS; Janet Chernow Wenger, RDMS; and Lauren C. Wood, RDMS.

Many thanks to Zara Jump, who not only provided detailed and original illustrations for us but also managed to do so while preparing for her first year of college. We are grateful for the opportunity Davies Publishing gave us to publish this book and appreciate the personal assistance from Michael Davies, Christina Moose, and Charlene Locke during the process.

We want to thank our families for their unwavering support, care, and patience during our year of writing and research. You cheered us on and helped us stay focused. Thank you for understanding our passion for this project and providing the momentum to bring it to a reality.

Finally, you—the budding or cross-training pediatric sonographer—have not only our best wishes for success but also our admiration for taking this big and important step in your career!

Julie Plaugher
Julie Plaugher, RDMS

Marielis Marrero Maldonado
Marielis Marrero Maldonado, RDMS

Publisher's Note

THIS MOCK EXAM is a question/answer/reference review of Pediatric Sonography for those candidates who plan to take the specialty examination for the Registered Diagnostic Medical Sonographer (RDMS) credential, administered by the American Registry for Diagnostic Medical Sonography (ARDMS). It is designed as an adjunct to your regular study and as a means of helping you determine your strengths and weaknesses so that you can study more effectively. This mock exam is also considered a CME activity; an SDMS-approved CME quiz worth 12 credits will be found in Part 20 of this book.

Facts about *Pediatric Sonography Review*

- This mock exam covers the material on the ARDMS exam content outline in effect as of 2019. Readers are advised to check the ARDMS website, www.ardms.org, for the latest updates. The mock exam itself is continuously updated and revised as necessary, and readers can check Davies' website for the latest Study Alerts and other product updates at http://www.daviespublishing.com/Product-Updates-C220.aspx.

- The mock exam focuses exclusively on the PS specialty exam to ensure thorough coverage of even the smallest subtopic on the exam. (For those preparing for the Sonography Principles and Instrumentation exam, see Davies' *Ultrasound Physics Review: SPI Edition*, available in both print and interactive formats at www.daviespublishing.com.)

- In preparing this mock exam, the authors have referred to the current ARDMS content outline as a guideline for coverage. At the same time, they have organized the content using a comprehensive, subject-driven approach to ensure that all important topics are fully addressed. The ARDMS exam content outline provides a generalized categorical overview together with very specific clinical tasks, but it can omit and assume the mastery of key intermediate topics you must know to pass the examination. Hence this hybrid approach gives you the best of both worlds.

- This mock exam contains 623 questions, many of which are accompanied by sonographic and other images, anatomic illustrations, and schematics—more than 250 in all.

- The answer key located in Part 19 contains not only the answers but also concise explanations that are abundant, clear, and authoritatively referenced for further study. We recommend that you have a standard pediatric ultrasound review text at your side when using this mock exam to study for the PS exam; you will see several of these referenced in the answer section and the "Suggested Readings" in Part 21.

- This mock examination has been approved by the Society of Diagnostic Medical Sonography (SDMS) as a CME activity. A CME application form, quiz, and full submission instructions are included in Part 20. Passing this quiz will qualify the applicant for 12 CME credits. A modest administrative processing fee applies at the time of submission, and more than one sonographer may use the forms to complete this activity for CME credit. These credits are accepted by ARDMS, its companion council the Alliance for Physician Certification and Advancement (APCA), the American Registry of Radiologic Technologists (ARRT), and other organizations toward meeting their CME requirements. Some credentials carry stipulations regarding specialty areas in which CME credits may be earned. Always check with the organization that governs your credential(s). All the credits in this activity may be applied to maintain the ARDMS PS credential.

▸ The expanded ARDMS exam content outline appears in Part 22. Under each task we have indexed mock exam questions related to that task, for your convenience in targeting your study on specific exam topics.

ARDMS Advanced Item Type (AIT) Questions

All the ARDMS exams now include Advanced Item Type (AIT) questions that assess practical sonography instrumentation skills. For the PS specialty exam, these AIT questions include what ARDMS calls "Hotspot" questions. Hotspot items display an image with the question and ask you to indicate the correct answer by marking directly on the image using your cursor. (To learn how to use the interface during the exam you can visit a handy YouTube video posted by ARDMS.) This type of question is called "advanced" because it involves a higher level of thinking and processing than you perform when answering a conventional multiple-choice question. In Davies' mock exam, similar questions are identified as "AIT—Hotspot" questions. These items ask you to identify what an arrow in the image is pointing at or to indicate the label on an image that corresponds to the correct answer.

Another type of AIT question, the Semi-Interactive Console (SIC) item, requires the examinee to use a semi-interactive console to correct a problem with the image presented. Currently these items do not appear on the PS exam, but as a bonus feature we have identified similar items as "AIT—SIC" questions.

Finally, PACSim items—case-based Picture Archive and Communication Simulation questions—are not included in this PS mock exam because currently this type of question is limited to the Ob/Gyn exam and the Physician in Vascular Interpretation (PVI) exam.

How to Use This Mock Exam

Pediatric Sonography Review effectively simulates the content of the PS exam. Current ARDMS standards call for 170 multiple-choice questions to be answered during a three-hour period. That is, you will have an average time of approximately one minute to answer each question. Timing your practice sessions according to the number of questions you need to finish will help you prepare for the pressure experienced by PS candidates taking this exam. It also helps to ensure that your practice scores accurately reflect your strengths and weaknesses so that you can study more efficiently in the limited time you are able to devote to preparation.

ARDMS test results are reported as a "scaled" score that ranges from a minimum of 300 to a maximum of 700. A scaled score of 555 is the passing score—the "passpoint" or "cutoff score" for all ARDMS examinations. Also known as the Angoff method, scaled scoring takes the difficulty of each question into account, which helps ensure the fairness of the exam.

We include below and strongly recommend that you read *Taking and Passing Your Exam*, by Don Ridgway, RVT, who offers practical tips for passing the ARDMS examinations.

Taking and Passing Your Exam

by Don Ridgway, RVT[*]

Preparing for Your Exam . . .

Study. And then study some more. Knowing your stuff is the most important factor in your success. Start early, set a regular study schedule, and stick to it. Make your schedule specific so you know exactly what to study on a particular day. Write it down. Establish realistic goals so that you don't build a mountain you can't climb.

As to what you study, don't just read aimlessly. Focus your efforts on what you need to know. Rely on a core group of dependable references, referring to others as necessary to firm up your understanding of specific topics. Let the ARDMS exam outline guide you. And use different but complementary study methods—texts, flashcards, and mock exams—to exercise those neural pathways.

Ease down on studying the week before. Wind down, reduce stress, build confidence, and rest up. Don't cram! And no studying the night before. You had your chance. Watch a movie, relax, go to bed early, and sleep well.

Organize your things the night before. Lay out comfortable clothes (including a sweater or sweatshirt in case the testing center is cold), your photo ID, car and house keys, glasses, prescriptions, directions to the test center, and any other personal items you might need. Remember that the only thing you can take into the testing room is you—there will be lockers for your personal items. Read about necessary documentation and examination admission compliance requirements for your exam at www.ardms.org. Be prepared!

The Day of Your Exam . . .

Eat lightly. You do not want to fall asleep during the exam. Go easy on the coffee or tea so your bladder doesn't distract you halfway through the exam.

Arrive early. Plan to arrive at the test center early, especially if you haven't been there before. Take directions, including the telephone number of the testing center in case you have to make contact en route. You don't need a wrong-offramp adventure.

Be confident. As you wait for the exam to begin, smile, lift both hands, wave them toward yourself, and say, "Bring it on."

---

[*]Don Ridgway is the author of *Introduction to Vascular Scanning: A Guide for the Complete Beginner* and editor of *Vascular Technology Review*. He is Professor Emeritus at Grossmont College in El Cajon, California.

During the Exam . . .

Read each question twice before answering. Guess how easy it is to get one word wrong and misunderstand the whole question!

Try to answer the question before looking at the choices. Formulating an answer before peeking at the possibilities minimizes the distraction of the incorrect answer choices, which in the test-making business are called—guess what?—distractors.

Knock off the easy ones first. First answer the questions you feel good about. Then go back for the more difficult items. Next, attack the really tough ones. Taking notes on long or tricky questions often can jog your memory or put the question in new light. For questions you just cannot answer with certainty, eliminate the obviously wrong answer choices and then guess.

Guessing. Passing the exam depends on the number of correct answers you make. Because unanswered questions are counted as incorrect, it makes sense to guess when all else fails. The ARDMS itself advises that it is to the candidate's advantage to answer all questions. Guessing alone improves your chances of scoring a point from zero (for an unanswered question) to 25% (for randomly picking one of four possible answers). Eliminating answer choices you know or suspect are wrong further improves your odds of success. For example, by using your knowledge and skill to eliminate two of the four answer choices before guessing, you increase your odds of scoring a point to 50%.

Pace yourself; watch the time. Work methodically and quickly to answer those you know, and make your best guesses at the gnarly ones. Leave no question unanswered.

Don't despair 50 minutes into the exam. At some point you may feel that things just aren't going well. Take 10 seconds to breathe deeply—in for a count of five, out for a count of five. Relax. Recall that you need to get only about three out of four answers correct to pass. If you've prepared reasonably well, a passing score is attainable even if you feel sweat running down your back.

Taking the Exam on Computer . . .

Some candidates express concern about taking the registry exam on a computer. Most folks find this to be pretty easy; some find it offputting, at least in prospect. But the computerized exams are quite convenient: You know whether or not you passed before you leave the testing center (compare that to waiting weeks and even months, as used to be the case), and if you don't pass the exam the first time, you can usually take it again after a few months. Another advantage: The illustrations are said to be clearer on computer than in the booklets at a Scantron-type exam.

Taking the test on computer is not complicated. The test center even has a tutorial to be sure you know what you need to do. You sit in a carrel with a computer and answer the multiple-choice questions by pointing and clicking with a mouse. There is a clock on the display letting you know how much time is left. Use it to pace yourself. A white board (today's equivalent of scratch paper) is available upon request, and it's a good idea to have one at your side for notes. You can mark questions for answering later. A display shows which questions have not been answered so you can return to them. When you have finished, you click on "DONE," and you find out immediately whether you passed.

It's nothing to be afraid of. The principles are the same as those for any exam. Be methodical and keep breathing.

Summary...

Preparing for the exam:
- Study.
- Use flashcards.
- Join a study group.
- Wind down a week before.
- Don't cram.
- Relax!

The day of your exam:
- Eat lightly; avoid too much caffeine.
- Arrive early.
- Take a sweater.
- Be confident!

During the exam:
- Read each question twice.
- Answer the question before looking at the answer choices.
- Answer the easy ones first.
- Guess when necessary.
- Pace yourself.
- Don't despair.

Taking the exam on computer:
- Just point and click.
- Take notes.
- Mark and return to the hard questions.
- Use the onscreen clock to pace yourself.
- Be methodical.
- Breathe!

Contents

Reviewers   v
Authors' Preface   vii
Publisher's Note   ix
Taking and Passing Your Exam   xi
Color Plates   xxiii

PART 1   Head   1

 Embryology and development

 Normal anatomy
  Newborn skull
  Brain lobes
  Ventricular system
  Posterior fossa
  Choroid plexus
  Cavum septi pellucidi
  Corpus callosum
  Basal ganglia
  Circle of Willis
  Tentorium cerebelli
  Massa intermedia
  Cerebral peduncles
  Middle cerebral artery
  Ependyma
  White matter
  Gray matter

 Associated lab values and hormones

 Ultrasound prep and protocol

 Normal ultrasound appearance

 Pathology
  Congenital
   Chiari malformation
   Dandy-Walker complex
   Holoprosencephaly
   Schizencephaly

  Lissenecephaly
  Hydranencephaly
  Agenesis of the corpus callosum
  Absent septum pellucidum
  Colpocephaly
  Septo-optic dysplasia
Obstruction abnormalities
  Congenital aqueductal stenosis
  Hydrocephalus
Cystic abnormalities
  Arachnoid cyst
  Choroid plexus cyst
  Connatal cyst
  Subependymal cyst
  Porencephaly
  Cystic encephalomalacia
Solid masses
  Benign
   Cerebellar astrocytoma
   Choroid plexus papilloma
  Malignant
   Ependymoma
   Glioma
Infection and inflammation
  TORCH infections
  Meningitis
Vascular abnormalities
  Intracranial hemorrhage
  Extracranial hemorrhage
  Vein of Galen malformation
  Lenticulostriatal vasculopathy
Injury and trauma
  Hypoxic-ischemic event
  Periventricular leukomalacia
  Caput succedaneum
  Hematoma
   Cephalohematoma
   Subgaleal hematoma
   Epidural hematoma
   Subdural hematoma
Diseases and syndromes
Miscellaneous

Procedures
 Extracorporeal membrane oxygenation (ECMO)

PART 2 Spine   27

    Embryology and development

    Normal anatomy
        Spinal cord
        Conus medullaris
        Filum terminale
        Cauda equina
        Ventriculus terminalis

    Associated lab values and hormones
        Alpha-fetoprotein

    Ultrasound prep and protocol

    Normal ultrasound appearance

    Pathology
        Congenital
            Filar cyst
            Spinal dysraphism
                Non–skin-covered
                Skin-covered
                Occulta
                Tethered cord
                Caudal regression syndrome
                Diastematomyelia
                Sacrococcygeal teratoma
        Obstruction abnormalities
        Cystic abnormalities
            Syringomyelia
            Hydromyelia
            Syringohydromyelia
        Solid masses
            Benign
                Lipoma
            Malignant
                Sacrococcygeal teratoma
        Infection and inflammation
        Vascular abnormalities
        Injury and trauma
            Cord compression
            Cord displacement
        Diseases and syndromes
        Miscellaneous
            Pseudomass
            Pilonidal sinus

    Procedures
        Lumbar puncture

PART 3 Neck and Face 37

Embryology and development
Normal anatomy
Salivary glands
- Parotid
- Submandibular
- Sublingual

Thyroid gland
Parathyroid glands

Associated lab values and hormones
Thyroid-stimulating hormone (TSH)
Parathyroid hormone (PTH)

Ultrasound prep and protocol
Normal ultrasound appearance
Pathology
Congenital
- Branchial cleft anomaly
- Lymphangiomas
- Fibromatosis colli

Obstruction abnormalities
Cystic abnormalities
- Ranula
- Duplication cyst
- Thyroglossal duct cyst

Solid masses
- Benign
  - Colloid follicles
  - Thyroid nodules
  - Thyroid adenoma
  - Parathyroid adenoma
- Malignant
  - Papillary thyroid carcinoma
  - Follicular carcinoma

Infection and inflammation
- Parotitis
- Lymphadenopathy

Vascular abnormalities
- Hemangioma

Injury and trauma
Diseases and syndromes
- Hashimoto's thyroiditis
- Graves' disease
- Primary hyperparathyroidism
- Secondary hyperparathyroidism

Miscellaneous
   Sialolithiasis
   Goiter

Procedures
  Biopsies
  Percutaneous drainage

PART 4   Chest   49

Embryology and development

Normal anatomy
  Thymus
  Diaphragm
  Pleura

Associated lab values and hormones

Ultrasound prep and protocol

Normal ultrasound appearance

Pathology
  Congenital
    Congenital pulmonary airway malformation (CPAM)
    Bronchopulmonary sequestration
    Bochdalek hernia
    Morgagni hernia
  Obstruction abnormalities
  Cystic abnormalities
  Solid masses
    Benign
      Thymoma
    Malignant
      Lymphoma
  Infection and inflammation
    Lung consolidation
  Vascular abnormalities
  Injury and trauma
    Diaphragmatic paralysis
  Miscellaneous
    Pleural effusion
    Atelectasis
    Gastroesophageal reflux

Procedures
  Thoracentesis

PART 5 Liver 55

Embryology and development

Normal anatomy
- *Segments*
- *Lobes*
- *Bile ducts*
- *Hepatic veins*
- *Portal veins*
- *Hepatic artery*

Associated lab values and hormones
- *Alanine transaminase (ALT)*
- *Aspartate transaminase (AST)*
- *Alkaline phosphatase (ALP)*
- *Albumin*
- *Bilirubin*

Ultrasound prep and protocol

Normal ultrasound appearance

Pathology
- *Congenital*
  - Hepatic fibrosis
- *Obstructive abnormalities*
- *Cystic abnormalities*
  - Liver cysts
  - Polycystic liver
- *Solid masses*
  - Benign
    - *Hemangiomas*
    - *Hemangioendothelioma*
    - *Adenomas*
    - *Mesenchymal hamartomas*
    - *Focal nodular hyperplasia*
  - Malignant
    - *Hepatoblastoma*
    - *Hepatocellular carcinoma*
    - *Undifferentiated embryonal sarcoma*
    - *Metastases*
- *Infection and inflammation*
  - Liver abscesses
  - Granuloma
- *Vascular abnormalities*
  - Budd-Chiari
  - Portal vein hypertension
  - Portosystemic collaterals
  - Portal vein thrombosis

Cavernous transformation of the portal vein
Veno-occlusive disease
Arteriovenous malformations
Injury and trauma
Hematomas
Diseases and syndromes
Hepatitis
Cirrhosis
Miscellaneous
Steatosis
Hepatomegaly
Portal venous gas

Procedures
Liver transplant
Biopsies
Percutaneous drainage
Elastography

PART 6   Gallbladder and Biliary Ducts   71

Embryology and development

Normal anatomy
Segments
Bile ducts

Associated lab values and hormones
Direct bilirubin
Indirect bilirubin
Alkaline phosphatase (ALP)

Ultrasound prep and protocol

Normal ultrasound appearance

Pathology
Congenital
Biliary atresia
Obstructive abnormalities
Choledocholithiasis
Jaundice
Cystic abnormalities
Choledochal cyst
Solid masses
Benign
Polyps
Malignant
Rhabdomyosarcoma

  Infection and inflammation
   Cholecystitis
   Cholangitis
  Vascular abnormalities
  Injury and trauma
  Diseases and syndromes
   Caroli disease
   Alagille syndrome
  Miscellaneous
   Gallbladder hydrops
   Air in the gallbladder
   Cholelithiasis
   Biliary sludge
 Procedures
  Endoscopic retrograde cholangiopancreatography (ERCP)
  Kasai procedure

PART 7 **Pancreas** 85

 Embryology and development

 Normal anatomy
  Segments
  Ducts
  Vascular landmarks

 Associated lab values and hormones
  Exocrine
  Endocrine

 Ultrasound prep and protocol

 Normal ultrasound appearance

 Pathology
  Congenital
   Congenital cysts
   Annular pancreas
   Pancreatic divisum
   Ectopic pancreas
   Congenital hyperinsulinism/nesidioblastosis
  Obstruction abnormalities
  Cystic abnormalities
   Pseudocyst
  Solid masses
   Benign
    Insulinoma
    Lymphangioma

      Malignant
         Adenocarcinoma
         Pancreatoblastoma
    Infection and inflammation
      Pancreatitis
    Vascular abnormalities
    Injury and trauma
    Diseases and syndromes
      Cystic fibrosis
      Schwachman-Diamond syndrome
    Miscellaneous

Procedures
    Endoscopic retrograde cholangiopancreatography (ERCP)
    Percutaneous drainage

PART 8   Spleen   95

Embryology and development

Normal anatomy

Associated lab values and hormones

Ultrasound prep and protocol

Normal ultrasound appearance

Pathology
    Congenital
      Polysplenia
      Asplenia
      Accessory spleen
      Wandering spleen
    Obstruction abnormalities
      Splenic vein thrombosis
    Cystic abnormalities
      Splenic cysts
    Solid masses
      Benign
         Lymphangioma
         Hemangioma
      Malignant
         Lymphoma
    Infection and inflammation
      Abscesses
    Vascular abnormalities
      Infarct
      Sequestration

Injury and trauma
    Hematomas
    Rupture/splenosis
Diseases and syndromes
    Sickle cell disease
Miscellaneous
    Calcifications
    Splenomegaly

Procedures
  Biopsies
  Percutaneous drainage

PART 9   Urinary Tract   101

Embryology and development

Normal anatomy
  Kidneys
  Ureters
  Bladder
  Vasculature

Associated lab values and hormones
  Blood urea nitrogen (BUN)
  Creatinine (CR)
  BUN/CR ratio

Ultrasound prep and protocol

Normal ultrasound appearance

Pathology
  Congenital
    Lobulated kidney
    Hypertrophied column of Bertin
    Junctional parenchymal defect of the kidney
    Dromedary hump
    Renal hypoplasia
    Renal agenesis
    Renal ectopia
    Horseshoe kidney
    Crossed-fused renal ectopia
    Duplex kidney
    Medullary sponge kidney
    Multicystic dysplastic kidney
    Polycystic kidney disease
    Ectopic ureter
    Vesicoureteral reflux
    Bladder exstrophy

    Posterior urethral valves
    Urachal abnormalities
    Cloacal anomalies
Obstruction abnormalities
    Hydronephrosis
    Megaureter
    Ureteropelvic junction obstruction
    Megacystis
Cystic abnormalities
    Renal cyst
    Ureterocele
Solid masses
    Benign
        Angiomyolipoma
        Mesoblastic nephroma
        Cystic nephroma
        Bladder diverticula
    Malignant
        Wilms tumor
        Renal cell carcinoma
        Lymphoma
        Nephroblastomatosis
        Rhabdoid tumors
Infection and inflammation
    Pyelonephritis
    Pyonephritis
    Pyonephrosis
    Xanthogranulomatous pyelonephritis
    Fungal infections
    Glomerulonephritis
Vascular abnormalities
    Renal vein thrombosis
    Renal artery stenosis
    Renal artery pseudoaneurysm
    Acute tubular necrosis
Injury and trauma
    Urinoma
    Fractured kidney
    Shattered kidney
Diseases and syndromes
    Eagle-Barrett syndrome
    Tuberous sclerosis
    Von Hippel–Lindau syndrome
    Acute renal failure
    Chronic renal failure

Miscellaneous
  Nephrocalcinosis
  Urolithiasis
  Neurogenic bladder
Procedures
  Biopsies
  Percutaneous drainage
  Renal transplant

PART 10 Adrenal Glands   127

Embryology and development

Normal anatomy

Associated lab values and hormones
  Cortisol
  Aldosterone
  Catecholamines

Ultrasound prep and protocol

Normal ultrasound appearance

Pathology
  Congenital
    Congenital adrenal hyperplasia
  Obstruction abnormalities
  Cystic abnormalities
  Solid masses
    Benign
      Pheochromocytoma
    Malignant
      Neuroblastoma
      Adrenocortical tumors
      Ganglioneuroblastoma
  Infection and inflammation
  Vascular abnormalities
  Injury and inflammation
    Adrenal hemorrhage
    Abscess
  Diseases and syndromes
    Wolman disease
    Cushing disease
  Miscellaneous

Procedures
  Biopsies
  Percutaneous drainage

PART 11 GI Tract and Mesentery 135

Embryology and development

Normal anatomy

Esophagus

Stomach

Small intestine

Large intestine

Appendix

Omentum

Mesentery

Associated lab values and hormones

Ultrasound prep and protocol

Normal ultrasound appearance

Pathology

Congenital

   Hypertrophic pyloric stenosis

   Duodenal atresia

   Midgut malrotation

   Imperforate anus

Obstruction abnormalities

   Volvulus

   Bezoars

   Intussusception

      Small bowel

      Large bowel

Cystic abnormalities

   Duplication cysts

Solid masses

   Benign

      Polyps

   Malignant

      Lymphoma

Infection and inflammation

   Appendicitis

   Necrotizing enterocolitis

Vascular abnormalities

   Median arcuate ligament syndrome (MALS)

Injury and trauma

Diseases and syndromes

   Crohn disease

   Hirschsprung disease

Miscellaneous

   Meckel's diverticulum

   Pylorospasm

Procedures

Air reduction enema

PART 12 Pediatric Hip   145
- **Embryology and development**
- **Normal anatomy**
- **Associated lab values and hormones**
- **Ultrasound prep and protocol**
- **Normal ultrasound appearance**
- **Pathology**
  - *Congenital*
    - Developmental dysplasia of the hip
  - *Obstruction abnormalities*
  - *Cystic abnormalities*
  - *Solid masses*
    - Benign
    - Malignant
  - *Infection and inflammation*
    - Transient synovitis
    - Osteomyelitis
    - Hip effusion
  - *Vascular abnormalities*
    - Avascular necrosis
  - *Injury and trauma*
  - *Diseases and syndromes*
    - Proximal femoral focal deficiency (PFFD)
  - *Miscellaneous*
- **Procedures**
  - Percutaneous drainage

PART 13 Female Pelvis   155
- **Embryology and development**
- **Normal anatomy**
  - *Uterus*
  - *Ovaries*
  - *Fallopian tubes*
- **Associated lab values and hormones**
  - *Estrogen*
  - *Progesterone*
  - *Follicle-stimulating hormone (FSH)*
  - *Luteinizing hormone (LH)*
  - *Alpha-fetoprotein (AFP)*
- **Ultrasound prep and protocol**
- **Normal ultrasound appearance**

Pathology
- *Congenital*
  - Müllerian anomalies
- *Obstruction abnormalities*
  - Hydrocolpos
  - Hematocolpos
  - Hydrometrocolpos
  - Hematometrocolpos
- *Cystic abnormalities*
  - Gartner's duct cyst
  - Peritoneal inclusion cyst
  - Ovarian cysts
    - *Follicular cyst*
    - *Corpus luteal cyst*
    - *Hemorrhagic cyst*
    - *Paraovarian cyst*
- Solid masses
  - Benign
    - *Dermoid/teratoma*
    - *Cystadenoma*
  - Malignant
    - *Rhabdomyosarcoma*
    - *Dysgerminoma*
    - *Malignant dermoid/teratoma*
    - *Endodermal sinus tumor*
    - *Granulosa cell tumor*
    - *Sertoli-Leydig tumor*
- *Infection and inflammation*
  - Pelvic inflammatory disease (PID)
  - Hydrosalpinx
  - Pyosalpinx
  - Tubo-ovarian abscess
  - Tubo-ovarian complex
- *Vascular abnormalities*
  - Torsion
- *Injury and trauma*
- *Diseases and syndromes*
  - Polycystic ovary syndrome (PCOS)
  - Gonadal dysgenesis
  - Intersex disorders
- *Miscellaneous*
  - Precocious puberty
  - Amenorrhea

Procedures
- *Biopsies*
- *Percutaneous drainage*

PART 14   **Male Pelvis, Scrotum, and Testes**   167

    Embryology and development
    Normal anatomy
      Scrotum
      Testes
    Associated lab values and hormones
      Testosterone
    Ultrasound prep and protocol
    Normal ultrasound appearance
    Pathology
      Congenital
        Cryptorchidism
        Anorchidism
        Monorchidism
        Appendix testis
        Hypospadias
        True hermaphroditism
      Obstruction abnormalities
      Cystic abnormalities
        Epididymal cyst
        Seminoma
      Solid masse
        Benign
          Leydig cell tumor
          Sertoli cell tumor
          Benign teratoma
        Malignant
          Gonadoblastoma
      Infection and inflammation
        Orchitis
        Epididymitis
      Vascular abnormalities
        Testicular torsion
        Torsion of the appendix testis
        Varicocele
      Injury and trauma
        Testicular rupture
      Miscellaneous
        Hydrocele
        Microlithiasis
    Procedures
      Biopsies
      Percutaneous drainage

PART 15 **Soft Tissue**   181

Normal ultrasound appearance
Dermis
Subcutaneous tissue
Fascia
Muscle
Joints

Use of the standoff pad

Imaging the contralateral side

Pathology
Congenital
  Hernia
Cystic abnormalities
  Popliteal cyst
  Ganglion cyst
  Pilonidal cyst
Solid mass
  Lipoma
Infection and injury
  Cellulitis
  Abscess
  Lymphadenopathy
  Hematoma
  Sports injury
Vascular abnormalities
  Hemangiomas
Miscellaneous
  Foreign bodies

PART 16 **Vasculature of the Extremities**   189

Normal anatomy
Upper extremity
Lower extremity
Superficial venous system
Deep venous system

Pathology
Deep venous thrombosis (DVT)
Arteriovenous malformation (AVM)
Arteriovenous fistula

PART 17 Physics and Instrumentation   193

    Transducer selection

    Image optimization

    Harmonics

    M-mode imaging

    3D/4D imaging

    Doppler imaging
- *Color Doppler*
- *Power Doppler*
- *Spectral Doppler*

    Artifacts
- *Gray-scale artifacts*
- *Color Doppler artifacts*
- *Spectral Doppler artifacts*

PART 18 Patient Care and Management   199

    Patient communication

    Physician communication

    Reporting and archiving

    Sterile procedure

    Infection control

PART 19 Answers, Explanations, and References   203

PART 20 Application for CME Credit   569

PART 21 Suggested Readings   605

PART 22 ARDMS Exam Content Outline: Tasks Cross-Referenced to Mock Exam Questions   607

Don't Forget to Register Your Book!

Register your book to get connected to study alerts, expert advice, exclusive promotions, and premium content. It's quick and easy! Register toll-free by phone at 1-877-792-0005 or at DaviesPublishing.com/book-registration. It will be helpful to have the last three digits of your book's ISBN at hand. Need help? Call us toll-free between 9 AM and 5 PM Pacific time. Thank you!

Color Plates

We have included this section of color images to enhance the black-and-white versions used with some of the questions and answers in this mock exam. These images go with the questions and/or answers referenced below, and you will see that the questions and answers also include a cross-reference to the color versions of the images that appear here. For fuller information, we encourage you to refer to the image in the context of its question as well as its corresponding answer in Part 19, "Answers, Explanations, and References."

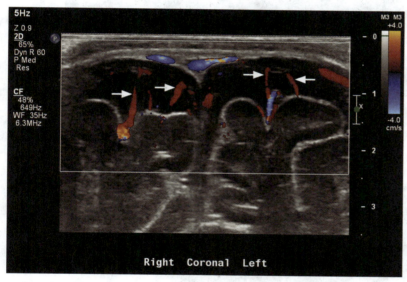

Color Plate 1 (page 21, question 61, and page 239, answer 61)

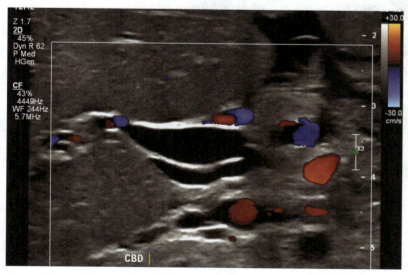

Color Plate 2 (page 73, question 218, and page 329, answer 218)

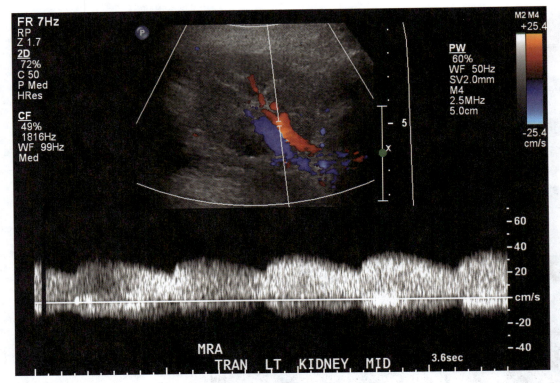

Color Plate 3 (page 126, question 390, and page 423, answer 390)

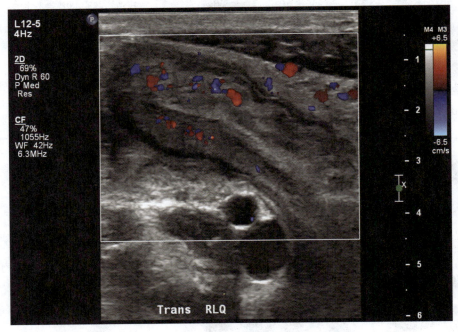

Color Plate 4 (page 136, question 419, and pages 439–440, answer 419)

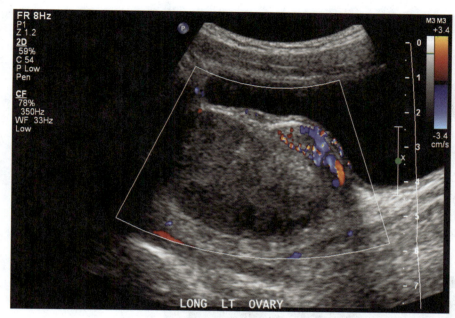

Color Plate 5 (pages 159–160, question 499, and pages 490–491, answer 499)

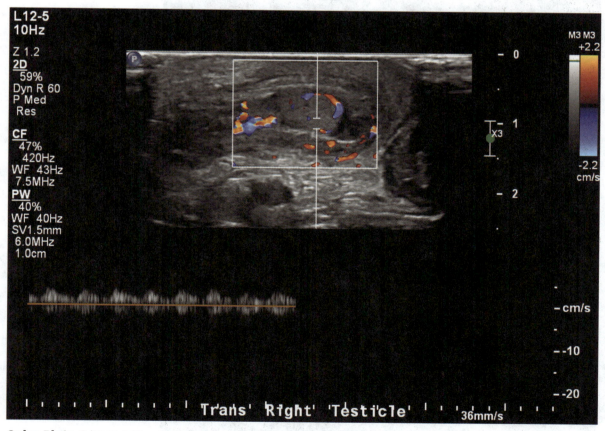

Color Plate 6 (page 168, question 525, and page 506, answer 525, image A)

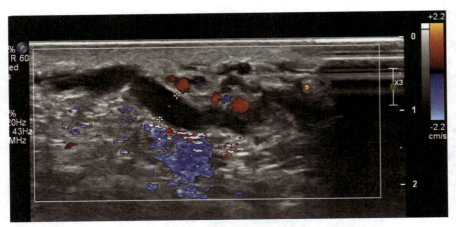

Color Plate 7 (page 174, question 540, and pages 517–518, answer 540)

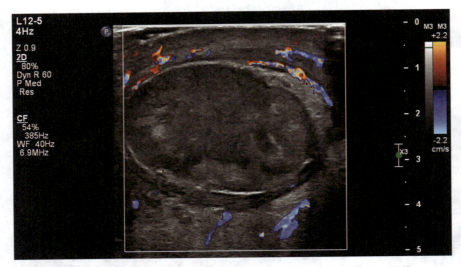

Color Plate 8 (page 177, question 552, and pages 523–524, answer 552)

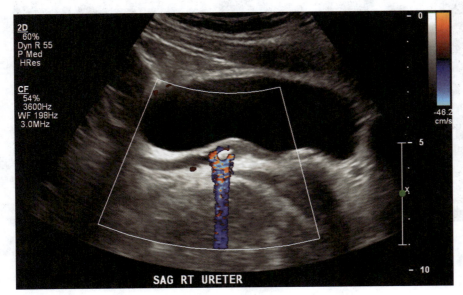

Color Plate 9 (page 197, question 607, pages 400–401, answer 354, and page 557, answer 607)

Pediatric Sonography Review

Ventricles of the Brain

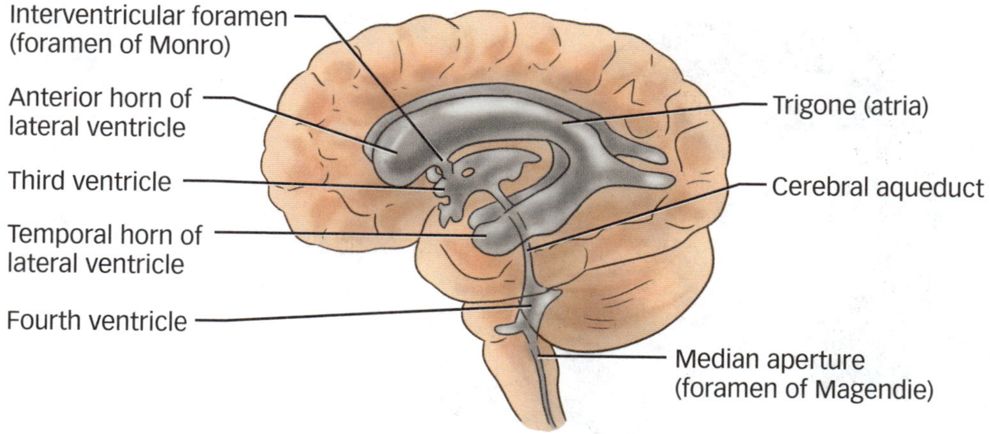

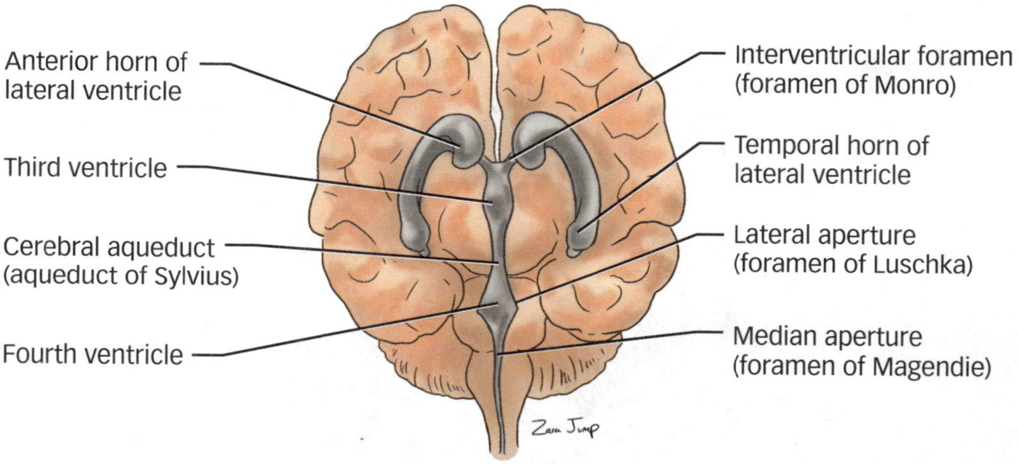

Locations of Hemorrhaging in the Skull

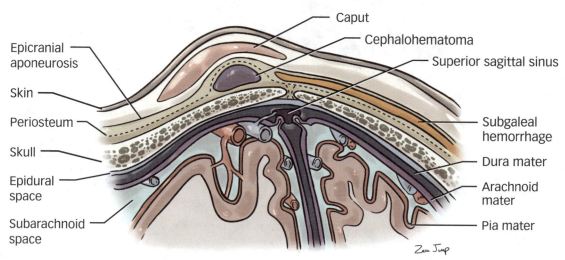

Color Plate 10 (pages 204–205, answer 2; page 207, answer 7; and page 244, answer 71)

Color Plate 11 (pages 215–216, answer 21; pages 218–219, answer 25; page 223, answer 33; page 224, answer 35; pages 227–228, answer 41; and page 239, answer 61)

The Salivary Glands

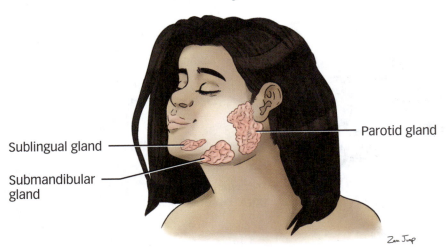

Color Plate 12 (page 267, answer 103; pages 268–269, answer 105; page 272, answer 112; page 277, answer 122; and page 284, answer 135)

The Abdominal Vasculature

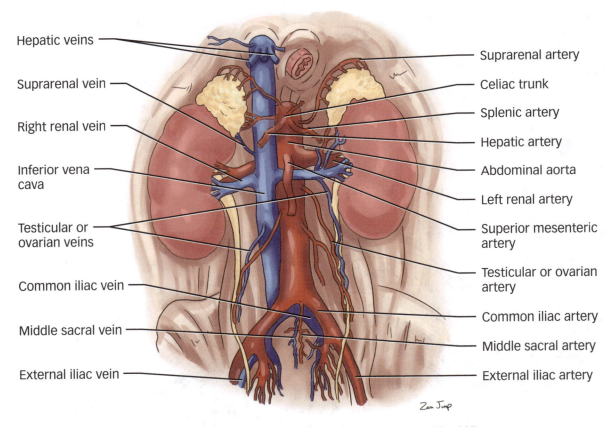

Color Plate 13 (pages 296–297, answer 158; page 302, answer 169; pages 306–307, answer 177; page 382, answer 320; and page 505, answer 523)

The Biliary Tree

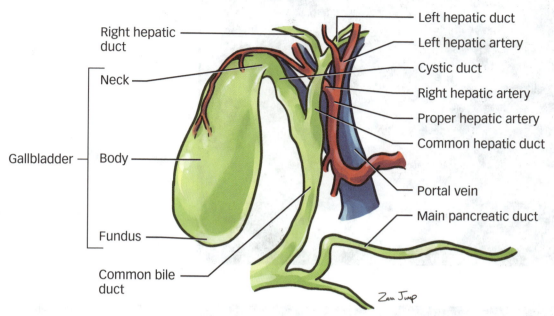

Color Plate 14 (page 305, answer 175; page 318, answer 198; page 336, answer 234; and page 341, answer 243)

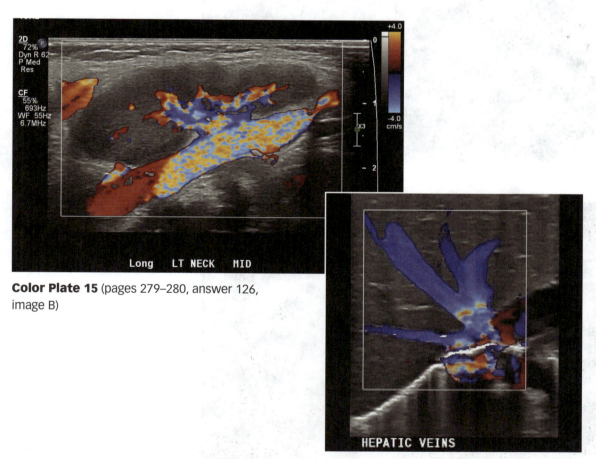

Color Plate 15 (pages 279–280, answer 126, image B)

Color Plate 16 (pages 306–307, answer 177, image B)

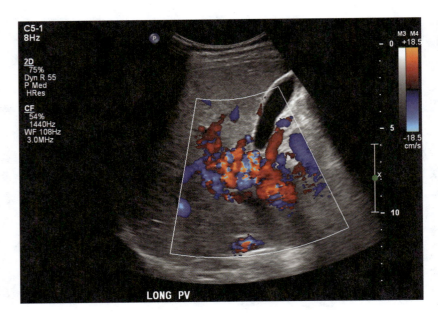

Color Plate 17 (pages 313–314, answer 190, image B)

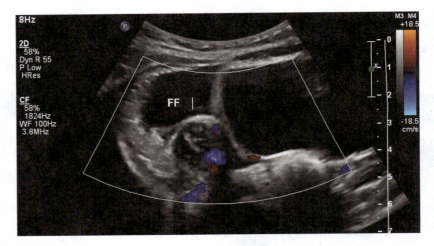

Color Plate 18 (pages 314–315, answer 192, image A)

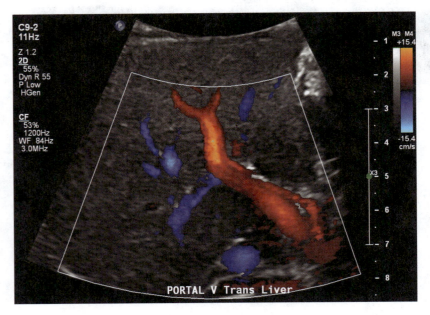

Color Plate 19 (page 324, answer 208, image B)

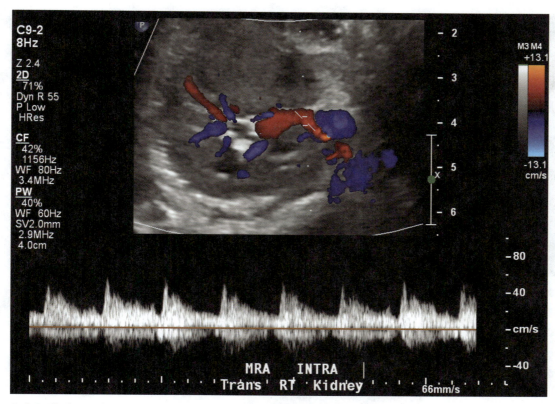

Color Plate 20 (pages 378–379, answer 314, image A)

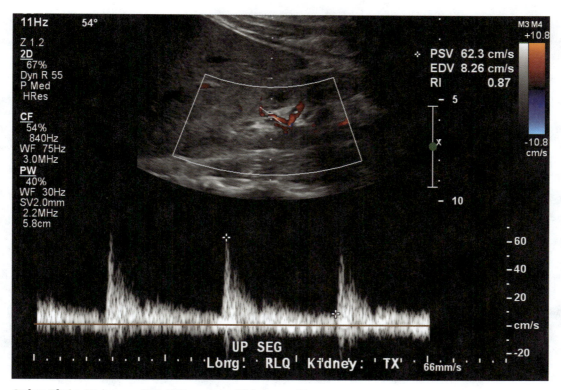

Color Plate 21 (pages 378–379, answer 314, image B)

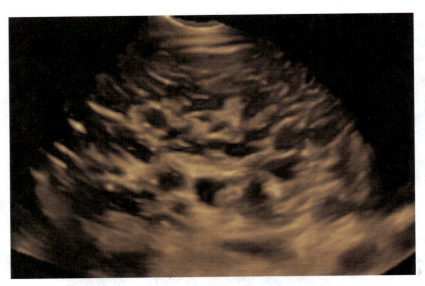

Color Plate 22 (pages 409–411, answer 369, image C)

Vasculature of the Kidney

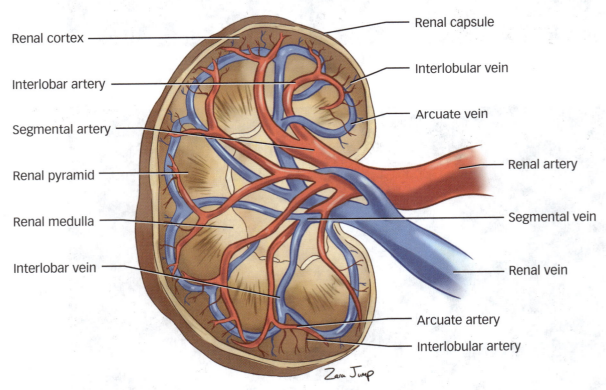

Color Plate 23 (page 422, answer 389)

The Gastrointestinal Tract

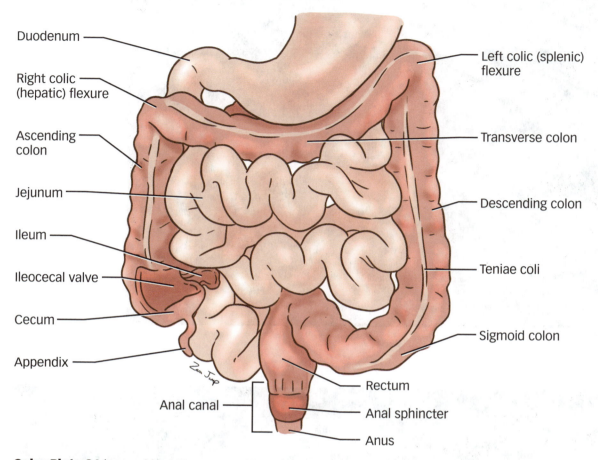

Color Plate 24 (pages 440–441, answer 420, and page 458, answer 446)

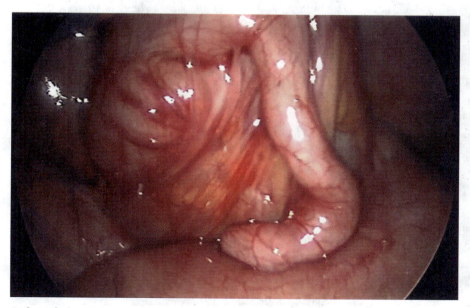

Color Plate 25 (pages 441–442, answer 421, image B)

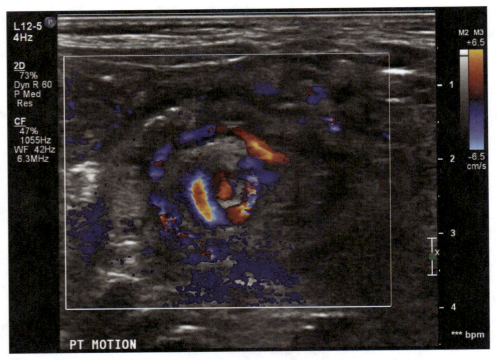

Color Plate 26 (pages 445–446, answer 427)

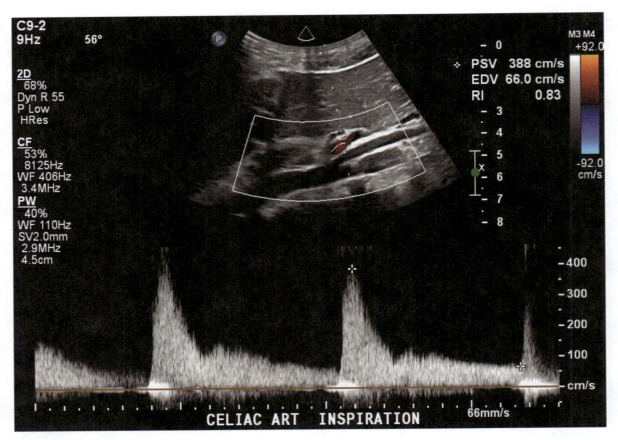

Color Plate 27 (page 456, answer 443)

Pediatric Sonography Review

The Pediatric Hip: Angle Measurements

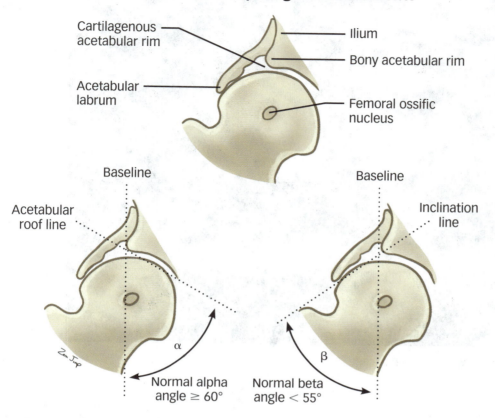

Color Plate 28 (page 459, answer 447)

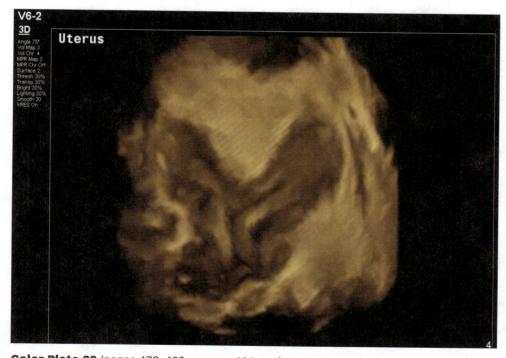

Color Plate 29 (pages 479–480, answer 481, and page 502, answer 518)

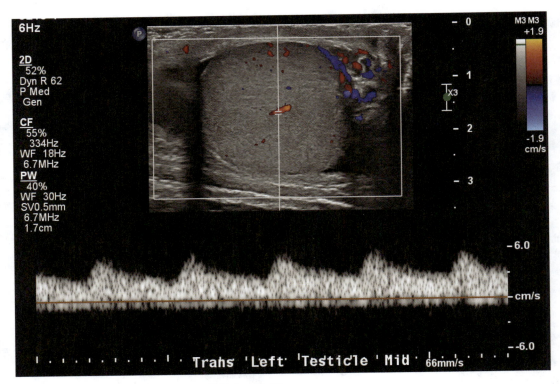

Color Plate 30 (page 506, answer 525, image B)

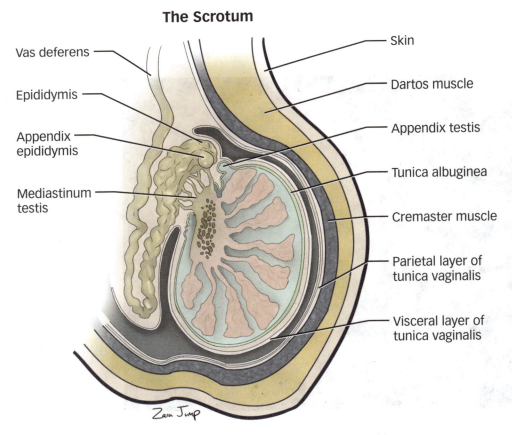

Color Plate 31 (page 507, answer 526; pages 510–511, answer 530; and pages 521–522, answer 548)

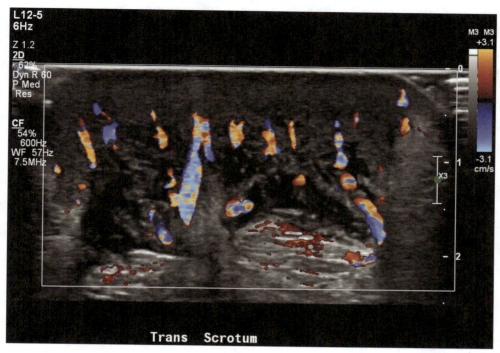

Color Plate 32 (pages 531–532, answer 565, image B)

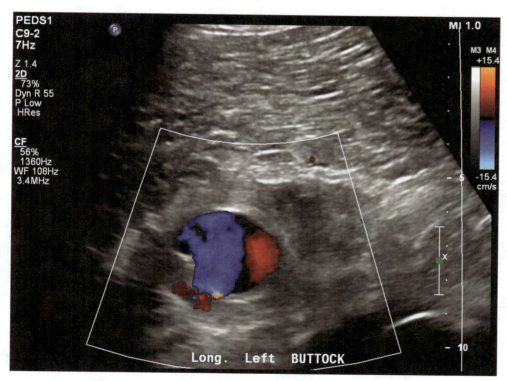

Color Plate 33 (pages 542–543, answer 583)

Vasculature of the Arms

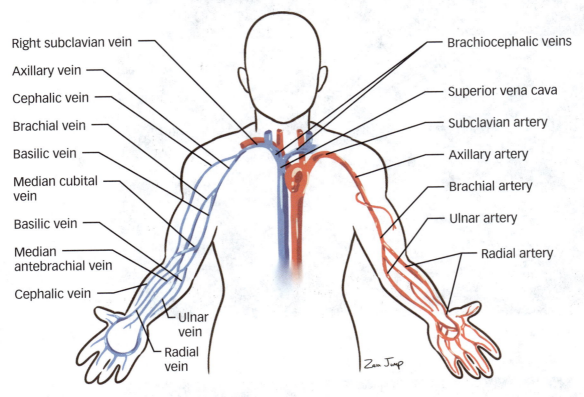

Color Plate 34 (pages 543–544, answer 584, and page 546, answer 590)

Vasculature of the Legs

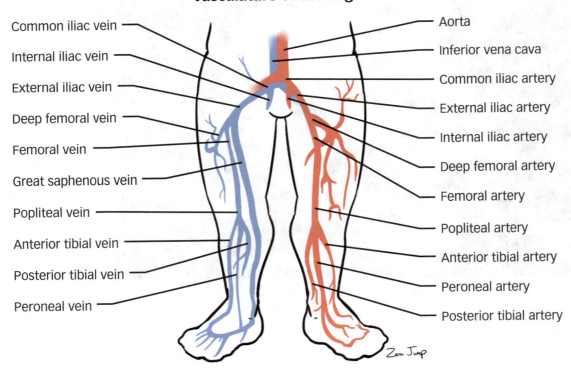

Color Plate 35 (page 544, answer 585, and page 547, answers 591–592)

PART 1

Head

Embryology and development

Normal anatomy

Associated lab values and hormones

Ultrasound prep and protocol

Normal ultrasound appearance

Pathology

Procedures

Note: The main topics of Part 1 are listed. For a complete study outline by topics and subtopics, see pages xv–xvi of the table of contents. The clinical tasks on the ARDMS exam outline are cross-referenced to the entire text of this mock exam starting on page 607.

1. When you are scanning through the anterior fontanelle in a midline sagittal plane, which of the following structures lies immediately cephalad to the cavum septi pellucidi (CSP)?
    A. Cingulate sulcus
    B. Third ventricle
    C. Corpus callosum
    D. Massa intermedia

2. You are scanning a full-term neonate due to an increased head circumference. You notice distention of the lateral and third ventricles without evidence of any other abnormality. What is the most likely cause of these findings?
    A. Vein of Galen aneurysm
    B. Congenital aqueductal stenosis
    C. Chiari malformation
    D. Cerebrospinal fluid (CSF) malabsorption

3. What is the name of the echogenic structure seen within the body of the lateral ventricle in the coronal plane of a normal head ultrasound?
    A. Bilateral grade 2 intraventricular hemorrhage (IVH)
    B. Choroid plexus papilloma
    C. Choroid plexus cyst
    D. Choroid plexus

4. The vein of Galen malformation forms from which of the following vessels?
    A. Primitive prosencephalic vein
    B. Pericallosal artery
    C. Great vein of Galen
    D. Straight sinus

5. You are performing an ultrasound scan of the head for TORCH infection, and you see multiple scattered calcifications in the periventricular area. This congenital infection is most likely:
    A. Cytomegalovirus (CMV)
    B. Toxoplasmosis
    C. Meningitis
    D. Herpes simplex virus (HSV)

6. In early brain development, what is the outcome when there is a failed or incomplete cleavage of the prosencephalon into the telencephalon and diencephalon?

    A. Hydranencephaly

    B. Lissencephaly

    C. Holoprosencephaly

    D. Schizencephaly

7. What is the most universally accepted measurement for evaluating the ventricular index of the lateral ventricles for dilatation?

    A. The distance between the lateral walls of the lateral ventricles divided by 2

    B. The distance from the falx to the lateral wall of the frontal horn of the lateral ventricle

    C. The distance from the medial wall of the lateral ventricle to the falx

    D. The distance between the medial walls of the lateral ventricles multiplied by 2

8. You obtained this image during neonatal screening of an asymptomatic infant. What is the most likely diagnosis given these findings?

    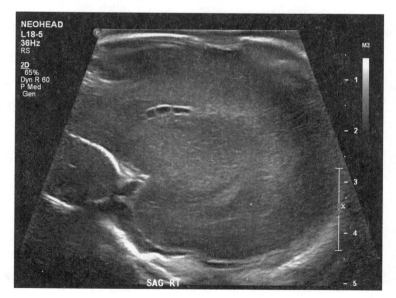

    A. Subependymal cysts

    B. Arachnoid cysts

    C. Choroid plexus cysts

    D. Connatal cysts

9. Meningitis in newborns is most commonly the result of what infection?
   A. Haemophilus influenzae
   B. Group B streptococcus
   C. Enterococcus
   D. Cytomegalovirus (CMV)

10. What is the term for a cystic lesion in the brain containing cerebrospinal fluid (CSF) and located between the two layers of arachnoid membranes in the posterior fossa?
    A. Cavum septi pellucidi (CSP)
    B. Porencephalic cyst
    C. Arachnoid cyst
    D. Dandy-Walker cyst

11. An infant with a myelomeningocele is referred for cranial ultrasound. During the scan, you see that the cerebellar vermis, medulla, and fourth ventricle are inferiorly displaced into the spinal canal. What condition would this represent?
    A. Dandy-Walker complex
    B. Holoprosencephaly
    C. Colpocephaly
    D. Arnold-Chiari malformation

12. What is the name for the group of structures, located deep in the cerebral hemispheres, that include the caudate nucleus, putamen, globus pallidus, substantia nigra, and subthalamic nucleus?
    A. Posterior fossa
    B. Brainstem
    C. Circle of Willis
    D. Basal ganglia

13. After focal tissue destruction, a cystic lesion continuous with the ventricular system is most likely:
    A. Porencephaly
    B. Colpocephaly
    C. Arachnoid cyst
    D. Hydrocephalus

14. Which grade of intraventricular hemorrhage (IVH) is shown in this coronal image obtained from a premature infant?

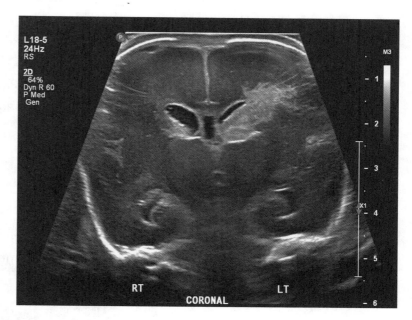

A. Grade 1
B. Grade 2
C. Grade 3
D. Grade 4

15. What brain structure are the arrows in this coronal image pointing to?

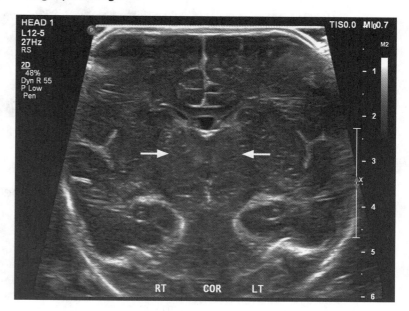

A. Massa intermedia

B. Corpus callosum

C. Pons

D. Thalamus

AIT—Hotspot*

16. Unilateral and single small choroid plexus cysts (<1 cm) are most often associated with:

    A. Trisomy 18

    B. Trisomy 21

    C. Ventriculomegaly

    D. Nothing of clinical significance

17. What type of event can cause the brain appearance seen in this coronal image of the brain of a full-term infant?

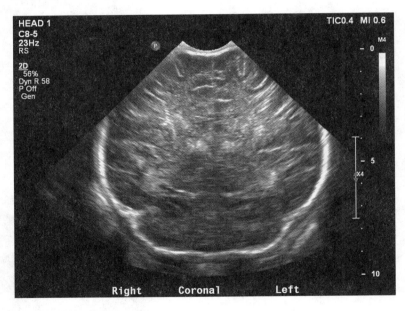

A. Hypoxic-ischemic injury

B. Cytomegalovirus (CMV)

C. Germinal matrix hemorrhage

D. Intraparenchymal hemorrhage

---

*Questions that are similar to the ARDMS Advanced Item Type (AIT) Hotspot items are marked throughout this mock exam. On the actual exam, Hotspot items require you to indicate the correct answer by marking directly on the image using your cursor. In this Davies mock exam, similar questions are marked **AIT—Hotspot**. These ask you to identify what an arrow in the image is pointing at or to indicate the label on an image that corresponds to the correct answer.

18. What fluid-containing cavity separates the two frontal horns of the lateral ventricles and lies anterior to the foramen of Monro?

    A. Third ventricle

    B. Fourth ventricle

    C. Cavum vergae

    D. Cavum septi pellucidi (CSP)

19. You are scanning the head of a full-term infant with microcephaly. During the examination, you notice an abnormally smooth brain. What is the most likely diagnosis?

    A. Schizencephaly

    B. Lissencephaly

    C. Intraparenchymal hemorrhage

    D. Hydranencephaly

20. What abnormality is this image demonstrating?

    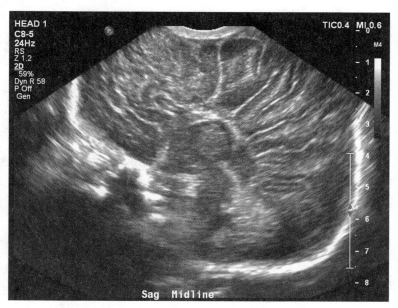

    A. Agenesis of the corpus callosum

    B. Agyria

    C. Holoprosencephaly

    D. Pachygyria

21. After confirmation by magnetic resonance imaging (MRI), this bleed was localized between the periosteum and the epicranial aponeurosis of the scalp. Which type of injury does this represent?

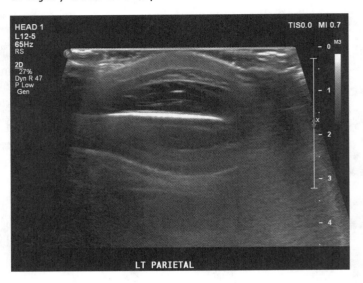

A. Cephalohematoma

B. Caput succedaneum

C. Subgaleal hematoma

D. Epidural hemorrhage

22. This image was obtained from a premature infant post placental abruption. What do these findings most likely represent?

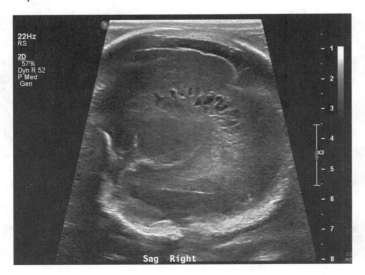

A. Periventricular blush

B. Grade 4 IVH

C. Periventricular leukomalacia (PVL)

D. Meningitis

23. The best images for evaluating the neonatal posterior fossa can be obtained through which of the following fontanelles?

    A. Anterior fontanelle
    B. Posterior fontanelle
    C. Sphenoidal fontanelle
    D. Mastoid fontanelle

24. Bilateral occlusion of the internal carotid arteries (ICAs) during fetal development can lead to:

    A. Hydranencephaly
    B. Alobar holoprosencephaly
    C. Cystic encephalomalacia
    D. Arachnoid cyst

25. A head ultrasound was done on this patient after forceps-assisted delivery. What is the most likely diagnosis for the finding (arrow) in this image?

    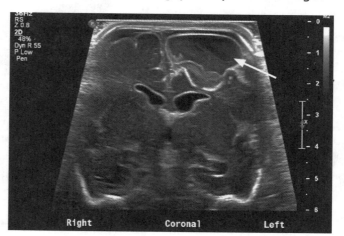

    A. Cephalohematoma
    B. Subdural hematoma
    C. Caput succedaneum
    D. Subgaleal hematoma

AIT—Hotspot

26. Which of the following brain neoplasms is the most frequently found within the first year of life?

    A. Ependymoma
    B. Teratoma
    C. Germinoma
    D. Ganglioma

27. What is most likely represented by the arrow in this image obtained from an infant with a maternal history of cytomegalovirus (CMV)?

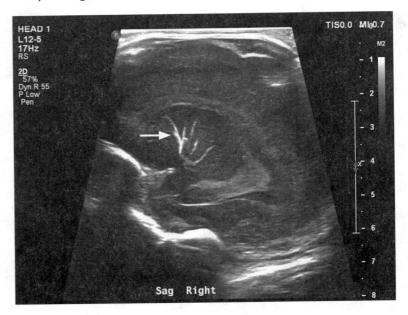

   A. Abscess
   B. Ventriculitis
   C. Lenticulostriate vasculopathy
   D. Cerebral infarction

AIT—Hotspot

28. What type of technique can be used to treat infants with acute reversible respiratory failure who do not respond to conventional treatment?
   A. Extracorporeal membrane oxygenation (ECMO)
   B. Therapeutic hypothermia and brain cooling
   C. Dialysis
   D. Tracheostomy

29. A hypervascular echogenic mass that arises from the trigone of the lateral ventricle is most likely a:
   A. Glioma
   B. Ependymoma
   C. Teratoma
   D. Choroid plexus papilloma

30. What abnormality is demonstrated in this image?

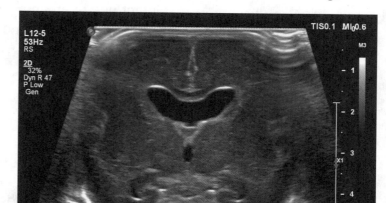

A. Absent corpus callosum
B. Enlarged third ventricle
C. Absent septum pellucidum
D. Enlarged massa intermedia

31. Which lobe of the brain is the arrow pointing to?

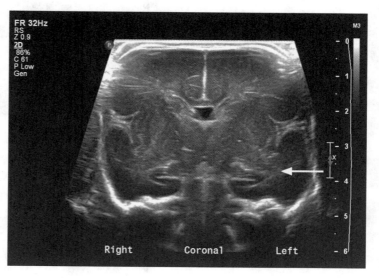

A. Frontal lobe
B. Occipital lobe
C. Temporal lobe
D. Parietal lobe

AIT—Hotspot

32. A "stat" head ultrasound is ordered on a premature infant due to an unexpected drop in hematocrit. What pathology are you trying to rule out?

   A. Malignant tumor
   B. Hemorrhage
   C. Hydrocephalus
   D. Infection

33. A head ultrasound is ordered on a newborn after scalp swelling was noticed on physical exam. Based on the image obtained and the physical findings, what is the most likely diagnosis?

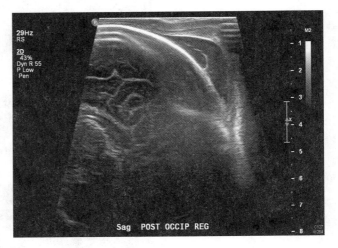

   A. Cerebral edema
   B. Epidural hematoma
   C. Subdural hematoma
   D. Caput succedaneum

34. What is seen on this routine 7-day ultrasound of a premature infant born at 26 weeks' gestational age?

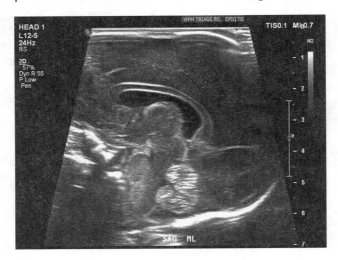

A. Lissencephaly

B. Ischemia

C. Cerebral edema

D. Normal brain

35. What is the name of a hemorrhage located between the skull and the dura mater?

    A. Subgaleal hemorrhage

    B. Epidural hemorrhage

    C. Subdural hemorrhage

    D. Subarachnoid hemorrhage

36. Brain tumors in neonates are usually located in what region?

    A. Suprasellar

    B. Intrasellar

    C. Supratentorial

    D. Infratentorial

37. What type of intraventricular hemorrhage (IVH) is demonstrated in this image?

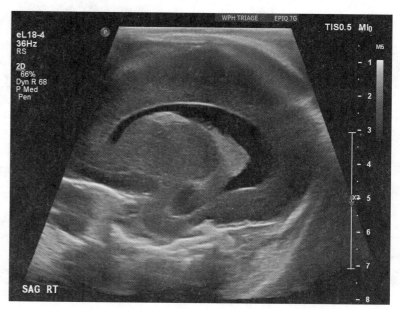

    A. Grade 1

    B. Grade 2

    C. Grade 3

    D. Grade 4

38. Which lobe of the brain is the most posterior?

    A. Parietal lobe

    B. Temporal lobe

    C. Occipital lobe

    D. Frontal lobe

39. What abnormality is represented in this axial image obtained from the mastoid fontanelle?

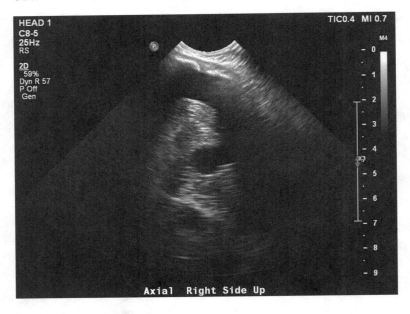

    A. Chiari malformation

    B. Dandy-Walker malformation

    C. Mega cisterna magna

    D. Subarachnoid cyst

40. Which scanning window is used to evaluate the blood flow velocity in the middle cerebral artery (MCA)?

    A. Mastoid fontanelle

    B. Anterior fontanelle

    C. Foramen magnum

    D. Temporal bone

41. What type of injury demonstrated in this coronal image cannot cross the midline suture lines and is located underneath the periosteum?

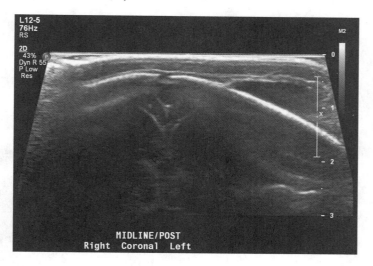

   A. Cephalohematoma
   B. Caput succedaneum
   C. Subgaleal hematoma
   D. Subarachnoid hemorrhage

42. Abnormal clefts or slits in the brain parenchyma that extend through the entire hemisphere are known as:
   A. Porencephaly
   B. Lissencephaly
   C. Hydranencephaly
   D. Schizencephaly

43. What type of intraventricular hemorrhage is demonstrated in this image?

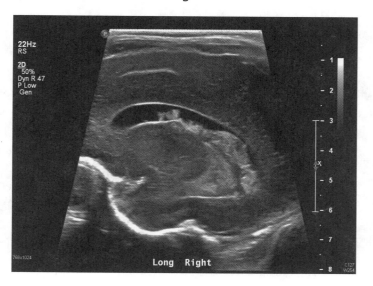

A. Grade 1
B. Grade 2
C. Grade 3
D. Grade 4

44. This image was obtained from a patient with a known intraventricular hemorrhage (IVH). What is the most likely diagnosis of the echogenic lesion of the cerebellum?

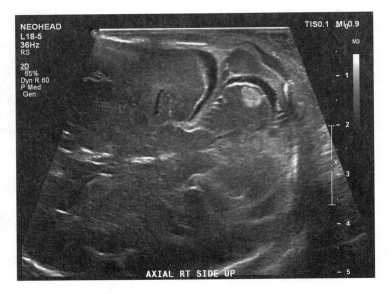

A. Cerebellar hemangioblastoma
B. Cerebellar hemorrhage
C. Cerebellar astrocytoma
D. Cerebellar liponeurocytoma

45. What type of abnormality can result from brain damage due to an ischemic insult?
A. Cystic encephalomalacia
B. Ventriculitis
C. Hydrocephalus
D. Schizencephaly

46. Which of the following abnormalities is associated with absence of the corpus callosum?
A. Vein of Galen aneurysm
B. Periventricular leukomalacia (PVL)
C. Colpocephaly
D. Intracranial hemorrhage

47. What type of intraventricular hemorrhage (IVH) is demonstrated in this image?

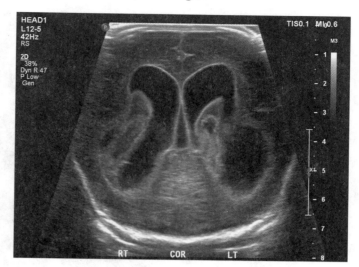

A. Grade 1

B. Grade 2

C. Grade 3

D. Grade 4

48. During early development, what primary vesicle of the brain forms the cerebrum, thalamus, and hypothalamus?

A. Mesencephalon

B. Prosencephalon

C. Rhombencephalon

D. Metencephalon

49. Which lobe of the brain is located superior to the temporal lobe and anterior to the occipital lobe?

A. Frontal lobe

B. Posterior lobe

C. Parietal lobe

D. Superior lobe

50. When you are performing a head ultrasound for macrocephaly in a full-term infant, what transducer would be the most adequate?

A. 8.5 MHz

B. 10.5 MHz

C. 12 MHz

D. 18 MHz

51. What structure does the star in this image of the posterior fossa represent?

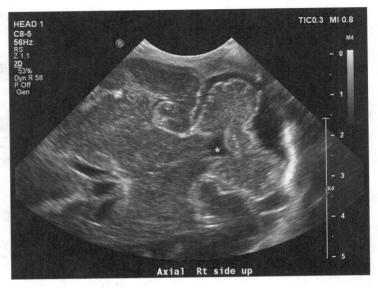

A. Cerebellar vermis
B. Fourth ventricle
C. Third ventricle
D. Cisterna magna

AIT—Hotspot

52. What differentiates a grade 2 from a grade 3 intraventricular hemorrhage (IVH)?
    A. Blood products within the brain parenchyma
    B. The extension of the bleed into the cortex
    C. Hemorrhage within the choroid plexus
    D. Ventricular distention

53. What primary vesicle of the brain becomes the pons, cerebellum, and medulla oblongata?
    A. Rhombencephalon
    B. Mesencephalon
    C. Prosencephalon
    D. Diencephalon

54. In this image, what structure is the arrow pointing to?

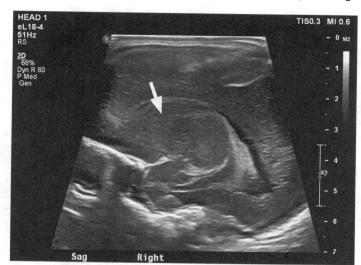

A. Putamen
B. Caudate nucleus
C. Tentorium
D. Pons

AIT—Hotspot

55. What is the main function of the choroid plexus?
    A. To regulate intracranial pressure
    B. To produce cerebrospinal fluid (CSF)
    C. To allow communication between the brain hemispheres
    D. To absorb CSF

56. The arrow in this image is pointing to what hypoechoic structure?

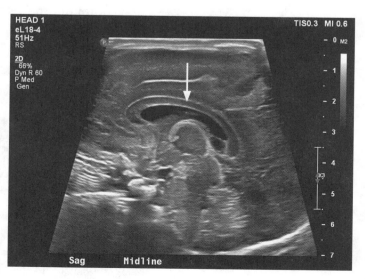

A. Cavum septi pellucidi (CSP)

B. Massa intermedia

C. Corpus callosum

D. Thalamus

AIT—Hotspot

57. What structure is the arrow pointing to in this image?

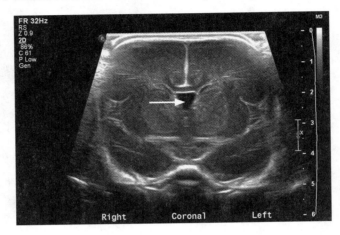

A. Cavum septi pellucidi (CSP)

B. Corpus callosum

C. Cavum vergae

D. Cavum veli interpositi

AIT—Hotspot

58. Which bones form the anterior fontanelle?

A. Occipital and temporal

B. Occipital and parietal

C. Frontal and temporal

D. Frontal and parietal

59. What pathology is represented in this image?

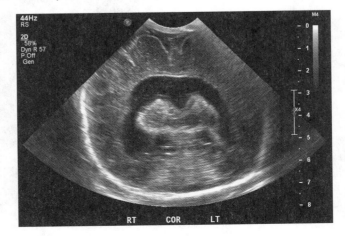

A. Porencephaly
B. Colpocephaly
C. Holoprosencephaly
D. Schizencephaly

60. What number in this image represents the medulla oblongata?

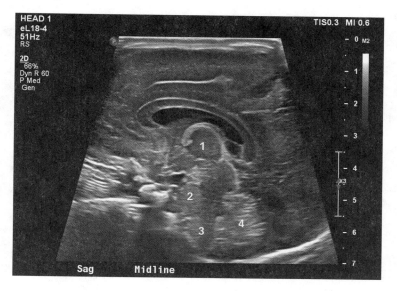

A. 1
B. 2
C. 3
D. 4

AIT—Hotspot

61. The fluid collection in this image is located within which space?

See Color Plate 1 on page xxxiii.

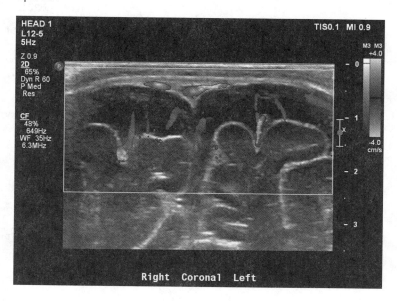

A. Subarachnoid space
B. Subgaleal space
C. Epidural space
D. Subdural space

62. Until what age is ultrasound the initial modality for evaluating the brain?
    A. 6 months
    B. 12 months
    C. 18 months
    D. 24 months

63. How many main sutures are there in the skull?
    A. 2
    B. 3
    C. 5
    D. 8

64. What is the most popular grading system for intraventricular hemorrhage (IVH)?
    A. Barkovich's
    B. Levene's
    C. Gille's
    D. Papile's

65. When a congenital malformation of the brain occurs during cytogenesis, which of the following malformations can be the result?
    A. Congenital neoplasms
    B. Chiari malformation
    C. Holoprosencephaly
    D. Tuberous sclerosis

66. Where is most of the white matter located in the brain?
    A. Deep in the brain
    B. Superficial in the brain
    C. Anteriorly in the brain
    D. Posteriorly in the brain

67. What structure is seen separating the cerebellum from the cerebrum in this image?

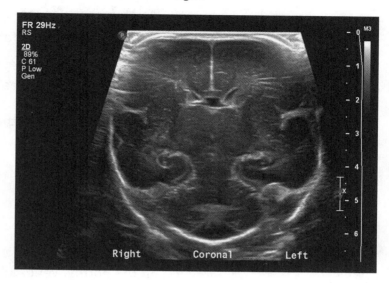

A. Cerebral peduncles
B. Tentorium cerebelli
C. Cerebellar vermis
D. Fourth ventricle

68. The arrow is pointing to what structure?

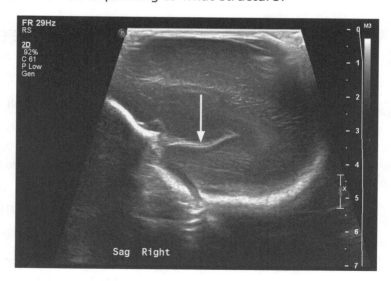

A. Cingulate sulcus
B. Cingulate gyrus
C. Interhemispheric fissure
D. Sylvian fissure

AIT—Hotspot

69. Which of the following is associated with absence of the septum pellucidum?
    A. Hemimegalencephaly
    B. Vein of Galen malformation
    C. Lissencephaly
    D. Septo-optic dysplasia

70. What is the name of the lining that borders the ventricles?
    A. Germinal matrix
    B. Pia mater
    C. Ependyma
    D. Tentorium cerebelli

71. In the normal ventricular circulation, where does the cerebrospinal fluid (CSF) go after passing through the third ventricle?
    A. Fourth ventricle
    B. Aqueduct of Sylvius
    C. Foramen of Monro
    D. Foramen of Magendie

72. What structure connects both sides of the thalamus?
    A. Massa intermedia
    B. Third ventricle
    C. Tentorium cerebelli
    D. Quadrigeminal cistern

73. What vessel bifurcates to form the middle cerebral artery (MCA)?
    A. External carotid artery (ECA)
    B. Internal carotid artery (ICA)
    C. Anterior cerebral artery (ACA)
    D. Posterior cerebral artery (PCA)

74. What number in the image represents the cerebral peduncles?

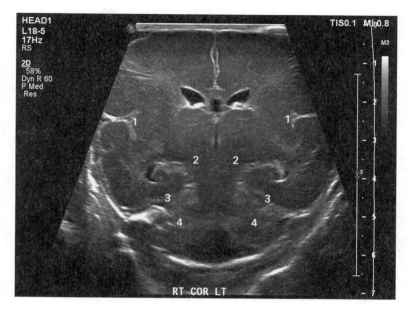

- A. 1
- B. 2
- C. 3
- D. 4

AIT—Hotspot

75. Which of the following arteries is NOT part of the circle of Willis?

    A. Middle cerebral artery (MCA)

    B. Anterior cerebral artery (ACA)

    C. Posterior cerebral artery (PCA)

    D. Anterior communicating artery (ACoA)

PART 2

Spine

Embryology and development

Normal anatomy

Associated lab values and hormones

Ultrasound prep and protocol

Normal ultrasound appearance

Pathology

Procedures

Note: The main topics of Part 2 are listed. For a complete study outline by topics and subtopics, see page xvii of the table of contents. The clinical tasks on the ARDMS exam outline are cross-referenced to the entire text of this mock exam starting on page 607.

76. The formation of the neural tube occurs during:
    A. Gastrulation
    B. Invagination
    C. Neurulation
    D. Ingression

77. Which of the following is the most common dorsal cutaneous stigma?
    A. Sacral dimple
    B. Skin tag
    C. Hair tuft
    D. Hemangioma

78. Which technique would be helpful in ruling out a pseudomass within the spinal canal?
    A. Adding color Doppler imaging
    B. Changing the patient's position
    C. Using a low-frequency transducer
    D. Increasing the gain

79. A 14-year-old reports to the ER with a history of pain while sitting, along with redness and swelling in his tailbone region. What is the most likely diagnosis given the findings in this image?

    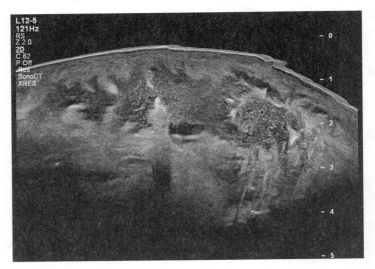

    A. Simple meningocele
    B. Pilonidal cyst
    C. Sacrococcygeal teratoma
    D. Pilonidal abscess

80. Which of the following is considered an abnormal level of termination for the conus medullaris?
    A. At or below L3
    B. At or below L2
    C. L1–L2 disk space
    D. L2–L3 disk space

81. What is the term for a fluid-filled sac within the central canal of the spinal cord?
    A. Filar cyst
    B. Syrinx
    C. Thecal sac
    D. Myelocystocele

82. The echogenic ovoid structure indicated by the arrow most likely represents:

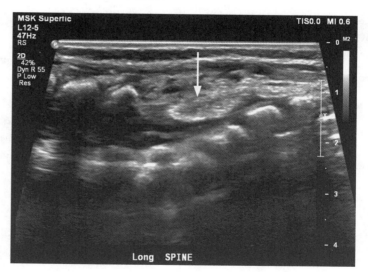

    A. Coccyx
    B. Cauda equina
    C. Lipoma
    D. Notochord

AIT—Hotspot

83. What is the echogenic, string-like extension from the conus medullaris called?
    A. Filum terminale
    B. Cauda equina
    C. Meninges
    D. Leptomeninges

84. Which transducer is optimal for ultrasound of the neonatal spine?
    A. 5 MHz curved array
    B. 8 MHz curved array
    C. 9 MHz curved array
    D. 12 MHz linear array

85. When elevated, which lab value is associated with an increased risk of neural tube defects?
    A. Folic acid
    B. Alpha-fetoprotein (AFP)
    C. Human chorionic gonadotropin (hCG)
    D. Inhibin-A

86. Which of the following is NOT associated with bony vertebral defects?
    A. Meningocele
    B. Lipomyelocele
    C. Sacrococcygeal teratoma
    D. Myelocystocele

87. Sterile sonography was performed to image an exposed (non-skin-covered), lumbosacral mass. What is the most likely diagnosis?
    A. Lipomyelocele
    B. Myelocystocele
    C. Myelomeningocele
    D. Sacrococcygeal teratoma

88. The last rib is normally located at the level of what vertebra?
    A. T11
    B. T12
    C. L1
    D. L2

89. The arrows in ultrasound image A and corresponding magnetic resonance image B are pointing at examples of what type of spinal dysraphism?

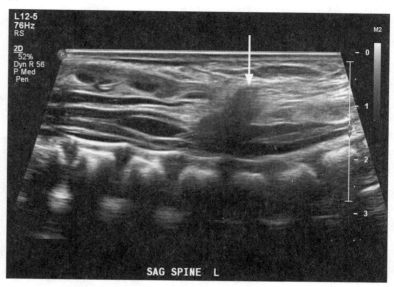

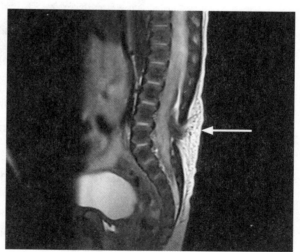

A. Spina bifida aperta

B. Occult spina bifida

C. Diastematomyelia

D. Caudal regression syndrome

AIT—Hotspot

90. The main difference between spina bifida aperta and occult spina bifida is the presence of:

    A. Meninges
    B. Bony defect
    C. Tethered cord
    D. Skin covering

91. As seen in this image, the blunted appearance of the spinal cord and lack of sacral vertebrae are associated with:

    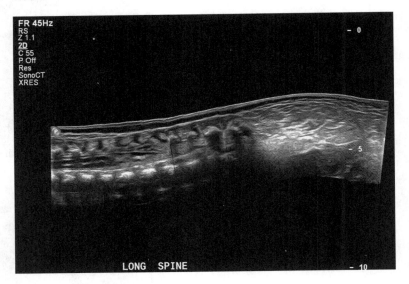

    A. Spina bifida aperta
    B. Tight filum syndrome
    C. Diastematomyelia
    D. Caudal regression syndrome

92. What minimally invasive procedure is performed to diagnose disorders of the brain and spinal cord?

    A. Lumbar puncture
    B. Epidural
    C. Laminotomy
    D. Quad screen

93. In this image, the conus medullaris terminates at what level?

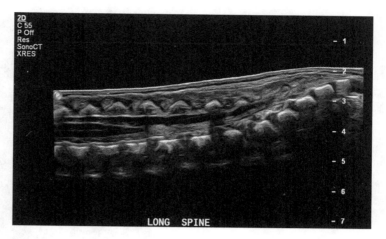

A. L1-L2
B. L2
C. L2-L3
D. L3

94. The presence of two symmetric hemicords is known as:
A. Notochord
B. Diastematomyelia
C. Dysraphism
D. Bicordism

95. What hypoechoic structure is represented by the number 2 in this image?

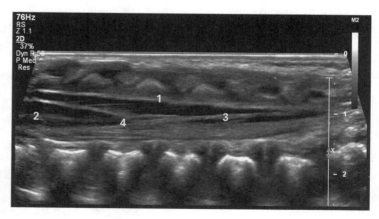

A. Conus medullaris
B. Dura mater
C. Filum terminale
D. Spinal cord

AIT—Hotspot

96. What pathology is most likely demonstrated in this transverse image of the spinal cord?

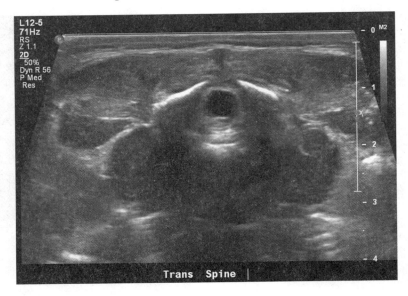

A. Hydromyelia
B. Enlarged thecal sac
C. Filar cyst
D. Meningocele

97. Spinal cord compression is often the result of:
A. Sacrococcygeal teratoma
B. Trauma
C. Pilonidal sinus
D. Caudal regression syndrome

98. What is most likely represented by the arrow in this ultrasound image?

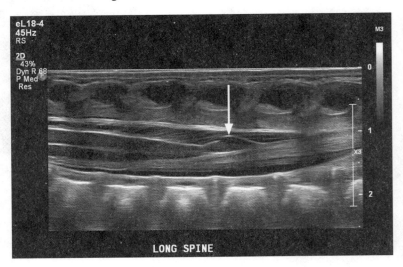

A. Syrinx

B. Ventriculus terminalis

C. Hydromyelia

D. Tight filum syndrome

AIT—Hotspot

99. What structure is indicated by the arrow?

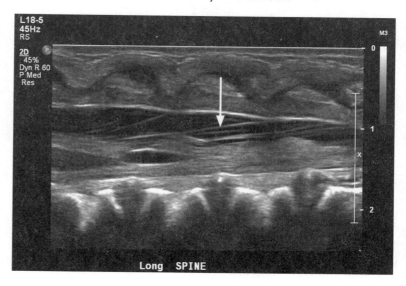

A. Nerve root

B. Filum

C. Filar cyst

D. Dura mater

AIT—Hotspot

100. What abnormality connects the skin to the neural components of the spine?

A. Pilonidal sinus

B. Sacrococcygeal teratoma

C. Dorsal dermal sinus

D. Sacral dimple

PART 3
Neck and Face

Embryology and development

Normal anatomy

Associated lab values and hormones

Ultrasound prep and protocol

Normal ultrasound appearance

Pathology

Procedures

Note: The main topics of Part 3 are listed. For a complete study outline by topics and subtopics, see pages xviii–xix of the table of contents. The clinical tasks on the ARDMS exam outline are cross-referenced to the entire text of this mock exam starting on page 607.

101. A patient presents to the ultrasound department complaining of a midline neck mass that moves when she swallows. On ultrasound you find the cystic structure seen just below the hyoid bone. What is the most likely diagnosis?

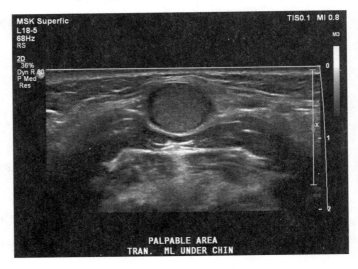

A. Thyroglossal duct cyst
B. Branchial cleft cyst
C. Ranula
D. Thyroid cyst

102. How many parathyroid glands are normally present?
A. 1
B. 2
C. 3
D. 4

103. Where would a salivary gland hemangioma most likely be encountered?
A. Sublingual gland
B. Submandibular gland
C. Parotid gland
D. Parathyroid gland

104. Which of the following is NOT a hormone associated with the thyroid?
A. Triiodothyronine (T3)
B. Thyroxine (T4)
C. Thyroid-stimulating hormone (TSH)
D. Parathyroid hormone (PTH)

105. This image was obtained by placing the transducer parallel and anterior to the ear. What structure is represented in this image?

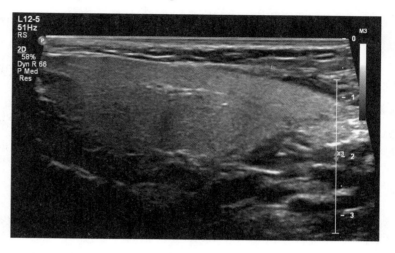

A. Submandibular gland
B. Parotid gland
C. Sublingual gland
D. Lymph node

106. A neonate presents with torticollis and a palpable mass in the right neck. Based on this image of the sternocleidomastoid muscle, what is the most likely diagnosis?

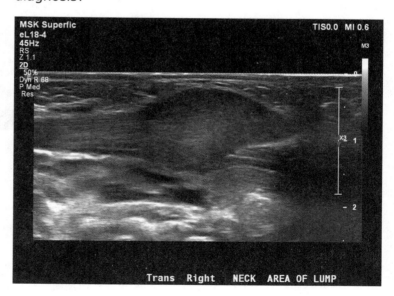

A. Fibromatosis colli
B. Aggressive fibromatosis
C. Nodular fasciitis
D. Inflammatory myofibroblastic tumor

107. Which of the following carcinomas of the thyroid is the most common in children?

    A. Acinar cell carcinoma

    B. Follicular carcinoma

    C. Papillary carcinoma

    D. Medullary carcinoma

108. Which of the following are NOT among the muscles that border the thyroid gland?

    A. Sternocleidomastoid muscles

    B. Strap muscles

    C. Masseter muscles

    D. Longus colli muscles

109. A child presents with hypercalcemia, pruritus, and bone pain. With ultrasound examination of the neck, these findings are seen. What is the most likely diagnosis?

    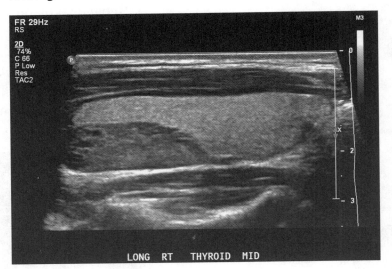

    A. Thyroid carcinoma

    B. Thyroid adenoma

    C. Parathyroid carcinoma

    D. Parathyroid adenoma

110. The obstruction of which of the following ducts can result in a ranula?

    A. Stensen duct

    B. Sublingual duct

    C. Wharton duct

    D. Wirsung duct

111. What vessel is the arrow identifying in this image?

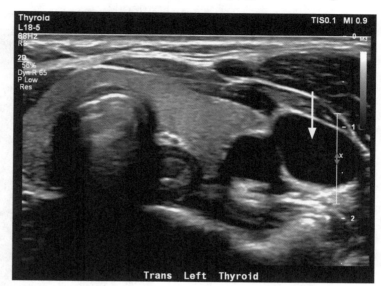

A. Common carotid artery (CCA)

B. Internal carotid artery (ICA)

C. External jugular vein

D. Internal jugular vein

AIT—Hotspot

112. Which of the following is the largest salivary gland?

A. Submandibular

B. Parotid

C. Sublingual

D. Thyroid

113. What is the normal echogenicity of the thyroid when compared to the adjacent muscle?

A. Hyperechoic and homogeneous

B. Hypoechoic and heterogeneous

C. Hypoechoic and homogeneous

D. Isoechoic and homogeneous

114. Which of the following is a target organ of parathyroid hormone (PTH)?

A. Kidneys

B. Spleen

C. Pancreas

D. Gallbladder

115. What structure is the arrow indicating in this transverse image?

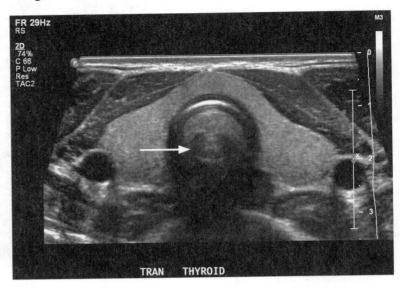

A. Esophagus

B. Trachea

C. Hyoid bone

D. Cervical spine

AIT—Hotspot

116. You are scanning a child due to a painless left facial mass and see this cystic structure just below and posterior to the ear. What is the most likely diagnosis?

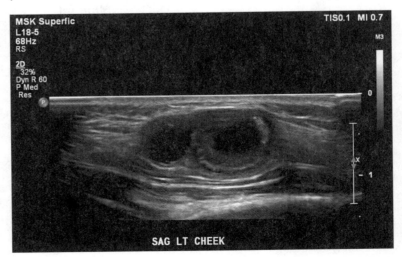

A. Branchial cleft cyst

B. Thyroglossal duct cyst

C. Cystadenoma

D. Ranula

117. Which of the following is a sonographic characteristic of a malignant thyroid nodule?

   A. Microcalcifications

   B. Comet-tail artifact

   C. Nodule size <1 cm

   D. Eggshell, large calcifications

118. An 8-year-old patient presents with a painful swollen cheek after being diagnosed with mononucleosis. During ultrasound examination of the region of interest, you see the finding in this image. What is the most likely diagnosis?

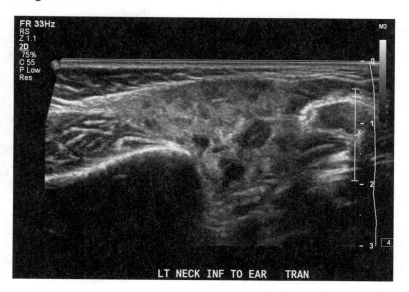

   A. Sialadenitis

   B. Sialolithiasis

   C. Bacterial parotitis

   D. Viral parotitis

119. *Sublingual* means:

   A. Under the tongue

   B. Under the mandible

   C. Under the nose

   D. Under the ear

120. The most common cause of congenital hypothyroidism is:

   A. Maternal thyrotoxicosis

   B. Thyroid dysgenesis

   C. Dyshormonogenesis

   D. Pituitary/hypothalamic hypothyroidism

121. Which bone forms the angle of the jaw?

    A. Zygoma

    B. Vomer

    C. Maxilla

    D. Mandible

122. Where would you place your transducer to obtain this image of the submandibular gland?

    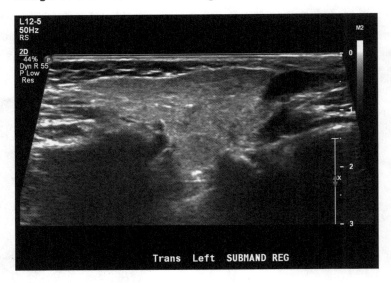

    A. Parallel and anterior to the ear

    B. Sagittal and midline under the chin

    C. Parallel and lateral to the horizontal portion of the mandible

    D. Perpendicular and anterior to the trachea

123. What is the most common cause of secondary hyperparathyroidism?

    A. Generalized parathyroid hyperplasia

    B. Parathyroid adenoma

    C. Parathyroid carcinoma

    D. Parathyroid cyst

124. What is the term used to describe the appearance of the thyroid gland seen in this transverse image?

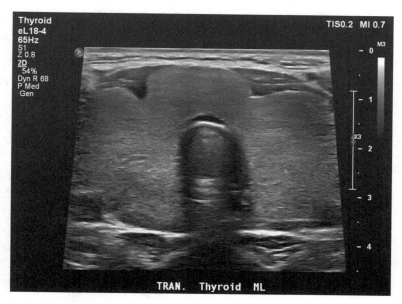

A. Thyroid inferno

B. Lymphocytic thyroiditis

C. Goiter

D. Multinodular goiter

125. A patient presents with a hyperechoic thyroid nodule that contains a hypoechoic rim with peripheral curvilinear calcifications and vascularity. The lesion is isolated and contains some cystic changes and a comet-tail artifact within. Based on the sonographic characteristics described, what is the most likely diagnosis?

A. Papillary carcinoma

B. Medullary carcinoma

C. Colloid cyst

D. Adenoma

126. Which of the following groups of facial or neck lymph nodes are most often involved in disease processes?

   A. Facial lymph nodes
   B. Retropharyngeal lymph nodes
   C. Lateral cervical lymph nodes
   D. Sublingual lymph nodes

127. What is the name of the midline structure that connects the two lobes of the thyroid?

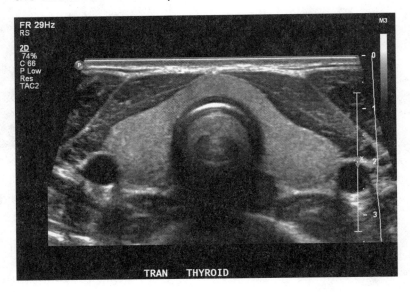

   A. Isthmus
   B. Pyramidal lobe
   C. Thyroid arch
   D. Accessory lobe

128. A benign congenital septated cystic mass arising from the parotid gland is most likely a:

   A. Lymphangioma
   B. Hemangioma
   C. Pleomorphic adenoma
   D. Cystadenoma

129. What is the most common autoimmune cause of hypothyroidism in children and adolescents?
    A. Focal thyroiditis
    B. Hashimoto's thyroiditis
    C. Graves' disease
    D. Acute suppurative thyroiditis

130. Which of the following abnormalities most commonly affects the submandibular gland?
    A. Hemangiomas
    B. Ranulas
    C. Mumps
    D. Sialolithiasis

131. In which of the following lesions would a fine needle biopsy NOT be recommended?
    A. Carotid bifurcation mass
    B. Enlarged cervical lymph node
    C. Cystic lesion of the neck
    D. Parathyroid neoplasm

132. Sonographically, which of the following findings will help to differentiate Graves' disease from Hashimoto's thyroiditis?
    A. Hypervascularity
    B. Nodular formation
    C. Enlarged gland
    D. Lobulated contours

133. What is the most common cause of primary hyperparathyroidism?
    A. Generalized parathyroid hyperplasia
    B. Multiple endocrine neoplasia (MEN) type I
    C. Parathyroid adenoma
    D. Parathyroid carcinoma

134. What structure (arrow) is seen in the posteromedial aspect of the left thyroid lobe?

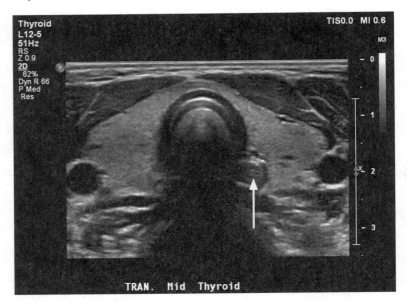

A. Parathyroid

B. Thyroid adenoma

C. Lymph node

D. Esophagus

AIT—Hotspot

135. Which of the following is the smallest of the major salivary glands?

A. Parotid

B. Submandibular

C. Sublingual

D. Thyroid

PART 4
Chest

Embryology and development

Normal anatomy

Associated lab values and hormones

Ultrasound prep and protocol

Normal ultrasound appearance

Pathology

Procedures

Note: The main topics of Part 4 are listed. For a complete study outline by topics and subtopics, see page xix of the table of contents. The clinical tasks on the ARDMS exam outline are cross-referenced to the entire text of this mock exam starting on page 607.

136. You need to scan an infant to rule out pleural effusion. Which of the following transducers is best for the evaluation of the pleural space?
    A. 17.5 MHz linear transducer
    B. 12.5 MHz linear transducer
    C. 8.5 MHz sector transducer
    D. 5.0 MHz curved transducer

137. Which of the following conditions can cause "hepatization" of the lungs?
    A. Atelectasis
    B. Congenital pulmonary airway malformation (CPAM)
    C. Empyema
    D. Pneumothorax

138. What is the appearance of a normal thymus in a neonate?
    A. Hyperechoic
    B. Hypoechoic
    C. Complex
    D. Not visualized on ultrasound

139. What type of congenital hernia occurs in the posterior portion of the diaphragm?
    A. Spigelian hernia
    B. Morgagni hernia
    C. Hiatal hernia
    D. Bochdalek hernia

140. In which portion of the mediastinum is the thymus located?
    A. Anterior
    B. Posterior
    C. Superior
    D. Middle

141. What pathology is represented in this image?

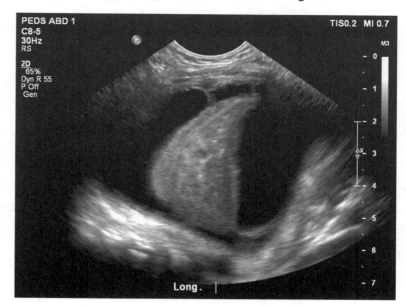

A. Empyema

B. Hemothorax

C. Transudative pleural effusion

D. Exudative pleural effusion

142. What is the name of the structure formed by muscle and connective tissue that separates the thoracic from the abdominal cavity?

A. Thymus

B. Pleura

C. Diaphragm

D. Mediastinum

143. While you are scanning a child for a palpable chest mass, color Doppler demonstrates a vessel arising directly from the aorta, feeding a thoracic mass. What is the most likely diagnosis?

A. Bronchopulmonary sequestration

B. Congenital pulmonary airway malformation (CPAM)

C. Teratoma

D. Pulmonary arteriovenous malformation (PAVM)

144. In which portion of the diaphragm do Morgagni hernias occur?

    A. Posterior
    B. Anterior
    C. Lateral
    D. Medial

145. Which of the following is considered one of the most common childhood malignant masses involving the mediastinum?

    A. Pleuropulmonary blastoma
    B. Congenital pulmonary airway malformation (CPAM)
    C. Thymoma
    D. Lymphoma

146. This image of the esophagus demonstrated retrograde flow of the fluid in real-time scanning. The patient was being scanned to rule out pyloric stenosis. What is the most likely diagnosis?

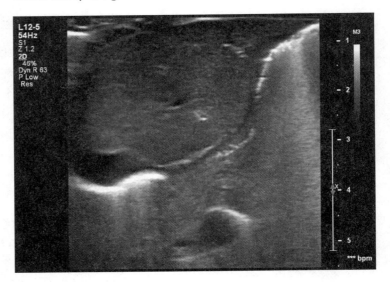

    A. Pyloric stenosis
    B. Midgut malrotation
    C. Esophageal atresia
    D. Gastroesophageal reflux

147. Which serous membrane of the chest covers the lungs?
    A. Synovial
    B. Peritoneum
    C. Pleura
    D. Pericardium

148. What abnormality can phrenic nerve injury cause?
    A. Diaphragmatic inversion
    B. Diaphragmatic paralysis
    C. Diaphragmatic eventration
    D. Diaphragmatic hernia

149. What is the name of the procedure that consists of aspirating fluid from the chest?
    A. Thoracentesis
    B. Paracentesis
    C. Amniocentesis
    D. Pericardiocentesis

150. You are performing chest ultrasound and see multiple tubular cystic areas. Upon Doppler interrogation you notice no color flow within these structures. What condition would this most likely represent?
    A. Atelectasis
    B. Lung consolidation
    C. Bronchopulmonary sequestration
    D. Pneumothorax

151. Which of the following is an anterior mediastinal mass?
    A. Neuroblastoma
    B. Ganglioneuroma
    C. Thymoma
    D. Ganglioneuroblastoma

152. A multicystic avascular mass seen within the lungs prenatally is most likely a:
    A. Lymphoma
    B. Thymic cyst
    C. Lymphangioma
    D. Congenital pulmonary airway malformation (CPAM)

153. What is the term used to describe the free movement between the visceral and parietal pleura during respiration?
    A. Visceroparietal pleural sign
    B. Sliding sign
    C. Gliding sign
    D. Pleural sign

154. Which of the following structures is NOT located within the mediastinum?
    A. Lungs
    B. Heart
    C. Thymus
    D. Esophagus

155. Which of the following conditions can lead to an exudative pleural effusion?
    A. Congestive heart failure
    B. Renal failure
    C. Cirrhosis
    D. Bacterial pneumonia

PART 5

Liver

Embryology and development

Normal anatomy

Associated lab values and hormones

Ultrasound prep and protocol

Normal ultrasound appearance

Pathology

Procedures

Note: The main topics of Part 5 are listed. For a complete study outline by topics and subtopics, see pages xx–xxi of the table of contents. The clinical tasks on the ARDMS exam outline are cross-referenced to the entire text of this mock exam starting on page 607.

156. What is the name of the connective tissue that encapsulates the liver?
    A. Gerota's fascia
    B. Glisson's capsule
    C. Peritoneum
    D. Mesentery

157. In fetal circulation, the fetal liver receives oxygenated blood from which vessel?
    A. Umbilical artery
    B. Umbilical vein
    C. Hepatic artery
    D. Hepatic vein

158. Identify the vessel marked with the number 1.

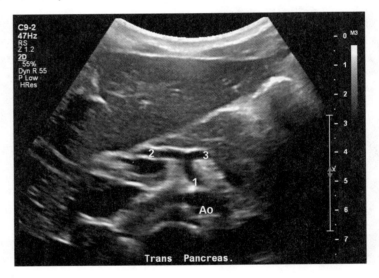

    A. Splenic artery
    B. Hepatic artery
    C. Celiac axis
    D. Superior mesenteric artery

AIT—Hotspot

159. What is the term used when the right lobe of the liver extends below the right kidney as a normal anatomic variant?
    A. Quadrate lobe
    B. Succenturiate lobe
    C. Caudate lobe
    D. Riedel lobe

160. Which of the following would NOT be elevated in the presence of liver damage?

    A. Albumin

    B. Alanine transaminase (ALT)

    C. Aspartate transaminase (AST)

    D. Alkaline phosphatase (ALP)

161. The condition in which the liver is located on the left side of the body is known as:

    A. Situs solitus

    B. Situs inversus

    C. Riedel lobe

    D. Hemihypertrophy

162. The anechoic linear structure seen in this postnatal ultrasound image is the remnant of the fetal umbilical vein that will become the:

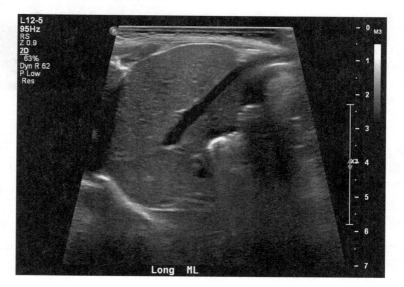

    A. Urachus

    B. Ligamentum venosum

    C. Falciform ligament

    D. Ligamentum teres

163. The normal portal vein diameter in pediatric patients should not exceed:

    A. 6 mm

    B. 8 mm

    C. 10 mm

    D. 12 mm

164. Which of the following liver abnormalities is usually congenital?

    A. Focal nodular hyperplasia (FNH)

    B. Cirrhosis

    C. Cavernous transformation

    D. Arteriovenous malformation (AVM)

165. What abnormality is seen located between the left lobe of the liver and the aorta?

    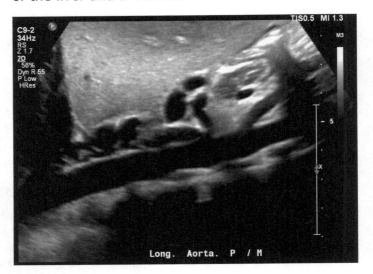

    A. Dilated bile ducts

    B. Gastroesophageal varices

    C. Cavernous transformation

    D. Budd-Chiari syndrome

166. The proper exam preparation for abdominal sonography is:

    A. Moderate hydration

    B. Fatty meal prior to exam

    C. Fasting

    D. Full bladder

167. When you are scanning the liver, which patient position is NOT ideal for optimal visualization?

    A. Supine

    B. Right lateral decubitus

    C. Left lateral decubitus

    D. Left posterior oblique

168. Which rare malignant liver tumor originates from the hepatic mesenchyme?
    A. Undifferentiated embryonal sarcoma
    B. Hepatoblastoma
    C. Hepatocellular carcinoma
    D. Hemangioendothelioma

169. What vessel carries blood from the spleen and mesentery to the liver?
    A. Hepatic vein
    B. Superior mesenteric vein
    C. Inferior mesenteric vein
    D. Portal vein

170. The condition associated with hepatic venous outflow obstruction is known as:
    A. Portal vein thrombosis
    B. Budd-Chiari syndrome
    C. Cavernous transformation
    D. Veno-occlusive disease

171. Which ligament courses between the caudate lobe and the lateral left lobe of the liver?
    A. Ligamentum venosum
    B. Falciform ligament
    C. Round ligament
    D. Ligamentum teres

172. What is the most common malignant liver tumor in children?
    A. Hepatocellular carcinoma
    B. Hepatoblastoma
    C. Embryonal sarcoma
    D. Liver metastases

173. What substance gives bile and feces their pigment?
    A. Bilirubin
    B. Red blood cells
    C. Protein
    D. Plasma

174. After infancy the normal liver echotexture, when compared to the right kidney, should be:
    A. Less echogenic than the right kidney cortex
    B. More echogenic than the right kidney cortex
    C. Less echogenic than the right kidney medulla
    D. More echogenic than the right kidney medulla

175. Which of the following is NOT a component of the biliary tree?
    A. Common bile duct
    B. Intrahepatic ducts
    C. Pancreatic duct
    D. Common hepatic duct

176. Which benign liver tumor is known to have a central stellate scar that appears echogenic on ultrasound?
    A. Focal nodular hyperplasia (FNH)
    B. Hemangioendothelioma
    C. Hemangioma
    D. Hamartoma

177. Identify the vessel labeled 2:

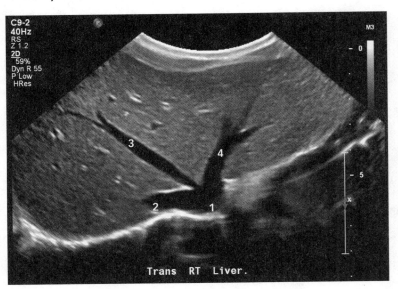

    A. Inferior vena cava (IVC)
    B. Mid hepatic vein
    C. Left hepatic vein
    D. Right hepatic vein

AIT—Hotspot

178. In the Couinaud classification of segmental anatomy, what segment is the caudate lobe of the liver?

   A. 1

   B. 3

   C. 5

   D. 7

179. What is the term for fatty infiltration of damaged hepatocytes?

   A. Cirrhosis

   B. Fibrosis

   C. Steatosis

   D. Hepatitis

180. Which of the following is NOT a sonographic sign of portal hypertension?

   A. Decreased portal vein inflow

   B. Portosystemic collaterals

   C. Increased portal vein diameter

   D. Decreased flow of the hepatic artery

181. Identify the vessel (arrow) in this image.

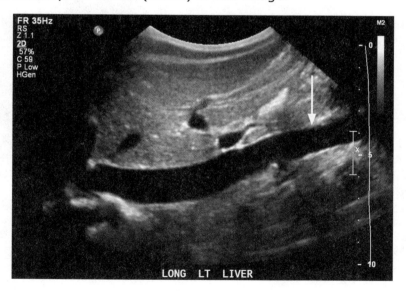

   A. Aorta

   B. Inferior vena cava (IVC)

   C. Portal vein

   D. Azygos vein

AIT—Hotspot

182. If present after early infancy, what clinical symptom is a concern for hepatobiliary disease?

    A. Vomiting

    B. Fever

    C. Jaundice

    D. Seizures

183. Which of the following is associated with cases of necrotizing enterocolitis (NEC) or infarcted bowel?

    A. Portal vein thrombosis

    B. Air in the portal vein

    C. Portal vein hypertension

    D. Portal vein obstruction

184. Which chronic disease process is identified by the nodular appearance and scarring of the liver parenchyma seen in this image?

    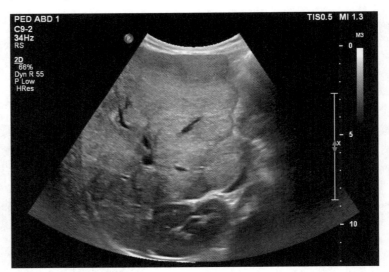

    A. Metastases

    B. Hydatid disease

    C. Hepatic granulomas

    D. Cirrhosis

185. Infestation by what parasite causes hydatid disease?

    A. *Echinococcus granulosus*

    B. Amoeba

    C. *Schistosoma*

    D. *Ascaris lumbricoides*

186. These focal infiltrating lesions (arrows), seen within the abdominal cavity following liver or kidney transplantation, indicate a complication known as:

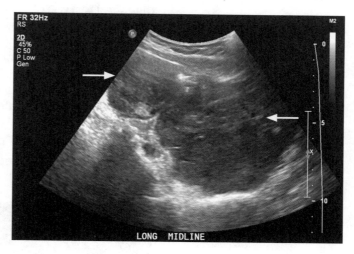

A. Seroma

B. Lymphoproliferative disorder

C. Biloma

D. Adrenal hemorrhage

AIT—Hotspot

187. What ligament is commonly seen as a hyperechoic linear focus at the junction of the right and left hepatic lobes in a transverse view of the liver?

A. Ligamentum teres

B. Ligamentum venosum

C. Falciform ligament

D. Round ligament

188. Prior to the Couinaud classification, what was defined as the division between the right and left lobes of the liver?

A. Left hepatic vein

B. Middle hepatic vein

C. Right hepatic vein

D. Portal vein

189. Which condition is associated with the inherited autosomal dominant diseases von Hippel–Lindau, tuberous sclerosis, and autosomal dominant polycystic kidney disease (ADPKD)?

    A. Polycystic liver

    B. Congenital hepatic fibrosis

    C. Cirrhosis

    D. Focal nodular hyperplasia

190. In chronic portal vein thrombosis, multiple tortuous vessels (arrow) will replace the portal vein. This condition is called:

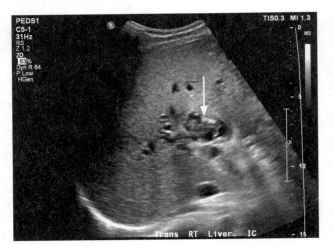

    A. Budd-Chiari syndrome

    B. Gastroesophageal varices

    C. Cavernous transformation

    D. Arteriovenous malformation

191. Which of the following is a cause of intrahepatic portal hypertension?

    A. Splenic vein thrombosis

    B. Cirrhosis

    C. Hepatic vein obstruction

    D. Congestive heart failure

192. The FAST sonogram is used to detect:

    A. Hemoperitoneum

    B. Ascites

    C. Tumors

    D. Infarction

193. Which liver malignancy most often follows preexisting liver disease?

   A. Hepatoblastoma

   B. Undifferentiated embryonal sarcoma

   C. Angiosarcoma

   D. Hepatocellular carcinoma

194. The liver condition in this image precedes cirrhosis and is known as:

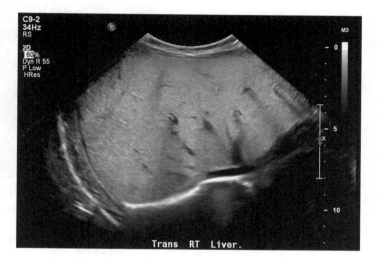

   A. Hepatic fibrosis

   B. Focal nodular hyperplasia (FNH)

   C. Metastatic disease

   D. Veno-occlusive disease

195. Which type of liver injury is a lenticular-shaped fluid collection that flattens or indents the liver beneath it?

   A. Parenchymal hematoma

   B. Subcapsular hematoma

   C. Hepatic laceration

   D. Hepatic fracture

196. Healthcare workers have an increased risk for which type of hepatitis?

   A. Hepatitis A

   B. Hepatitis B

   C. Hepatitis C

   D. Hepatitis E

197. The procedure that can most accurately diagnose diffuse liver disease is:

   A. Abscess drainage

   B. Contrast ultrasound

   C. Elastography

   D. Percutaneous biopsy

198. What structure is indicated by the number 3?

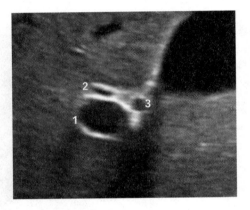

   A. Common bile duct

   B. Portal vein

   C. Hepatic artery

   D. Inferior vena cava (IVC)

AIT—Hotspot

199. Which of the following is the result of an inflammatory response of the liver?

   A. Granulomas

   B. Hemangiomas

   C. Lipomas

   D. Sarcomas

200. Which rare, benign pediatric liver tumor arises from the periportal connective tissue?

   A. Hemangioma

   B. Hemangioendothelioma

   C. Mesenchymal hamartoma

   D. Adenoma

201. Arteries traveling toward the liver in a preprandial patient should display:

    A. Hepatofugal high-resistance flow
    B. Hepatofugal low-resistance flow
    C. Hepatopetal high-resistance flow
    D. Hepatopetal low-resistance flow

202. What is the most likely diagnosis for this mass (arrows) in a 1-year-old with symptoms of abdominal mass, jaundice, and anorexia?

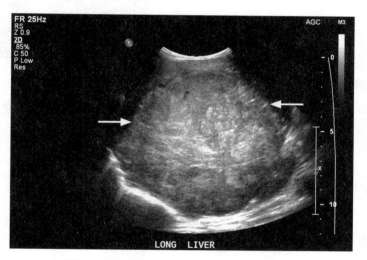

    A. Focal nodular hyperplasia (FNH)
    B. Hepatoblastoma
    C. Cirrhosis
    D. Undifferentiated embryonal sarcoma

AIT—Hotspot

203. What noninvasive procedure measures liver stiffness?

    A. Elastography
    B. Contrast-enhanced ultrasound
    C. Abdominal vascular study
    D. Liver function tests

204. Which structure is marked with the number 2?

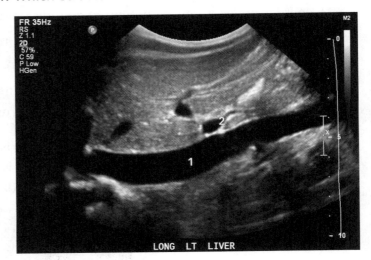

A. Gallbladder

B. Common bile duct

C. Inferior vena cava

D. Portal vein

AIT—Hotspot

205. This incidental finding (arrow) in a 14-year-old male during an abdominal ultrasound is most likely:

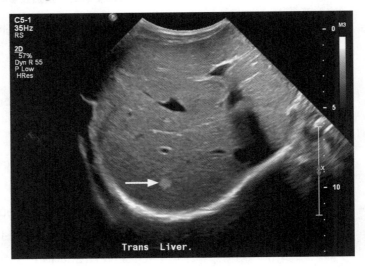

A. Hemangioendothelioma

B. Hemangioma

C. Hepatoblastoma

D. Mesenchymal hamartoma

AIT—Hotspot

206. Which technical issue would NOT be a cause of an absent Doppler signal?

   A. High wall filter

   B. High pulse repetition frequency (PRF)

   C. Low Doppler gain

   D. 30-degree vessel-beam angle

AIT—SIC*

207. Which hepatic neoplasm is associated with preexisting metabolic liver disease?

   A. Adenoma

   B. Hamartoma

   C. Hemangioma

   D. Lymphoma

208. Which vessel is indicated by the number 2?

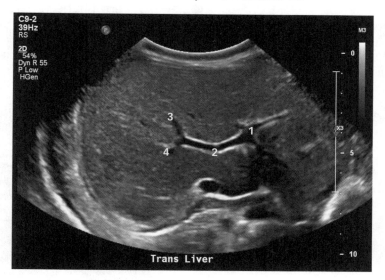

   A. Main portal vein

   B. Left portal vein

   C. Right portal vein

   D. Posterior branch of the right portal vein

AIT—Hotspot

---

*Questions marked **AIT—SIC** are similar to ARDMS Advanced Item Type (AIT) questions called "Semi-Interactive Console" items. These require you to use your cursor to adjust controls on an onscreen console to correct a problem with the image presented. The console is "semi-interactive" because only some of the controls can be "adjusted." AIT—SIC items are currently limited to the Sonography Principles and Instrumentation (SPI) examination and as of this printing do not appear on the Pediatric Sonography exam, but as a bonus feature we have identified similar items in this mock exam.

209. Which type of liver abnormality will appear thick-walled and contain air?

   A. Hemangioma
   B. Lymphoma
   C. Hepatic cyst
   D. Pyogenic abscess

210. Which of the following is NOT a cause of hepatomegaly?

   A. Inflammation
   B. Portal vein thrombosis
   C. Vascular congestion
   D. Biliary obstruction

211. Name the condition caused by obstruction of small sublobular hepatic veins that is not normally visualized with ultrasound:

   A. Portal hypertension
   B. Arteriovenous malformation
   C. Budd-Chiari syndrome
   D. Veno-occlusive disease

212. The hypoechoic, focal liver masses in this infant's liver are most likely:

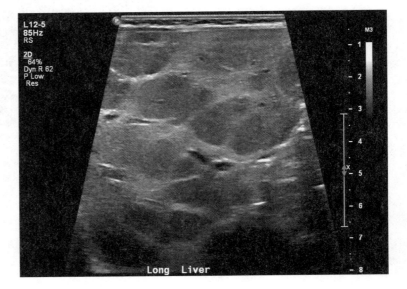

   A. Hemangioendotheliomas
   B. Hemangiomas
   C. Hepatoblastomas
   D. Polycystic liver

PART 6

Gallbladder and Biliary Ducts

Embryology and development

Normal anatomy

Associated lab values and hormones

Ultrasound prep and protocol

Normal ultrasound appearance

Pathology

Procedures

Note: The main topics of Part 6 are listed. For a complete study outline by topics and subtopics, see pages xxi–xxii of the table of contents. The clinical tasks on the ARDMS exam outline are cross-referenced to the entire text of this mock exam starting on page 607.

213. Which enzyme, when elevated, may indicate gallbladder or liver problems?

    A. Amylase

    B. Alkaline phosphatase (ALP)

    C. Albumin

    D. Aldosterone

214. What is the name of the hyperechoic linear structure located between the gallbladder and the right portal vein?

    A. Ligamentum teres

    B. Ligamentum venosum

    C. Interlobar fissure

    D. Cystic duct

215. What is the term for the folding of the gallbladder fundus, seen here?

    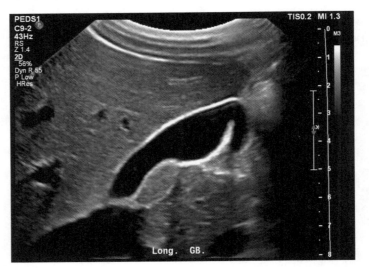

    A. Junctional fold

    B. Septate gallbladder

    C. Gallbladder fissure

    D. Phrygian cap

216. What is the most common indication for pediatric gallbladder and biliary tree imaging?

    A. Jaundice

    B. Abdominal pain

    C. Nausea and vomiting

    D. Family history of gallstones

217. Which hepatic vein courses in the same plane as the gallbladder fossa?

   A. Right hepatic vein

   B. Middle hepatic vein

   C. Left hepatic vein

   D. Left portal vein

218. An infant is scanned for persistent jaundice. A fluid-filled structure (arrow) is seen within the porta hepatis and continuous with the common bile duct. What is the most likely diagnosis?

See Color Plate 2 on page xxxiii.

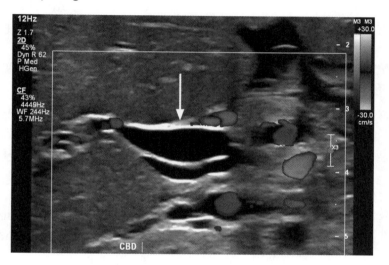

   A. Choledocholithiasis

   B. Fluid filled duodenum

   C. Choledochal cyst

   D. Hydropic gallbladder

AIT—Hotspot

219. What is the primary cause of acalculous cholecystitis?

   A. Cholestasis

   B. Trauma

   C. Gallstones

   D. Cholangitis

220. Which patient positions are most commonly used for imaging the gallbladder?

   A. Supine and right lateral decubitus

   B. Supine and left lateral decubitus

   C. Supine and prone

   D. Supine and right posterior oblique

221. What is the end product of the metabolic breakdown of hemoglobin?

    A. Biliverdin

    B. Red blood cells

    C. Hematocrit

    D. Bilirubin

222. The common hepatic duct is formed by the union of the:

    A. Cystic duct and common bile duct

    B. Main right and left hepatic ducts

    C. Intrahepatic bile ducts and common bile duct

    D. Common bile duct and pancreatic duct

223. Which of the following is a sonographic sign of air within the gallbladder?

    A. Reverberation and ring-down artifact

    B. Clean shadowing

    C. Ring-down artifact without shadowing

    D. Posterior enhancement

224. The normal gallbladder wall of a fasting patient should not measure more than:

    A. 1 mm

    B. 2 mm

    C. 3 mm

    D. 4 mm

225. Based on this image, what is the patient's most likely condition?

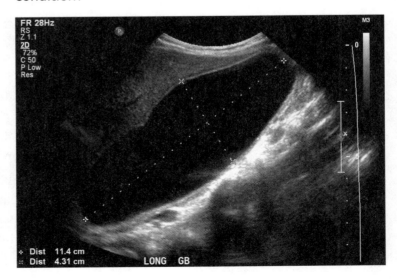

A. Chronic cholecystitis

B. Biliary atresia

C. Micro gallbladder

D. Hydropic gallbladder

226. Infection within the bile ducts is known as:
    A. Cholecystitis
    B. Cholangitis
    C. Cholestasis
    D. Choledocholithiasis

227. Where are biliary rhabdomyosarcomas most commonly found?
    A. Gallbladder
    B. Cystic duct
    C. Porta hepatis
    D. Common bile duct

228. Which of the following is the most common cause of jaundice in adolescents?
    A. Air in the gallbladder
    B. Choledochal cyst
    C. Biliary atresia
    D. Hepatitis

229. Which imaging modality has a 95% specificity for finding gallbladder pathology?
    A. Magnetic resonance imaging (MRI)
    B. Computed tomography (CT)
    C. Nuclear medicine
    D. Ultrasound

230. What is the LEAST likely location for an ectopic gallbladder?
    A. Retroperitoneal
    B. Suprahepatic
    C. Retrohepatic
    D. Intrahepatic

231. What is one way to differentiate side-lobe artifacts from sludge?

   A. Increase the power.
   B. Turn on the color Doppler.
   C. Increase the gain.
   D. Change the position of the patient.

AIT—SIC

232. The hypoechoic outline (arrow) seen along the outer edge of the gallbladder wall is most likely:

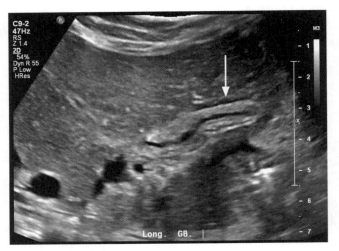

   A. Pericholecystic fluid
   B. Intrahepatic duct
   C. Ligamentum venosum
   D. Interlobar fissure

AIT—Hotspot

233. The surgical treatment for biliary atresia known as the Kasai procedure uses what portion of the intestine for draining bile from the liver?

   A. Stomach
   B. Duodenum
   C. Jejunum
   D. Ileum

234. What is the name of the duct (arrow) that drains the gallbladder?

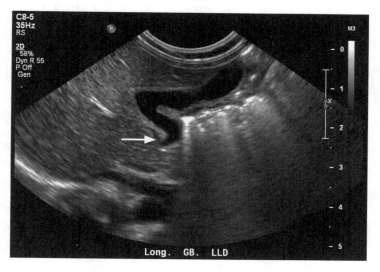

A. Cystic duct

B. Common hepatic duct

C. Common bile duct

D. Intrahepatic duct

AIT—Hotspot

235. Which hereditary disorder consists of an insufficient number of interlobular bile ducts?

A. Caroli disease

B. Cystic fibrosis

C. Biliary atresia

D. Alagille syndrome

236. A patient arrives for abdominal ultrasound an hour postprandial. The gallbladder in this image is most likely:

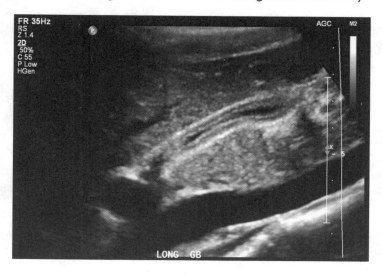

A. Perforated

B. Contracted

C. Inflamed

D. Septated

237. Stones within the biliary ducts are known as:

    A. Cholestasis

    B. Cholecystitis

    C. Choledocholithiasis

    D. Cholangitis

238. Which congenital anomaly results in common bile duct dilatation and biliary obstruction?

    A. Alagille syndrome

    B. Cholecystitis

    C. Choledocholithiasis

    D. Choledochal cyst

239. Which of the following is NOT a gallbladder segment?

    A. Head

    B. Body

    C. Fundus

    D. Neck

240. Ultrasound of the gallbladder is performed on a 16-year-old with a positive Murphy's sign, along with elevated alkaline phosphatase (ALP) and white blood cells (WBC). This image represents what finding?

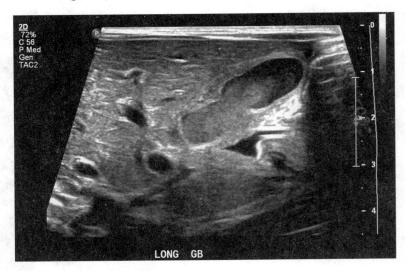

A. Choledocholithiasis

B. Chronic cholecystitis

C. Acute cholecystitis

D. Acalculous cholecystitis

241. Which congenital anomaly is associated with biliary atresia?

A. Gallbladder agenesis

B. Gallbladder duplication

C. Ectopic gallbladder

D. Septate gallbladder

242. Most gallstones in children occur as a result of:

A. Biliary atresia

B. Underlying disease

C. Low cholesterol

D. Gallbladder hydrops

243. The common bile duct is located between the junction of the cystic duct with the common hepatic duct and the:

A. Intrahepatic duct

B. Main right hepatic duct

C. Main left hepatic duct

D. Main pancreatic duct

244. Congenital cystic dilatation of the intrahepatic biliary tree is known as:

A. Alagille syndrome

B. Caroli disease

C. Cystic fibrosis

D. Biliary atresia

245. What procedure can be performed to remove ductal stones or place a stent within a bile duct?

A. Kasai procedure

B. Cholescintography

C. Endoscopic retrograde cholangiopancreatography (ERCP)

D. Magnetic resonance cholangiopancreatography (MRCP)

246. This echogenic, linear indention (arrow) is representative of a:

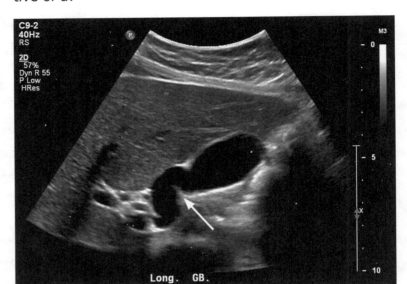

A. Phrygian cap
B. Sludge
C. Septate gallbladder
D. Junctional fold

AIT—Hotspot

247. Neonates undergoing total parenteral nutrition (TPN) are at a higher risk for developing gallstones secondary to:
A. Bile stasis
B. Cholangitis
C. Anemia
D. Malnutrition

248. You see a nonshadowing, echogenic structure adhered to the anterior gallbladder wall. It does not move when you shift the patient into a left lateral decubitus position. What is the most likely diagnosis?
A. Gallstone
B. Sludge
C. Air in the gallbladder wall
D. Polyp

249. Which of the following is NOT a sign of gallbladder perforation?
    A. Pericholecystic abscess
    B. Interruption of the gallbladder wall
    C. Thin gallbladder wall
    D. Small gallbladder size

250. Which two signs help to differentiate between acute and chronic cholecystitis?
    A. Wall thickness and lab values
    B. Murphy's sign and wall hyperemia
    C. Murphy's sign and lab values
    D. Wall thickness and hyperemia

251. Which of the following is a cause of gallbladder wall thickening?
    A. Anemia
    B. Splenomegaly
    C. Hypoalbuminemia
    D. Fasting

252. After turning a patient onto his left side, you noted this echogenic material (arrow) within the gallbladder lumen layers in the most dependent portion. What is the most consistent diagnosis?

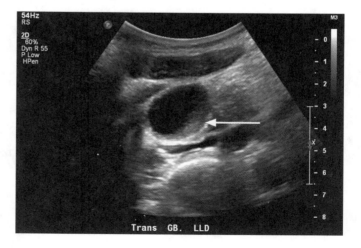

    A. Gallstones
    B. Air within the gallbladder
    C. Gallbladder polyp
    D. Sludge

AIT—Hotspot

253. Which sonographic finding increases the risk of malignancy when it accompanies a polypoid mass within the gallbladder?
    A. Sludge
    B. Wall thickening
    C. Ductal dilatation
    D. Hydrops

254. The most common pediatric complication occurring with gallstone disease is:
    A. Cholangitis
    B. Perforation
    C. Pancreatitis
    D. Choledocholithiasis

255. When sludge combines to form a mobile nonshadowing, echogenic ball it is known as:
    A. Tumorous
    B. Topical
    C. Tortuous
    D. Tumefactive

256. Which of the following is NOT a primary part of the biliary tree?
    A. Liver
    B. Pancreas
    C. Gallbladder
    D. Bile ducts

257. This sonographic finding (arrow), along with a small or absent gallbladder, has a specificity as high as 100% for:

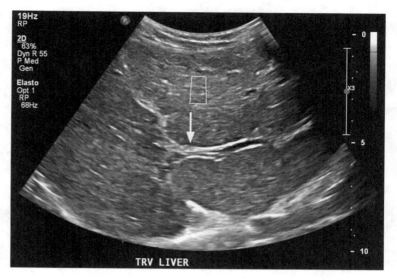

A. Biliary atresia

B. Portal vein thrombosis

C. Caroli disease

D. Choledochal cyst

AIT—Hotspot

258. In children and adolescents, the common bile duct should measure less than:

A. 1 mm

B. 2 mm

C. 4 mm

D. 6 mm

PART 7

Pancreas

Embryology and development

Normal anatomy

Associated lab values and hormones

Ultrasound prep and protocol

Normal ultrasound appearance

Pathology

Procedures

Note: The main topics of Part 7 are listed. For a complete study outline by topics and subtopics, see pages xxii–xxiii of the table of contents. The clinical tasks on the ARDMS exam outline are cross-referenced to the entire text of this mock exam starting on page 607.

259. Which portion of the pancreas lies posterior to the splenic vein?
    A. Uncinate process
    B. Head
    C. Body
    D. Tail

260. Which of the following is the most common endocrine tumor of the pancreas?
    A. Lymphangioma
    B. Adenocarcinoma
    C. Pancreatoblastoma
    D. Insulinoma

261. The endocrine component of the pancreas releases substances into the bloodstream known as:
    A. Hormones
    B. Enzymes
    C. Islet cells
    D. Proteins

262. What imaging modality is considered best for the evaluation of the pancreatic abnormalities?
    A. Ultrasound (US)
    B. Computed tomography (CT)
    C. Magnetic resonance imaging (MRI)
    D. Endoscopic ultrasound (EUS)

263. For imaging the pancreas in children, the best transducer selection would be:
    A. Curved 8 MHz
    B. Curved 9.5 MHz
    C. Curved 5 MHz
    D. Linear 12 MHz

264. What is the most common location of inflammatory spread and fluid collections from the pancreas?
    A. Pelvis
    B. Greater omentum
    C. Subphrenic space
    D. Anterior perirenal space

265. The diffuse proliferation of islet cells is a rare disorder known as:

   A. Hyperglycemia

   B. Insulinoma

   C. Congenital hyperinsulinism/nesidioblastosis

   D. Schwachman-Diamond syndrome

266. What is the vessel labeled 1?

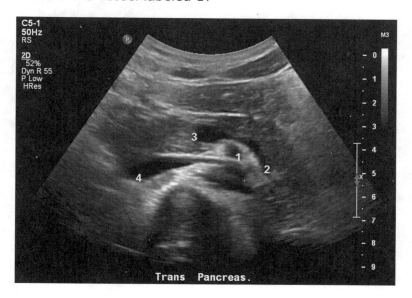

   A. Superior mesenteric artery (SMA)

   B. Splenic vein

   C. Portal vein

   D. Inferior vena cava (IVC)

AIT—Hotspot

267. The diameter of the pediatric main pancreatic duct should not exceed:

   A. 1 mm

   B. 2 mm

   C. 3 mm

   D. 4 mm

268. What is the most common complication of acute pancreatitis?

   A. Organ failure

   B. GI bleeding

   C. Pseudocyst

   D. Decreased calcium levels

269. What is the term for the segment of the pancreas labeled 3?

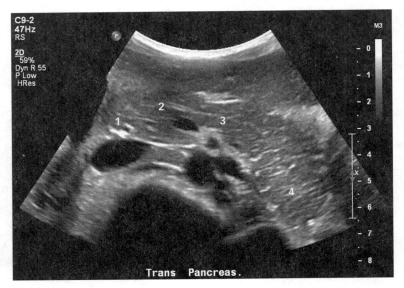

A. Head
B. Neck
C. Tail
D. Body

AIT—Hotspot

270. The exocrine functions of the pancreas aid in what process?

A. Digestion
B. Control of blood sugar
C. Production of white blood cells
D. Detoxification

271. Which of the following best characterizes the type of pancreatic cyst associated with von Hippel–Lindau disease or autosomal dominant polycystic kidney disease (ADPKD)?

A. Acquired
B. Secondary
C. Isolated
D. Congenital

272. Which of these conditions causes an increased echogenicity of the pancreas?
    A. Necrotizing pancreatitis
    B. Acute pancreatitis
    C. Cystic fibrosis
    D. Annular pancreas

273. What is the standard dimension for measuring the pancreas?
    A. Sagittal
    B. Anteroposterior
    C. Transverse
    D. Volume

274. What is another name for the main pancreatic duct?
    A. Duct of Wirsung
    B. Duct of Santorini
    C. Dorsal duct
    D. Ventral duct

275. What vessel is labeled 3?

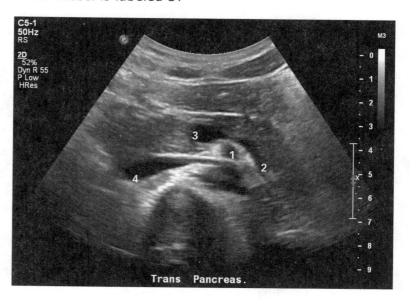

    A. Superior mesenteric artery (SMA)
    B. Splenic vein
    C. Portal vein
    D. Inferior vena cava (IVC)

AIT—Hotspot

276. Which of the following is a congenital pancreatic mass containing chylous fluid?
    A. Lymphoma
    B. Teratoma
    C. Insulinoma
    D. Lymphangioma

277. What is the most common location for an ectopic pancreas?
    A. Umbilicus
    B. GI tract
    C. Liver
    D. Spleen

278. In the sagittal plane, the head of the pancreas can be located directly inferior to which lobe of the liver?
    A. Left
    B. Right
    C. Caudate
    D. Quadrate

279. Which congenital anomaly could cause duodenal obstruction?
    A. Annular pancreas
    B. Pancreas divisum
    C. Ectopic pancreas
    D. Dorsal pancreatic agenesis

280. Which hereditary disorder results in thickened secretions in the lungs and digestive system?
    A. Schwachman-Diamond syndrome
    B. Von Hippel–Lindau disease
    C. Tuberous sclerosis
    D. Cystic fibrosis

281. One of the sonographic differences between a pancreatoblastoma and an adenocarcinoma is:
    A. Echogenicity
    B. Presence of metastasis
    C. Size
    D. Presence of ascites

282. Which vessel is labeled 2?

A. Superior mesenteric artery (SMA)

B. Splenic vein

C. Portal vein

D. Inferior vena cava (IVC)

AIT—Hotspot

283. What is the best acoustic window for visualizing the pancreas?

A. Left lobe of the liver

B. Right lobe of the liver

C. Stomach

D. Spleen

284. Which of the following is the most common congenital anomaly of the pancreas?

A. Annular pancreas

B. Congenital cysts

C. Pancreas divisum

D. Ectopic pancreas

285. Which pancreatic neoplasm is an infantile exocrine malignancy?

A. Pancreatoblastoma

B. Insulinoma

C. Adenocarcinoma

D. Lymphoma

286. A 10-year-old is involved in a bicycle accident and shows an upper abdominal contusion caused by falling on the handlebars. Which of the following would NOT be a concern in this case?

   A. Pancreatitis

   B. Insulinoma

   C. Hematoma

   D. Laceration

287. Which of the following is NOT a lab value used to assess the pancreas?

   A. Bilirubin

   B. Amylase

   C. Lipase

   D. Glucose

288. In a normal patient, how would the echogenicity of the pancreas appear in relation to that of the liver?

   A. Less than the liver

   B. More than the liver

   C. Isoechoic to the liver

   D. Anechoic to the liver

289. What is the term for the segment of the pancreas labeled 4?

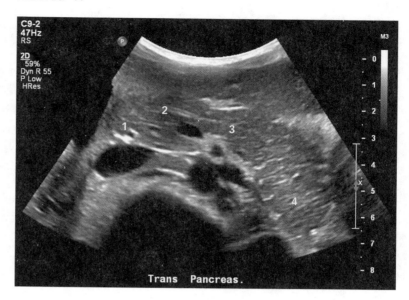

A. Head
B. Neck
C. Body
D. Tail

AIT—Hotspot

PART 8
Spleen

Embryology and development

Normal anatomy

Associated lab values and hormones

Ultrasound prep and protocol

Normal ultrasound appearance

Pathology

Procedures

Note: The main topics of Part 8 are listed. For a complete study outline by topics and subtopics, see pages xxiii–xxiv of the table of contents. The clinical tasks on the ARDMS exam outline are cross-referenced to the entire text of this mock exam starting on page 607.

290. Which of the following is NOT a component of the spleen?
    A. Red blood cells
    B. Smooth muscle
    C. White pulp
    D. Lymphoid tissue

291. Cat scratch fever can result in lymphadenopathy and:
    A. Abscess
    B. Cyst
    C. Hemangioma
    D. Lymphangioma

292. The arrows in this image identify the most common primary neoplasm of the pediatric spleen. What is this neoplasm?

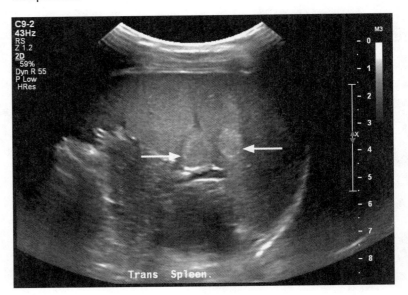

    A. Lymphangioma
    B. Hemangioma
    C. Lymphoma
    D. Hamartoma

AIT—Hotspot

293. The splenic vein and artery course transversely:
    A. Posterior to the pancreatic tail
    B. Anterior to the stomach
    C. Posterior to the left kidney
    D. Inferior to the transverse colon

294. The congenital condition in which the gastrosplenic and splenorenal ligaments are longer than normal results in:
    A. Sequestration
    B. Splenosis
    C. Wandering spleen
    D. Accessory spleen

295. Which of the following is a cause of splenomegaly?
    A. Heterotaxy
    B. Infarct
    C. Tuberous sclerosis
    D. Mononucleosis

296. A lethargic child with sickle cell anemia reports to the ER complaining of left upper quadrant pain. On ultrasound, the spleen is enlarged and contains heterogeneous areas. What would be the initial concern?
    A. Sarcoidosis
    B. Peliosis
    C. Infection
    D. Acute sequestration

297. In the presence of both non-Hodgkin and Hodgkin disease, which is the most common pediatric malignancy of the spleen?
    A. Hamartoma
    B. Metastasis
    C. Lymphoma
    D. Leukemia

298. A child with leukemia presents with abdominal pain. The ultrasound findings seen in this image are concerning for which splenic disorder?

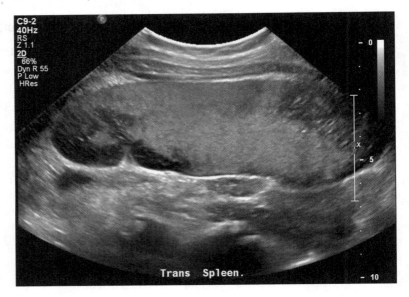

A. Infection

B. Infarction

C. Hematoma

D. Seqestration

299. Which lab value is NOT associated with the spleen?

A. Potassium

B. Hemoglobin

C. White blood cells

D. Platelets

300. The difference between congenital and post-traumatic splenic cysts is the presence of:

A. Blood flow

B. Posterior enhancement

C. Irregular borders

D. Epithelial lining

301. The sonographic appearance of the normal spleen should be:

A. Less echogenic than the liver

B. Less echogenic than the adrenal gland

C. More echogenic than the renal cortex

D. More echogenic than the pancreas

302. Splenic tissue found elsewhere in the body following trauma is known as:
    A. Sequestration
    B. Splenosis
    C. Polysplenia
    D. Wandering spleen

303. This small isoechoic structure (arrow) found adjacent to the splenic hilum is known as:

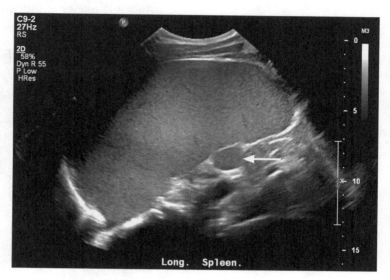

    A. Lymphangioma
    B. Polysplenia
    C. Splenic lobule
    D. Accessory spleen

AIT—Hotspot

304. Which of the following is NOT a sonographic finding in trauma involving the spleen?
    A. Fractures
    B. Peritoneal inclusion cyst
    C. Subcapsular hematoma
    D. Pleural effusion

305. Which congenital anomaly is associated with other thoracic and abdominal abnormalities?
    A. Spleen lobule
    B. Wandering spleen
    C. Asplenia
    D. Accessory spleen

306. A benign congenital malformation with the appearance of a multiloculated, hypoechoic mass is most consistent with a:

    A. Lymphangioma
    B. Complex cyst
    C. Lymphoma
    D. Hemangioma

307. This patient presents with fever, left shoulder pain, and left upper quadrant pain. What is the most likely diagnosis?

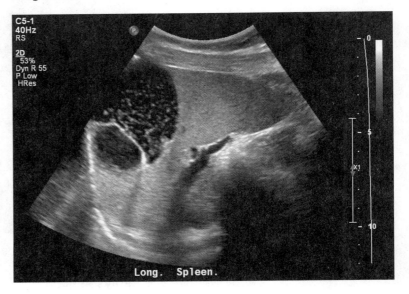

    A. Splenic cyst
    B. Pyogenic abscess
    C. Fungal abscess
    D. Lymphangioma

308. In children, splenic vein thrombosis is usually a result of:

    A. Infarction
    B. Portal vein thrombosis
    C. Trauma
    D. Pancreatitis

309. What is a function of the white pulp of the spleen?

    A. Regulates blood pressure
    B. Filters red blood cells
    C. Initiates the immune response
    D. Stores blood

PART 9

Urinary Tract

Embryology and development

Normal anatomy

Associated lab values and hormones

Ultrasound prep and protocol

Normal ultrasound appearance

Pathology

Procedures

Note: The main topics of Part 9 are listed. For a complete study outline by topics and subtopics, see pages xxiv–xxvi of the table of contents. The clinical tasks on the ARDMS exam outline are cross-referenced to the entire text of this mock exam starting on page 607.

310. What muscle lies medial to the kidneys?

    A. Latissimus dorsi

    B. Oblique

    C. Quadratus lumborum

    D. Psoas major

311. What is the term for two complete collecting systems within one kidney?

    A. Duplex kidney

    B. Crossed-fused ectopia

    C. Ureterocele

    D. Ectopic ureter

312. The inner portion of the kidney that contains the renal pyramids is called the:

    A. Sinus

    B. Medulla

    C. Column

    D. Cortex

313. The arrow in this image is pointing to the normal renal variant known as a:

    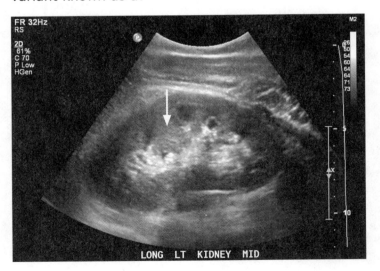

    A. Fetal lobulation

    B. Junctional parenchymal defect

    C. Hypertrophied column of Bertin

    D. Dromedary hump

AIT—Hotspot

314. The resistive index (RI) of a normal renal artery in a 10-year-old should not exceed:

   A. 0.5

   B. 0.7

   C. 0.9

   D. 1.0

315. Oligohydramnios, a "keyhole sign," and bilateral hydronephrosis are visualized on prenatal ultrasound. These findings are most consistent with what condition?

   A. Posterior urethral valves (PUV)

   B. Ureteropelvic junction (UPJ) obstruction

   C. Vesicoureteral reflux (VUR)

   D. Multicystic dysplastic kidney (MCDK)

316. In comparison to the right kidney, the left kidney lies slightly:

   A. Anterior

   B. Posterior

   C. Superior

   D. Inferior

317. What is the name of the fascia that covers the kidneys and adrenal glands?

   A. Scarpa's fascia

   B. Gerota's fascia

   C. Extraperitoneal fascia

   D. Psoas fascia

318. What is the name of the multiple channels that collect urine prior to drainage into the renal pelvis?

   A. Glomeruli

   B. Nephrons

   C. Pyramids

   D. Calyces

319. What is the name of the multiple hyperechoic masses (arrow) commonly seen with tuberous sclerosis?

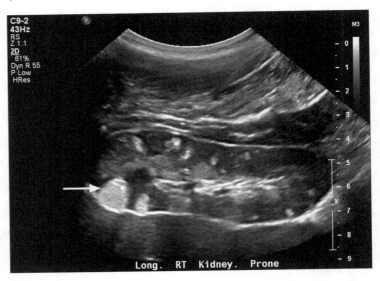

A. Lymphomas
B. Fungal balls
C. Angiomyolipomas
D. Rhabdomyomas

AIT—Hotspot

320. Where are the main renal veins located in relation to the renal arteries?
   A. Lateral
   B. Medial
   C. Posterior
   D. Anterior

321. Which tubular nephric structures of an embryo give rise to the adult kidneys?
   A. Mesonephroi
   B. Pronephroi
   C. Metanephroi
   D. Wolffian ducts

322. What is the most common unilateral cystic kidney finding in utero?

   A. Autosomal dominant polycystic kidney disease (ADPKD)

   B. Autosomal recessive polycystic kidney disease (ARPKD)

   C. Simple renal cyst

   D. Multicystic dysplastic kidney (MCDK)

323. Indicated by the arrow, this cystic projection is known as a:

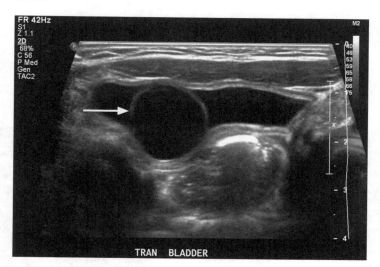

   A. Ureterocele

   B. Ectopic ureter

   C. Urachal cyst

   D. Bladder diverticula

AIT—Hotspot

324. The term for cysts located in the center of the kidney is:

   A. Parenchymal

   B. Cortical

   C. Extrarenal

   D. Parapelvic

325. The merging of the rectum, vagina, and urethra into one channel is known as:

   A. Urogenital sinus

   B. Persistent cloaca

   C. Patent urachus

   D. Megalourethra

326. A normal bladder wall measurement should not exceed:

   A. 3 mm

   B. 4 mm

   C. 5 mm

   D. 6 mm

327. This image was obtained from a patient with ultrasound findings of both kidneys on one side of the abdomen. What is the most likely diagnosis?

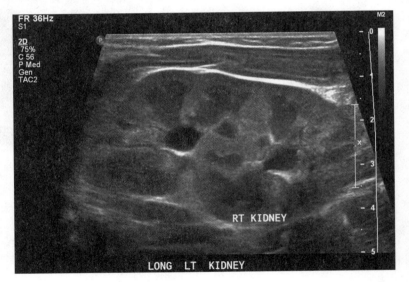

   A. Pelvic kidney

   B. Crossed-fused ectopia

   C. Horseshoe kidney

   D. Duplex kidney

328. Which kidney is most often used in a donor kidney transplant?

   A. Right

   B. Left

   C. Either

   D. The healthiest kidney

329. Which of the following is NOT a sonographic sign of renal artery stenosis?

   A. Low velocity at the site of the stenosis
   B. Discrepancy in renal size
   C. Elevated resistive index (RI) proximal to the stenosis
   D. Turbulence distal to the stenosis

330. A 3-year-old presents with abdominal distention, pain, and hematuria. What is the most likely diagnosis of the mass (arrow) demonstrated in this image?

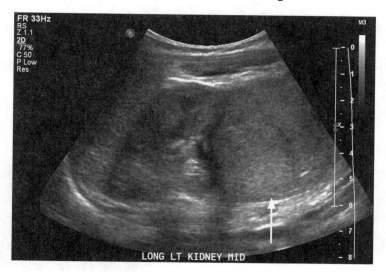

   A. Renal cell carcinoma
   B. Cystic nephroma
   C. Wilms tumor
   D. Lymphoma

AIT—Hotspot

331. Which sonographic characteristic can be seen when renal vein thrombosis is present?

   A. Decreased echogenicity of the kidneys
   B. Steady flow through the renal vein
   C. Distinct corticomedullary junction
   D. Renal arteries with a higher resistance

332. A child presents with an E. coli infection, fever, and vomiting. Both kidneys are enlarged, and the renal parenchyma is echogenic. What is the most likely condition?

   A. Pyonephritis

   B. Pyelonephritis

   C. Glomerulonephritis

   D. Fungal balls

333. Which sonographic characteristic would NOT be typical of a Wilms tumor?

   A. Echogenic

   B. Smooth, well-defined borders

   C. Solid

   D. Hypoechoic

334. What is the term for this extrarenal collection (arrow) caused by obstruction or trauma?

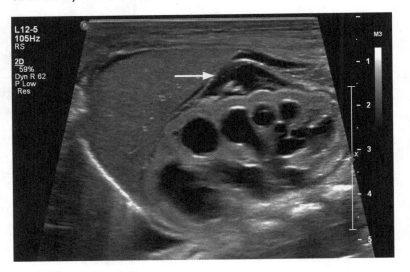

   A. Peripelvic cyst

   B. Abscess

   C. Urinoma

   D. Hematoma

AIT—Hotspot

335. Staghorn calculi are most commonly seen in which type of infection?
    A. Xanthogranulomatous pyelonephritis
    B. Fungal infections
    C. Pyonephritis
    D. Glomerulonephritis

336. As renal failure progresses and becomes chronic, the kidneys will appear:
    A. Edematous
    B. Hydronephrotic
    C. Hypoechoic
    D. Hyperechoic

337. Two months after a renal transplant, a recipient presents to the emergency room with right lower quadrant pain. The perinephric fluid collection seen on ultrasound most likely represents:

    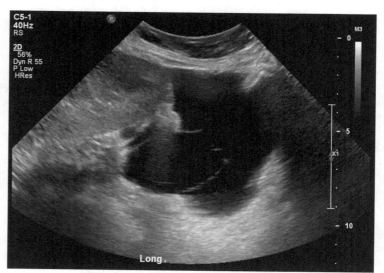

    A. Hematoma
    B. Lymphocele
    C. Hydronephrosis
    D. Urinoma

338. The dilatation of the renal pelvis and calyces seen in this image is known as:

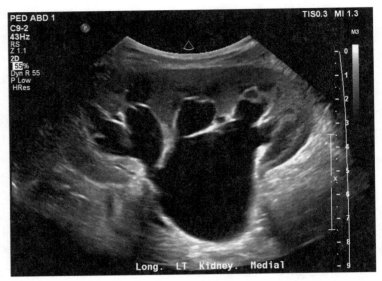

A. Reflux

B. Posterior urethral valves (PUV)

C. Hydronephrosis

D. Urinoma

339. During the percutaneous biopsy of a native kidney, the patient is placed in what position?

A. Prone

B. Supine

C. Right lateral decubitus

D. Left lateral decubitus

340. The renal hilum does NOT contain the:

A. Renal vein

B. Ureter

C. Calyces

D. Renal artery

341. Common indications for a renal sonogram include a urinary tract infection, congenital abnormalities, and:

A. Ear malformations

B. Sacral dimple

C. Hypotension

D. Headache

342. In this image, the kidney margin demonstrates:

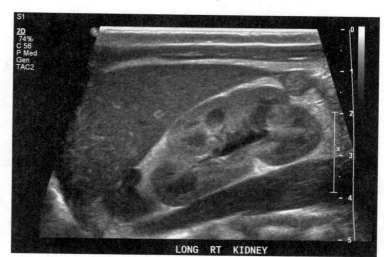

A. Junctional parenchymal defects
B. Dromedary humps
C. Hypertrophied columns of Bertin
D. Fetal lobulations

343. The purpose of a percutaneous nephrostomy drainage is to:
A. Catheterize the bladder
B. Obtain a biopsy sample
C. Relieve built-up pressure
D. Remove calculi

344. The artifact that is most diagnostic or most convincing of urolithiasis is:
A. Posterior enhancement
B. Acoustic shadowing
C. Reverberation
D. Ring-down artifact

345. You are performing a renal ultrasound exam and visualize a nonshadowing, echogenic mass within the collecting system of the right kidney. What would this finding most likely represent?
A. Nephrocalcinosis
B. Fungal ball
C. Medullary sponge kidney
D. Angiomyolipoma

346. Which of the following conditions is NOT associated with a neurogenic bladder?
    A. Prune belly syndrome
    B. Traumatic paraplegia
    C. Sacral agenesis
    D. Spina bifida

347. The urachus lies midline, superior and anterior to the peritoneum within the:
    A. Pouch of Douglas
    B. Anterior cul-de-sac
    C. Morison's pouch
    D. Space of Retzius

348. Which malignancy is most commonly found in older children or adults?
    A. Nephroblastoma
    B. Renal cell carcinoma
    C. Rhabdoid tumor
    D. Nephroblastomatosis

349. Renal size of more than 2 standard deviations below the expected mean for age is known as:
    A. Renal hyperplasia
    B. Renal agenesis
    C. Renal hypoplasia
    D. Renal ectopia

350. Which inherited disease is associated with renal cysts, pheochromocytomas, and an increased incidence of renal cell carcinoma?
    A. Autosomal recessive polycystic kidney disease (ARPKD)
    B. Multicystic dysplastic kidney disease (MCDK)
    C. Glomerulocystic disease
    D. Von Hippel–Lindau disease

351. Released after muscle activity as a waste product in the blood, this marker increases when kidney function slows down. Which is it?

    A. Blood urea nitrogen (BUN)

    B. Creatinine (CR)

    C. BUN/CR ratio

    D. Glomerular filtration rate (GFR)

352. What is the most likely diagnosis for a large, heterogeneous mass seen within the upper pole of the kidney (arrow) in a 3-month-old infant?

    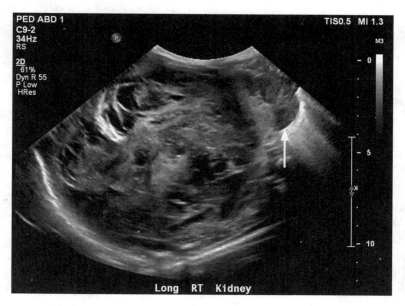

    A. Wilms tumor

    B. Renal cell carcinoma

    C. Lymphoma

    D. Mesoblastic nephroma

AIT—Hotspot

353. What abnormality is being demonstrated by the appearance of this kidney?

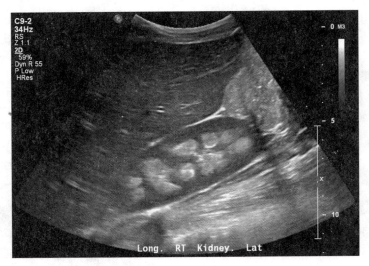

A. Urolithiasis

B. Nephrocalcinosis

C. Nephrolithiasis

D. Staghorn calculi

354. High-scale color Doppler can be used to demonstrate a twinkling artifact and assist in the diagnosis of what pathology?

A. Stones

B. Cysts

C. Abscesses

D. Hematomas

355. A 6-year-old with hematuria and hypertension is referred for a renal biopsy after sonography identifies enlarged kidneys with cortical echogenicity greater than that of the liver. What is the most likely cause?

A. Xanthogranulomatous pyelonephritis (XGP)

B. Glomerulonephritis

C. Nephrocalcinosis

D. Multicystic dysplastic kidney (MCDK)

356. What is the primary imaging modality for suspected renal trauma?
    A. Computed tomography (CT)
    B. Magnetic resonance imaging (MRI)
    C. Sonography
    D. Nuclear medicine

357. A 14-year-old presents with fever, abdominal pain, and lymphadenopathy. What is the most likely mass indicated by the arrows?

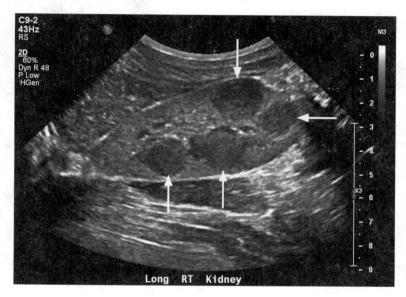

    A. Neuroblastoma
    B. Angiomyolipoma
    C. Lymphoma
    D. Cystic nephroma

AIT—Hotspot

358. The maximum anteroposterior measurement of the normal neonatal renal pelvis should not exceed:
    A. 10 mm
    B. 7 mm
    C. 5 mm
    D. 3 mm

359. What is the arrow pointing to in this image?

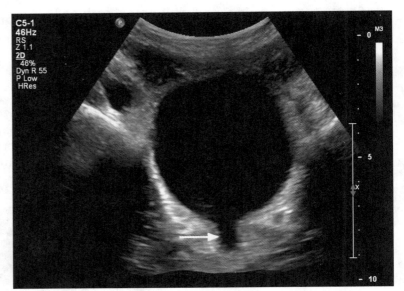

A. Ectopic ureter
B. Ureterocele
C. Dilated posterior urethra
D. Bladder diverticulum

AIT—Hotspot

360. Where is a Hutch diverticulum found?
A. Kidney
B. Bladder
C. Ureter
D. Urethra

361. Which of the following is NOT among the triad of abnormalities associated with prune belly syndrome?
A. Bilateral renal agenesis
B. Hypoplastic/absent abdominal wall muscles
C. Urinary tract anomalies
D. Cryptorchidism

362. This image was obtained when the sonographer was scanning an infant with an inflamed, wet umbilicus. What is the most likely diagnosis?

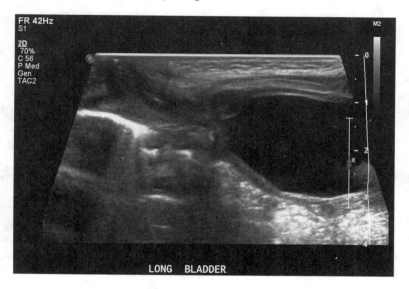

A. Persistent cloaca

B. Urachal cyst

C. Umbilical hernia

D. Patent urachus

363. When intrarenal pseudoaneurysms occur following percutaneous needle biopsy, what renal arteries are usually involved?

A. Main renal artery

B. Segmental arteries

C. Arcuate arteries

D. Interlobar arteries

364. The condition identified by an abnormally large, distended, and smooth-walled bladder is known as:

A. Bladder exstrophy

B. Neurogenic bladder

C. Hypertrophic bladder

D. Megacystis

365. A child with a known history of obstructive uropathy presents with a recent fever and flank pain. What is the most likely diagnosis of the pathology indicated by the arrow?

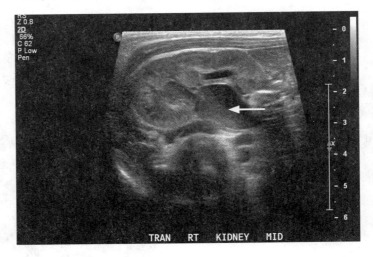

A. Pyelonephritis

B. Pyonephrosis

C. Fungal ball

D. Cystitis

AIT—Hotspot

366. Which condition is incompatible with life?

   A. Bilateral renal agenesis

   B. Eagle-Barrett syndrome

   C. Autosomal recessive polycystic kidney disease (ARPKD)

   D. Autosomal dominant polycystic kidney disease (ADPKD)

367. What is the name of the central band of tissue (arrow) that connects the two kidneys in a horseshoe kidney?

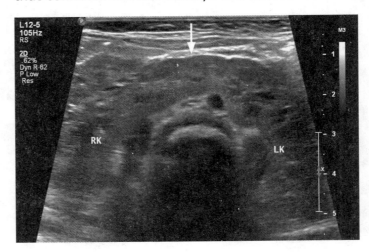

A. Moiety
B. Isthmus
C. Bridge
D. Renunculus

AIT—Hotspot

368. What is the condition associated with angiomyolipomas?
    A. Eagle-Barrett syndrome
    B. Henoch-Schönlein purpura
    C. Von Hippel–Lindau syndrome
    D. Tuberous sclerosis

369. What is the name for the bilateral renal cystic disease, seen in this image, that is associated with periportal hepatic fibrosis and Caroli syndrome?

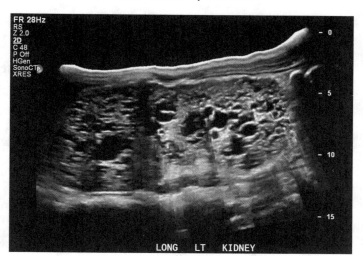

A. Multicystic dysplastic kidney (MCDK)
B. Autosomal dominant polycystic kidney disease (ADPKD)
C. Autosomal recessive polycystic kidney disease (ARPKD)
D. Medullary cystic disease

370. What type of obstructive uropathy is demonstrated in this image?

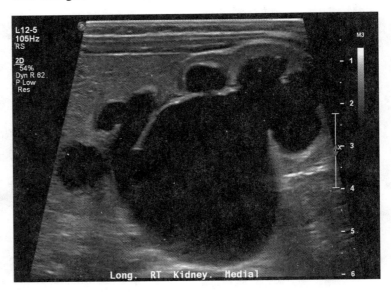

A. Vesicoureteral reflux (VUR)

B. Posterior urethral valves (PUV)

C. Ureterovesical junction (UVJ)

D. Ureteropelvic junction (UPJ) obstruction

371. What normal variant is demonstrated as a bulge in the middle of the lateral portion of the left kidney?

A. Hypertrophied column of Bertin

B. Dromedary hump

C. Junctional parenchymal defect

D. Fetal lobulation

372. When performing a renal ultrasound on a 6-week-old infant, which transducer frequency would you use?

A. 12 MHz

B. 9 MHz

C. 8 MHz

D. 5 MHz

373. What anatomic structure is indicated by the arrow?

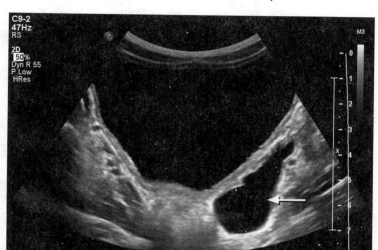

A. Bladder diverticula
B. Ureterocele
C. Megaureter
D. Hydronephrosis

AIT—Hotspot

374. Prior to the appointment, how would a patient be instructed to prepare for a renal ultrasound exam?
   A. Fast for 12 hours.
   B. Drink 32 ounces of water.
   C. Expect to undergo sedation.
   D. There is no routine exam preparation.

375. The end product of protein metabolism that is released through the kidneys is known as:
   A. Protein
   B. Creatinine (CR)
   C. Blood urea nitrogen (BUN)
   D. Urine

376. In this kidney, the arrows point out pathology representative of what disorder?

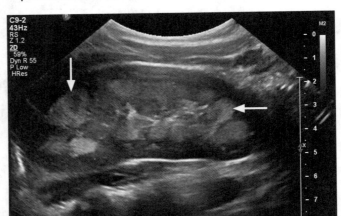

A. Medullary sponge kidney
B. Multicystic dysplastic kidney (MCDK)
C. Nephroblastomatosis
D. Urolithiasis

AIT—Hotspot

377. Which of these sonographic characteristics is associated primarily with acute renal failure?

A. Thinned renal parenchyma
B. Large, edematous kidneys
C. Decreased blood urea nitrogen (BUN) and creatinine (CR) levels
D. Small, echogenic kidneys

378. Which congenital anomaly is demonstrated in this image?

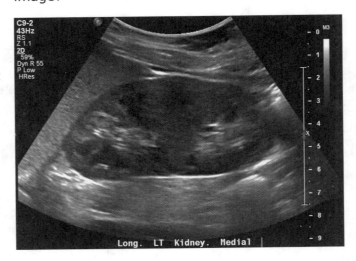

A. Horseshoe kidney

B. Hypertrophied column of Bertin

C. Cortical fusion defect

D. Duplex kidney

AIT—Hotspot

379. What defect results from failure of midline closure of the infraumbilical abdominal wall?

    A. Bladder exstrophy

    B. Patent urachus

    C. Bladder diverticula

    D. Megacystis

380. Of the four categories of renal trauma, which category is considered the most severe?

    A. Fractured kidney

    B. Avulsion

    C. Shattered kidney

    D. Laceration

381. Which of the following is considered to be a precursor to Wilms tumor?

    A. Mesoblastic nephroma

    B. Nephroblastoma

    C. Neuroblastoma

    D. Nephroblastomatosis

382. This image of a unilateral small kidney with multiple noncommunicating cysts most likely represents:

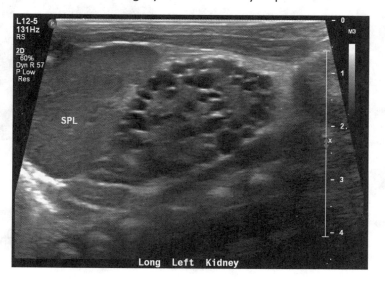

A. Autosomal recessive polycystic kidney disease (ARPKD)

B. Multicystic dysplastic kidney (MCDK)

C. Autosomal dominant polycystic kidney disease (ADPKD)

D. Glomerulocystic disease

383. The most common cause of acute renal failure is:

    A. Glomerulonephritis
    B. Xanthogranulomatous pyelonephritis (XGP)
    C. Henoch-Schönlein purpura
    D. Acute tubular necrosis (ATN)

384. When a ureter enters the bladder at an insertion point other than the normal location, it is considered:

    A. Eccentric
    B. Ectopic
    C. Aberrant
    D. Irregular

385. What is the most likely diagnosis for this rare, highly aggressive malignant tumor arising from the renal medulla and most commonly found in younger infants?

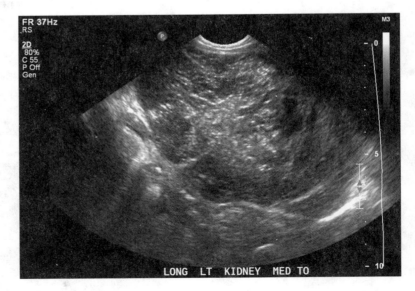

    A. Lymphoma
    B. Wilms tumor
    C. Rhabdoid tumor
    D. Renal cell carcinoma

386. What anomaly appears as an echogenic triangular focus or line within the renal cortex?
    A. Junctional parenchymal defect
    B. Fetal lobulations
    C. Hypertrophied column of Bertin
    D. Dromedary hump

387. Voiding cystourethrography (VCUG) is commonly performed to diagnose:
    A. Ureteral jets
    B. Vesicoureteral reflux (VUR)
    C. Ureteropelvic junction (UPJ) obstruction
    D. Hydronephrosis

388. This benign multiloculated mass (arrow) within the lower pole of the kidney is most likely a:

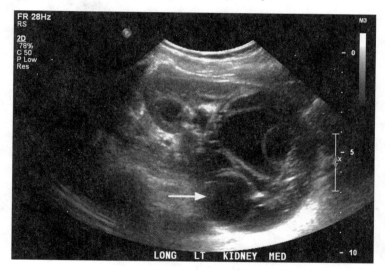

    A. Nephroblastoma
    B. Angiomyolipoma
    C. Rhabdoid tumor
    D. Cystic nephroma

AIT—Hotspot

389. Which renal arteries course between the renal pyramids?
    A. Segmental
    B. Interlobar
    C. Interlobular
    D. Arcuate

390. This image demonstrates a slow rise to peak systolic velocity, yielding a rounded appearance to the waveform upon Doppler interrogation. Which of the following terms applies to this waveform?

See Color Plate 3 on page xxxiv.

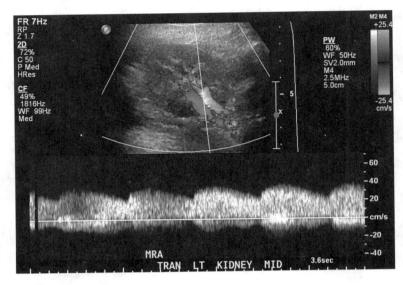

A. Early systole
B. Late systole
C. Tardus parvus
D. Acceleration time

PART 10

Adrenal Glands

Embryology and development

Normal anatomy

Associated lab values and hormones

Ultrasound prep and protocol

Normal ultrasound appearance

Pathology

Procedures

Note: The main topics of Part 10 are listed. For a complete study outline by topics and subtopics, see page xxvi of the table of contents. The clinical tasks on the ARDMS exam outline are cross-referenced to the entire text of this mock exam starting on page 607.

391. Which of the following does the adrenal medulla produce?
    A. Adrenocorticotropic hormone (ACTH)
    B. Creatinine (CR)
    C. Catecholamines
    D. Cortisol

392. In relation to the left kidney, the left adrenal gland lies:
    A. Anterolateral
    B. Anteromedial
    C. Posterolateral
    D. Posteromedial

393. An abdominal ultrasound is ordered for a 20-month-old outpatient for complaints of malaise and weight loss. What is the most likely diagnosis base on this image?

    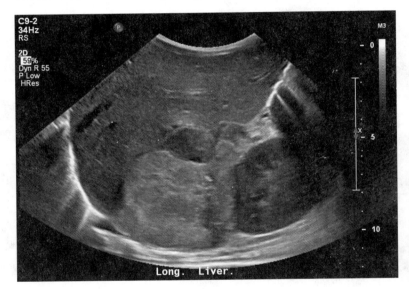

    A. Neuroblastoma
    B. Wilms tumor
    C. Hepatoblastoma
    D. Nephroblastoma

394. Cortisol, produced by the adrenal cortex, aids in all EXCEPT:
    A. Raising blood sugar
    B. Regulating the body's response to stress
    C. Reducing the immune response
    D. Absorbing calcium

395. In this image, the normal newborn adrenal medulla appears:

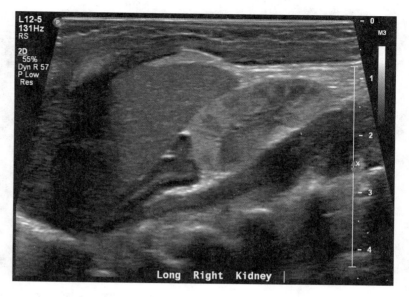

   A. Heterogeneous
   B. Anechoic
   C. Hypoechoic
   D. Hyperechoic

396. The right adrenal gland is posterior and lateral to what structure?
   A. Quadratus lumborum
   B. Inferior vena cava (IVC)
   C. Right kidney
   D. Tail of the pancreas

397. What is the term used to describe decreased levels of potassium?
   A. Hypokalemia
   B. Hypoglycemia
   C. Hypotension
   D. Hyposecretion

398. What abnormality seen in this image is associated with the traumatic delivery of a newborn?

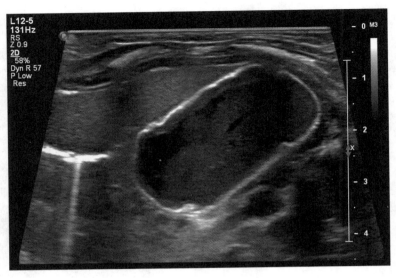

A. Adrenal hyperplasia
B. Adrenal hypoplasia
C. Adrenal hemorrhage
D. Adrenal infection

399. Which of the following can cause ambiguous genitalia in female infants?
A. Congenital adrenal hyperplasia (CAH)
B. Adrenocortical tumors
C. Neuroblastoma
D. Wolman disease

400. Which of the following assists in regulating blood pressure?
A. Adrenaline
B. Sodium
C. Creatinine (CR)
D. Aldosterone

401. Neuroblastoma is associated with all of the following EXCEPT:
A. Displacement of abdominal vessels
B. Malaise
C. Venous lakes
D. Abdominal mass

402. The shape of the adrenal gland in this image can be described as all of the following EXCEPT:

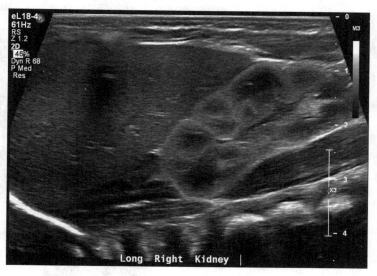

   A. Wishbone-shaped
   B. Y-shaped
   C. Inverted V–shaped
   D. C-shaped

403. Which of the following is NOT a zone or layer of the adrenal cortex?
   A. Glomerulosa
   B. Medullaris
   C. Fasciculata
   D. Reticularis

404. The adrenal medulla produces three types of catecholamines. Which of the following is NOT a catecholamine?
   A. Epinephrine (adrenaline)
   B. Norepinephrine
   C. Cortisol
   D. Dopamine

405. A sonographic finding that helps differentiate between a neuroblastoma and a Wilms tumor is:
   A. A well-defined mass
   B. Invasion or displacement of vessels
   C. Lymphadenopathy
   D. A solid mass

406. This hypoxic neonate presented with a left abdominal mass and anemia. Given the findings in this postnatal sonogram, what is the most probable diagnosis?

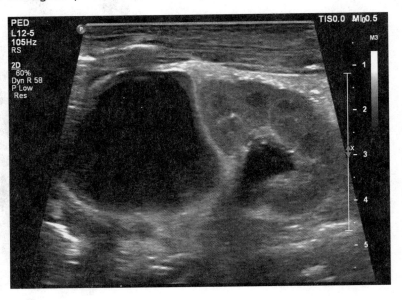

A. Adrenal cyst

B. Adrenal hemorrhage

C. Adrenocortical adenoma

D. Adrenal hypertrophy

407. What is the rare, and usually fatal, inherited disease that causes lipids (fats) to build up within body organs and the adrenal glands to become enlarged and calcified?

A. Wolman

B. Cushing

C. Addison

D. Beckwith-Wiedemann

408. In relation to the adrenal medulla, the adrenal cortex appears:

A. Isoechoic

B. Hypoechoic

C. Cystic

D. Hyperechoic

409. The arrows in this image demonstrate what characteristic of neuroblastoma?

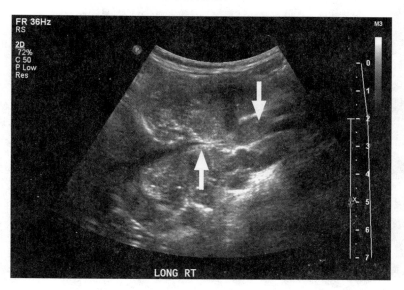

A. Liver metastasis

B. Pinpoint calcifications within the tumor

C. Encasement of the inferior vena cava (IVC)

D. Lobulated borders

AIT—Hotspot

410. The overproduction of cortisol by the adrenal cortex causes what syndrome?

A. Wolman

B. Addison

C. Beckwith-Wiedemann

D. Cushing

411. The adrenal tumor associated with hypertensive episodes, paroxysmal headache, and catecholamine secretion is:

A. Ganglioneuroblastoma

B. Pheochromocytoma

C. Neuroblastoma

D. Adenoma

412. What is the typical sonographic appearance of an adrenal cyst?
    A. Simple
    B. Complex
    C. Round
    D. Loculated

413. A neonate presents with an abdominal mass, fever, and leukocytosis. What is the most likely cause?
    A. Adrenal hemorrhage
    B. Adrenal adenoma
    C. Adrenal abscess
    D. Adrenal hyperplasia

414. Which adrenal tumor is associated with a "blueberry muffin" appearance of the skin and occurs in the neonatal period?
    A. 4S neuroblastoma
    B. Pheochromocytoma
    C. Ganglioneuroblastoma
    D. Adenoma

415. Which sonographic characteristic is NOT associated with cortisol-producing adenomas?
    A. Less than 5 cm in diameter
    B. Echogenic
    C. Demonstrating vascularity
    D. Heterogeneous

416. Which adrenal tumor may also be found in the mediastinum, head, or neck?
    A. Ganglioneuroblastoma
    B. Adrenal myelolipoma
    C. Adrenal adenoma
    D. Hemangioendothelioma

PART 11
GI Tract and Mesentery

Embryology and development

Normal anatomy

Associated lab values and hormones

Ultrasound prep and protocol

Normal ultrasound appearance

Pathology

Procedures

Note: The main topics of Part 11 are listed. For a complete study outline by topics and subtopics, see page xxvii of the table of contents. The clinical tasks on the ARDMS exam outline are cross-referenced to the entire text of this mock exam starting on page 607.

417. Which portion of the esophagus can be evaluated with ultrasound?

   A. Pharynx

   B. Thoracic portion

   C. Cervical portion

   D. Gastroesophageal junction

418. You are scanning a 4-year-old patient due to abdominal pain and see a peristalsing target structure in the left upper quadrant that measures 1.5 cm. With continuous evaluation this structure appears to resolve. What is the most likely diagnosis?

   A. Transient small-bowel intussusception

   B. Ileocolic intussusception

   C. Appendicitis

   D. Crohn disease

419. A 16-year-old patient presents to the emergency room with symptoms of chronic abdominal pain, weight loss, anorexia, diarrhea, and fever of unknown origin. Ultrasound is performed, and this image of the right lower quadrant is obtained. What is the most likely diagnosis based on the clinical symptoms and these findings?

See Color Plate 4 on page xxxiv.

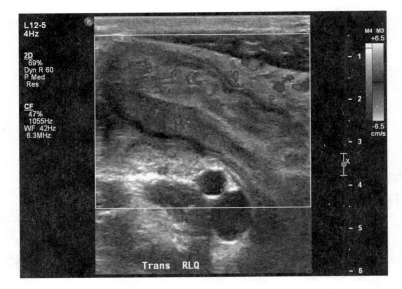

   A. Appendicitis

   B. Ileus

   C. Crohn disease

   D. Intussusception

420. What is the name of the most distal segment of the small bowel?

   A. Jejunum
   B. Ileum
   C. Duodenum
   D. Cecum

421. Which of the following landmarks is helpful when evaluating the appendix on ultrasound?

   A. Lower pole of the right kidney
   B. Psoas muscle
   C. Ascending colon
   D. Right lobe of the liver

422. What pathology is demonstrated in this image of an infant that presented with projectile vomiting?

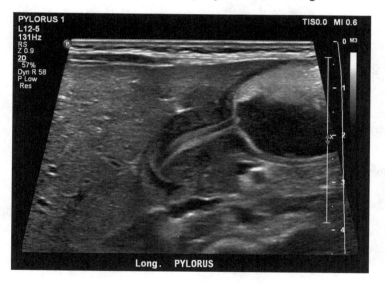

   A. Midgut malrotation
   B. Duodenal atresia
   C. Gastroesophageal reflux
   D. Hypertrophic pyloric stenosis

423. Which of the following conditions is associated with large-bowel obstruction?

   A. Henoch-Schönlein purpura
   B. Hirschsprung disease
   C. Cystic fibrosis
   D. Kawasaki disease

424. What is represented by the echogenic inner layer seen in this gastrointestinal duplication cyst?

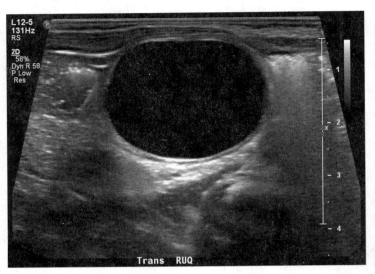

A. Mucosal layer
B. Muscular layer
C. Serosal layer
D. Fibrinous layer

425. Which of the following techniques is helpful in assessing the stomach?
A. Scan the patient in erect position.
B. Maintain patient fasting for 3 hours.
C. Distend the stomach with clear fluid.
D. Turn the patient into a left lateral decubitus position.

426. An inflamed blind-ending, fluid-filled tubular structure that arises from the ileum most likely indicates:
A. Appendicitis
B. Normal appendix
C. Meckel diverticulum
D. Crohn disease

427. A duodenal obstruction caused by intestinal malrotation is known as:
A. Midgut volvulus
B. Annular pancreas
C. Duodenal atresia
D. Pyloric stenosis

428. What pathology is shown in this image of a toddler with intermittent abdominal pain, vomiting, and bloody, "currant jelly" stools?

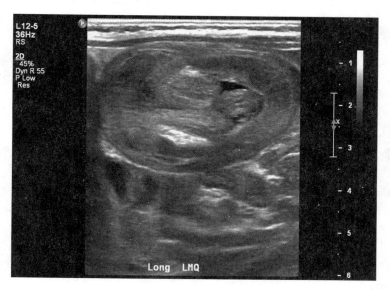

A. Appendicitis

B. Intussusception

C. Crohn disease

D. Ileus

429. A 12-year-old patient presents to the emergency room with acute periumbilical pain, fever, and an elevated white blood cell count (WBC). You obtained this image while interrogating the right lower quadrant and noticed tenderness in this area. What is the most likely diagnosis based on clinical symptoms and imaging findings?

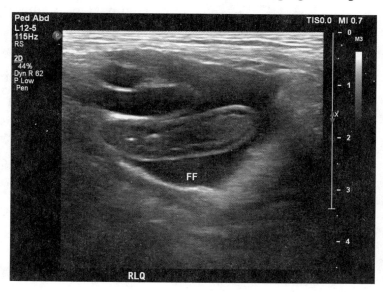

A. Intussusception

B. Crohn disease

C. Ileus

D. Appendicitis

430. What is the name of the peritoneal fold that connects the lesser curvature of the stomach and the liver?

    A. Mesentery

    B. Morison's pouch

    C. Greater omentum

    D. Lesser omentum

431. Which of the following is the most common type of bezoar in older children?

    A. Lactobezoar

    B. Phytobezoar

    C. Trichobezoar

    D. Foreign-body bezoar

432. Which of the following conditions is NOT associated with a "double bubble" sign?

    A. Duodenal diverticulum

    B. Duodenal atresia

    C. Severe duodenal stenosis

    D. Duodenal diaphragms (webs)

433. Which of the following measurements of the pyloric channel length and muscle wall thickness is considered abnormal?

    A. Muscle thickness of 2.5 mm

    B. Muscle thickness of 3 mm

    C. Channel length of 10 mm

    D. Channel length of 16 mm

434. Which of the following is NOT a cause of small-bowel mechanical obstruction?

    A. Ileus

    B. Intussusception

    C. Volvulus

    D. Duplication cyst

435. Which of the following is the most common malignant tumor of the small intestine in childhood?

    A. Non-Hodgkin lymphoma

    B. Hodgkin lymphoma

    C. Leiomyosarcoma

    D. Adenocarcinoma

436. What is the most common treatment for intussusception in younger children?

    A. Surgical reduction

    B. Endoscopic reduction

    C. Air reduction enema

    D. Surgical bowel resection

437. You are scanning an infant who presented with bilious vomiting. During the examination you see a fluid-filled proximal duodenum and these imaging findings in the mesenteric vessels. Which of the following conditions do you suspect?

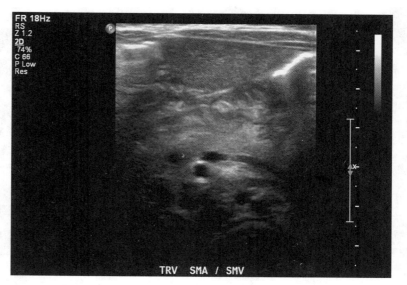

    A. Pyloric stenosis

    B. Annular pancreas

    C. Midgut malrotation

    D. Duodenal web

438. A double peritoneal fold that connects the intestines to the posterior abdominal wall is known as the:

   A. Visceral peritoneum

   B. Mesentery

   C. Lesser omentum

   D. Greater omentum

439. A 6-week-old infant presents to the emergency room with nonbilious projectile vomiting and a positive "olive sign." Which of the following pathologies is characterized by these clinical symptoms?

   A. Volvulus

   B. Duodenal atresia

   C. Midgut malrotation

   D. Pyloric stenosis

440. This transperineal image is showing a measurement between the skin line and the rectum. Which of the following conditions would require you to measure this distance?

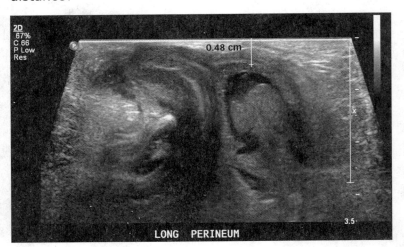

   A. Imperforate anus

   B. Rectovaginal fistula

   C. Cloaca

   D. Rectal mass

441. While scanning an infant for nonbilious projectile vomiting, you see an elongated pylorus with a muscle wall thickness up to 2.5 mm. During prolonged observation, the pylorus decreases in length and thickness, and fluid is seen passing through the canal. What is the most likely diagnosis?
   A. Hypertrophic pyloric stenosis
   B. Pylorospasm
   C. Gastroesophageal reflux
   D. Anisotropic effect

442. Premature patients are at a higher risk of developing which of the following diseases?
   A. Intussusception
   B. Pseudomembranous colitis
   C. Necrotizing enterocolitis
   D. Imperforate anus

443. When you are evaluating for median arcuate ligament syndrome (MALS) in the pediatric population, which of the following velocities obtained from the celiac artery during expiration would you use to determine an abnormal peak systolic velocity (PSV)?
   A. 75 cm/sec or greater
   B. 100 cm/sec or greater
   C. 200 cm/sec or greater
   D. 350 cm/sec or greater

444. Which of the following lesions is the most common primary benign tumor of the bowel in childhood?
   A. Duplication cyst
   B. Lymphoma
   C. Hemangioma
   D. Polyp

445. While scanning a patient for diffuse abdominal pain, you see this portion of the intestine and notice that peristalsis is absent. Which of the following pathologies is most likely to be diagnosed based on these findings?

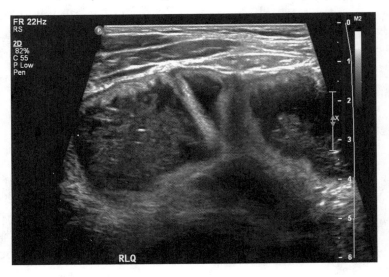

A. Crohn disease

B. Appendicitis

C. Ileus

D. Intussusception

446. Which portion of the large intestine is the cecum connected to?

A. Ascending colon

B. Transverse colon

C. Descending colon

D. Sigmoid colon

PART 12
Pediatric Hip

Embryology and development

Normal anatomy

Associated lab values and hormones

Ultrasound prep and protocol

Normal ultrasound appearance

Pathology

Procedures

Note: The main topics of Part 12 are listed. For a complete study outline by topics and subtopics, see page xxviii of the table of contents. The clinical tasks on the ARDMS exam outline are cross-referenced to the entire text of this mock exam starting on page 607.

447. Which scanning plane is used to evaluate and measure for developmental dysplasia of the hip (DDH)?
    A. Sagittal
    B. Coronal
    C. Transverse
    D. Oblique

448. A 5-year-old comes into the ER with hip pain, fever, and limping. What is the most likely diagnosis?
    A. Hip dysplasia
    B. Hip sprain
    C. Hip dislocation
    D. Hip effusion

449. What is the name of the harness used for treating DDH?
    A. Ortolani
    B. Barlow
    C. Pavlik
    D. Graf

450. Compared to bone, the infant femoral head is cartilaginous and:
    A. Hyperechoic
    B. Isoechoic
    C. Hypoechoic
    D. Anechoic

451. The angle in this image marked α is considered normal when it is greater than or equal to:

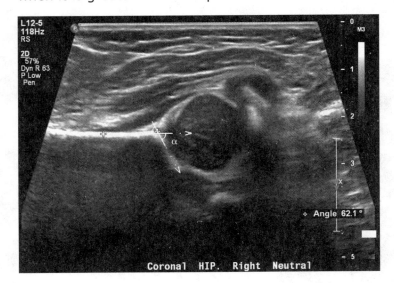

A. 30 degrees

B. 45 degrees

C. 50 degrees

D. 60 degrees

452. Femoral head coverage should be at least:

    A. 30%

    B. 40%

    C. 50%

    D. 90%

453. What is the name of the fibrofatty tissue that fills the space between the abnormal acetabulum and the femoral head?

    A. Pulvinar

    B. Hip capsule

    C. Triradiate cartilage

    D. Iliopsoas tendon

454. What do the calipers indicate on this image of the right hip?

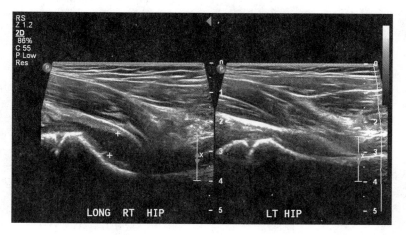

    A. Hip dysplasia

    B. Popliteal cyst

    C. Cellulitis

    D. Hip effusion

AIT—Hotspot

455. Who discovered the first method and technique for measuring hip dysplasia?
    A. Griffin
    B. Graf
    C. Grady
    D. Gregor

456. What is the maneuver performed during a physical exam involving a 90-degree flexion and frog-leg abduction of the hip?
    A. Ortolani
    B. Barlow
    C. Pavlik
    D. Graf

457. The harness used to treat DDH holds the legs in what position?
    A. Flexed and abducted
    B. Flexed and adducted
    C. Neutral and abducted
    D. Neutral and adducted

458. Identify the scan plane to use when you suspect hip effusion:
    A. Lateral
    B. Transverse
    C. Posterior
    D. Anterior

459. Which of the following is a risk factor for congenital hip dysplasia (DDH)?
    A. Family history
    B. Male gender
    C. Polyhydramnios
    D. Vertex presentation

460. What is the name of the maneuver whereby the infant hip is flexed, adducted, and pushed posteriorly?
    A. Ortolani
    B. Barlow
    C. Pavlik
    D. Graf

461. What is the one clinical sign that could help differentiate transient synovitis from osteomyelitis?
    A. Fever
    B. Hip pain
    C. Swelling
    D. Hip effusion

462. The examination to detect developmental dysplasia of the hip should be performed prior to:
    A. 4 weeks of age
    B. 6 weeks of age
    C. 8 weeks of age
    D. 12 weeks of age

463. How would you describe the femoral head shown in this image?

    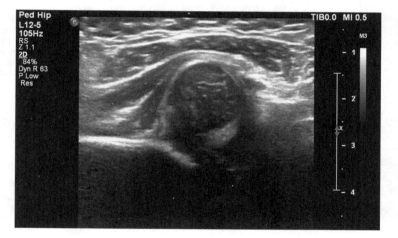

    A. Dislocated
    B. Subluxed
    C. Minimally covered
    D. Normal

464. In what pediatric age group does transient synovitis most commonly occur?
    A. Infants
    B. Toddlers
    C. Children
    D. Teenagers

465. What muscle lies immediately anteromedial to the hip capsule?

   A. Rectus femoris

   B. Psoas major

   C. Iliacus

   D. Iliopsoas

466. What is the best transducer for evaluation of the hip joint?

   A. 3D

   B. 5 MHz

   C. 8 MHz

   D. 12 MHz

467. If a hip joint is not correctly positioned in a harness during treatment, the most severe complication would be:

   A. Dislocation

   B. Subluxation

   C. Avascular necrosis (AVN)

   D. Osteomyelitis

468. The beta angle is the angle between the ilium and the:

   A. Acetabulum

   B. Labrum

   C. Ischium

   D. Femur

469. This image indicates which Graf classification of hip dysplasia?

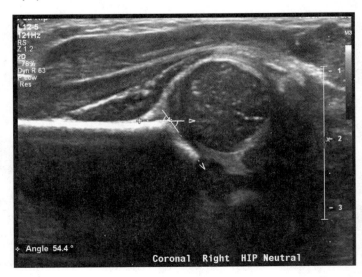

A. Type I
B. Type II
C. Type III
D. Type IV

470. What hypoechoic structure (arrow) lies centrally within the acetabulum on a transverse view of the infant hip joint?

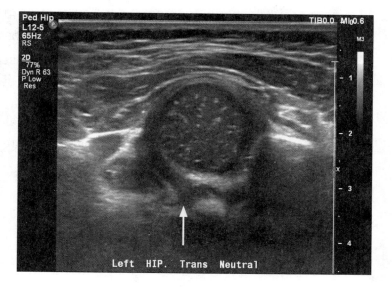

A. Iliopsoas muscle
B. Triradiate cartilage
C. Ilium
D. Labrum

AIT—Hotspot

471. Imaging of an infant for developmental dysplasia of the hip (DDH) should be done with the patient in primarily what position?
    A. Left lateral decubitus
    B. Right lateral decubitus
    C. Supine
    D. Prone

472. The alpha angle is the angle formed by the ilium and the:
    A. Ischium
    B. Acetabulum
    C. Labrum
    D. Femur

473. What advantage does radiography offer over ultrasound for evaluation of a 9-month-old for hip dysplasia?
    A. Allows for better hip stability
    B. Maintains patient cooperation
    C. Better visualizes the ossified femoral head
    D. Accommodates the presence of a harness

474. Developmental dysplasia of the hip (DDH) is the abnormal development of the:
    A. Acetabulum and femur
    B. Acetabulum and ischium
    C. Ilium and femur
    D. Ilium and ischium

475. Which bone is NOT one of the bones that make up the acetabulum?
    A. Pubis
    B. Ilium
    C. Labrum
    D. Ischium

476. In this radiograph what is the name of the structure labeled B?

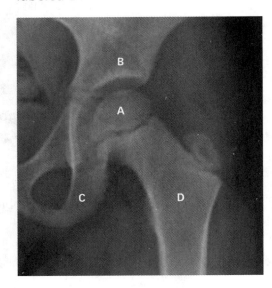

    A. Pubis
    B. Femur
    C. Ischium
    D. Ilium

AIT—Hotspot

477. The femoral head coverage documented on this image is:

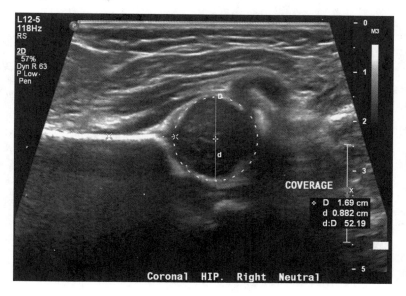

A. Dislocated
B. Subluxed
C. Shallow
D. Normal

478. Which congenital abnormality is usually characterized by a unilateral short lower extremity?

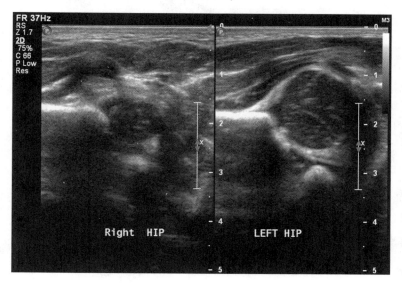

A. Dislocated hip
B. Developmental dysplasia of the hip (DDH)
C. Proximal focal femoral deficiency (PFFD)
D. Idiopathic avasuclar necrosis

PART 13
Female Pelvis

Embryology and development

Normal anatomy

Associated lab values and hormones

Ultrasound prep and protocol

Normal ultrasound appearance

Pathology

Procedures

Note: The main topics of Part 13 are listed. For a complete study outline by topics and subtopics, see page xxviii–xxix of the table of contents. The clinical tasks on the ARDMS exam outline are cross-referenced to the entire text of this mock exam starting on page 607.

479. In neonates and infants, which portion of the uterus is often the largest?
    A. Fundus
    B. Body
    C. Cervix
    D. Endometrium

480. When elevated, which hormone triggers ovulation?
    A. Follicle-stimulating hormone (FSH)
    B. Luteinizing hormone (LH)
    C. Estrogen
    D. Progesterone

481. What is the modality of choice for the diagnosis of uterine anomalies?
    A. Computed tomography (CT) scan
    B. Contrast-enhanced ultrasound (CEUS)
    C. Sonohysterography
    D. 3D ultrasound

482. Which phase of the endometrial cycle occurs after ovulation?
    A. Proliferative
    B. Secretory
    C. Menstrual
    D. Luteal

483. The ovaries are suspended within which ligament?
    A. Broad ligament
    B. Round ligament
    C. Cardinal ligament
    D. Inguinal ligament

484. Which cystic structure is NOT affected by the menstrual cycle?
    A. Physiologic cyst
    B. Corpus luteal cyst
    C. Peritoneal inclusion cyst
    D. Functional cyst

485. The most common pediatric ovarian malignancies are:
   A. Germ cell tumors
   B. Sex cord–stromal tumors
   C. Epithelial carcinomas
   D. Cystadenocarcinomas

486. Which female hormone is produced within the ovary?
   A. Luteinizing hormone (LH)
   B. Estrogen
   C. Follicle-stimulating hormone (FSH)
   D. Alpha-fetoprotein (AFP)

487. A cyst located along the anterior upper wall of the vagina is typically a/an:
   A. Inclusion cyst
   B. Nabothian cyst
   C. Cystadenoma
   D. Gartner duct cyst

488. The oviducts are also known as:
   A. Fallopian tubes
   B. Follicles
   C. Ovaries
   D. Gonads

489. In cases of precocious puberty, sonography is NOT important for:
   A. Measuring ovarian volume
   B. Evaluating the adrenal glands
   C. Assessing the presence of follicles
   D. Evaluating the size and shape of the uterus

490. The basalis layer of the endometrium:
   A. Stays intact throughout the menstrual cycle
   B. Thickens in the proliferative phase
   C. Thickens in the secretory phase
   D. Is closest to the uterine cavity

491. This image demonstrates:

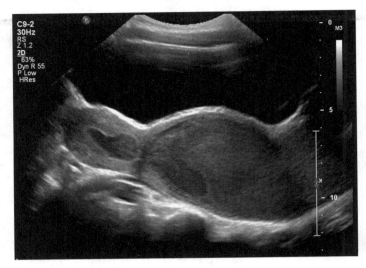

   A. Hydrometrocolpos
   B. Hydrocolpos
   C. Hematocolpos
   D. Hematometrocolpos

492. Uterine fusion defects are associated with:
   A. Precocious puberty
   B. Renal anomalies
   C. Cardiac anomalies
   D. Biliary atresia

493. Elevated alpha-fetoprotein levels may be found with which type of malignant ovarian tumor?
   A. Teratoma
   B. Endodermal sinus tumor
   C. Granulosa cell tumor
   D. Sertoli-Leydig tumor

494. For transabdominal pelvic sonography of a pediatric patient, a well-distended bladder:
   A. Is unnecessary
   B. Eliminates the need for vaginal sonography
   C. Displaces the bowel out of the pelvis
   D. Displaces the ovaries medially

495. What is the name for the dominant follicle within an ovary?
    A. Graafian
    B. Corpus luteum
    C. Functional
    D. Physiologic

496. Which type of cyst can be seen with pelvic inflammatory disease (PID)?
    A. Cystadenoma
    B. Cystic teratoma
    C. Peritoneal inclusion cyst
    D. Para-ovarian cyst

497. Amenorrhea, hirsutism, and obesity are clinical signs of:
    A. Stein-Leventhal syndrome
    B. Turner syndrome
    C. Noonan syndrome
    D. Mayer-Rokitansky-Küster-Hauser syndrome

498. What is the most common benign ovarian mass in females of all ages?
    A. Para-ovarian cyst
    B. Dysgerminoma
    C. Cystadenoma
    D. Functional cyst

499. An adolescent girl presents to the ER complaining of an acute onset of pelvic pain, nausea, and vomiting. A pelvic ultrasound was ordered and this image was obtained. What is the most likely diagnosis?

See Color Plate 5 on page xxxv.

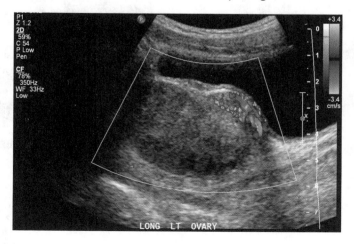

A. Precocious puberty
B. Ovarian torsion
C. Dermoid
D. Polycystic ovary

500. The most common congenital müllerian fusion anomaly of the uterus is:
A. Bicornuate uterus
B. Uterus didelphys
C. Septate uterus
D. Arcuate uterus

501. Postmenarcheal ovaries are located:
A. Posterior and lateral to the uterus
B. Superior and medial to the uterus
C. Superior and lateral to the fallopian tubes
D. Inferior and lateral to the fallopian tubes

502. Abnormal endometrial glands found within the myometrium of the uterus constitute a condition known as:
A. Leiomyoma
B. Adenomyosis
C. Endometritis
D. Endometrioma

503. The pathology represented in this image of an adolescent patient is most likely the result of:

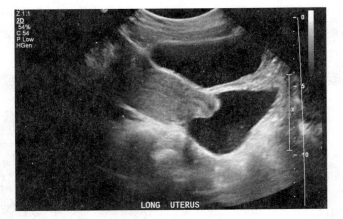

A. Ovarian cyst
B. Rhabdomyosarcoma
C. Gartner duct cyst
D. Vaginal obstruction

504. Which type of leiomyoma involves the endometrium?
    A. Submucosal
    B. Subserosal
    C. Intramural
    D. Pedunculated

505. Which of the following would NOT be included among the differential diagnoses for a hemorrhagic cyst?
    A. Cystic teratoma
    B. Appendiceal abscess
    C. Lymphadenopathy
    D. Ectopic pregnancy

506. Which of the following is the most common malignancy of the pediatric uterus or vagina?
    A. Adenocarcinoma
    B. Rhabdomyosarcoma
    C. Granulosa cell tumor
    D. Sertoli-Leydig tumor

507. Which of the following would NOT be a cause of primary amenorrhea?
    A. Pituitary lesions
    B. Polycystic ovary syndrome (PCOS)
    C. Arcuate uterus
    D. Hypothalamic lesions

508. The left ovarian vein drains into the:
    A. Left renal vein
    B. Left internal iliac vein
    C. Left common iliac vein
    D. Inferior vena cava (IVC)

509. In cases of intersex disorders, ultrasound plays an important role in identifying which organ(s)?
    A. Ovaries
    B. Testes
    C. Adrenal glands
    D. Uterus

510. Which pituitary hormone promotes the maturation of follicles?

    A. Luteinizing hormone (LH)

    B. Follicle-stimulating hormone (FSH)

    C. Estrogen

    D. Progesterone

511. A 14-year-old is scanned due to a palpable midline mass. Sonography demonstrates the complex midline mass seen in this image. What is the most likely diagnosis?

    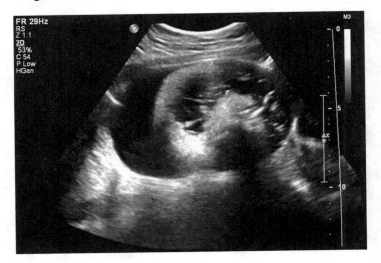

    A. Cystic teratoma

    B. Uterine fibroid

    C. Para-ovarian cyst

    D. Pyosalpinx

512. The endometrium is thinnest during which phase of the endometrial cycle?

    A. Secretory

    B. Proliferative

    C. Menstrual

    D. Ovulatory

513. Which malignant ovarian neoplasm may cause precocious puberty?

    A. Malignant teratoma

    B. Dysgerminoma

    C. Endodermal sinus tumor

    D. Granulosa cell tumor

514. The uterine arteries originate from the:
    A. Common iliac arteries
    B. Aorta
    C. Internal iliac arteries
    D. Renal arteries

515. The difference between physiologic and functional cysts is the:
    A. Lining
    B. Contents
    C. Age of the patient
    D. Size

516. The corpus luteum releases which hormone to help prepare the body for pregnancy?
    A. Follicle-stimulating hormone (FSH)
    B. Human chorionic gonadotropin (hCG)
    C. Estrogen
    D. Progesterone

517. A 16-year-old reports to the ER with right lower quadrant pain and tests positive for gonorrhea. What is the most likely diagnosis for this complex mass?

    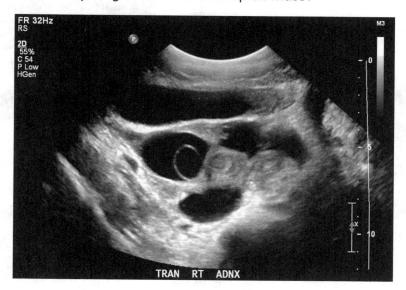

    A. Appendicitis
    B. Pelvic inflammatory disease (PID)
    C. Dermoid cyst
    D. Hemorrhagic cyst

518. What is the name of the fusion anomaly that results in two complete uteri, cervices, and vaginas?

   A. Uterus didelphys
   B. Bicornuate uterus
   C. Arcuate uterus
   D. Unicornuate uterus

519. Which of the following is the LEAST common pediatric ovarian mass?

   A. Hemorrhagic cyst
   B. Cystic teratoma
   C. Functional cyst
   D. Cystadenoma

520. What is the term for the structure indicated by the arrow?

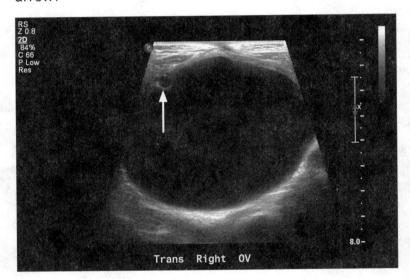

   A. Oocyte
   B. Theca-lutein cyst
   C. Graafian follicle
   D. Daughter cyst

AIT—Hotspot

521. Which of the following is NOT a component of the vascular pedicle of the ovary?

    A. Fallopian tube
    B. Broad ligament
    C. Round ligament
    D. Ovarian artery

522. What is the fusion anomaly in this image that consists of two symmetric uterine horns communicating with each other caudally?

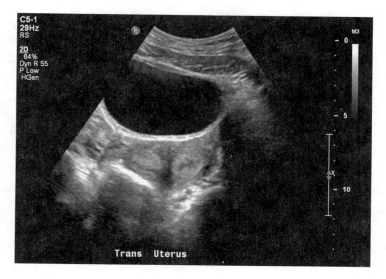

    A. Uterus didelphys
    B. Bicornuate uterus
    C. Septate uterus
    D. Uterine agenesis

PART 14

Male Pelvis, Scrotum, and Testes

Embryology and development

Normal anatomy

Associated lab values and hormones

Ultrasound prep and protocol

Normal ultrasound appearance

Pathology

Procedures

Note: The main topics of Part 14 are listed. For a complete study outline by topics and subtopics, see page xxx of the table of contents. The clinical tasks on the ARDMS exam outline are cross-referenced to the entire text of this mock exam starting on page 607.

523. What vessel does the left testicular vein drain into?

   A. Inferior vena cava

   B. Left common iliac vein

   C. Left renal vein

   D. Left adrenal vein

524. A testis that has been twisted for 6 hours will most likely appear:

   A. Hypoechoic

   B. Hyperechoic

   C. Heterogeneous

   D. Normal

525. What type of parameter adjustment is needed to improve the quality of this spectral Doppler image?

See Color Plate 6 on page xxxv.

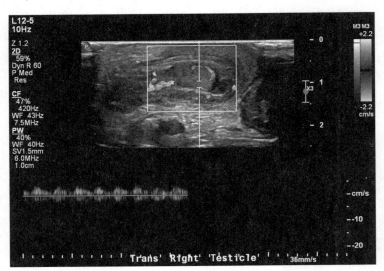

   A. Decrease gain.

   B. Increase wall filter.

   C. Decrease pulse repetition frequency.

   D. Increase pulse repetition frequency.

AIT—SIC

526. Which of the following muscles, in conjunction with the cremaster muscle, allows for the contraction and relaxation of the scrotum?

   A. Raphe

   B. Internal oblique

   C. External spermatic

   D. Dartos

527. In this longitudinal image of the scrotum, what structure is identified by the arrow?

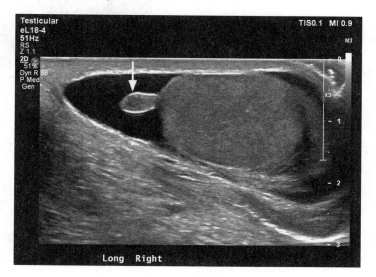

   A. Epididymal head

   B. Testicular appendage

   C. Scrotolith

   D. Epididymal tail

AIT—Hotspot

528. Which of the following conditions is often seen with epididymitis?

   A. Orchitis

   B. Intratesticular neoplasm

   C. Testicular torsion

   D. "Bell-clapper" deformity

529. What abnormality is shown in this image of the inguinal canal?

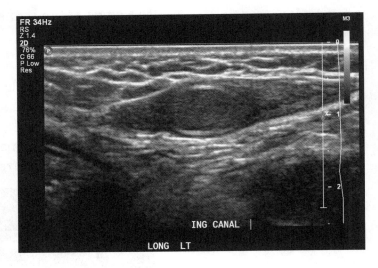

A. Testicular torsion
B. Cryptorchidism
C. Crossed testicular ectopia
D. Polyorchidism

530. Hydroceles form between which layers?

A. Internal and external spermatic fascia
B. Internal spermatic fascia and tunica vaginalis
C. Visceral tunica vaginalis and tunica albuginea
D. Visceral and parietal layers of the tunica vaginalis

531. What pathology is demonstrated in this image of the inguinal canal?

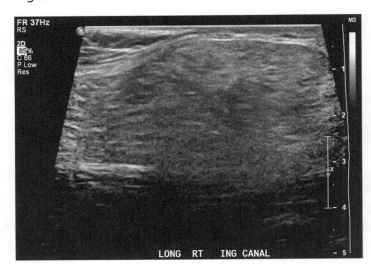

A. Varicocele

B. Epididymitis

C. Hydrocele

D. Hernia

532. What would be the normal echogenicity of the testes of a 10-year-old patient?

    A. High-level echoes

    B. Low-level echoes

    C. Medium-level echoes

    D. Anechoic

533. What is the most likely diagnosis of this pediatric primary paratesticular malignant neoplasm?

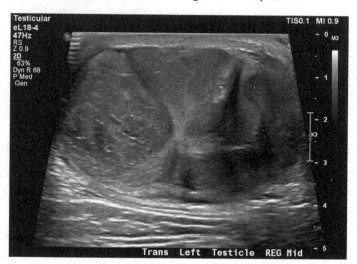

    A. Embryonal rhabdomyosarcoma

    B. Adenomatoid tumor

    C. Neurofibroma

    D. Seminoma

534. Which of the following conditions can cause a left varicocele?

    A. Epididymo-orchitis

    B. Hydrocele

    C. Bell-clapper deformity

    D. Nutcracker syndrome

535. This image was obtained from an adolescent patient with symptoms of gradual acute scrotal pain and edema. What is the most likely diagnosis?

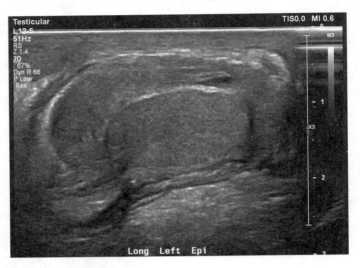

A. Orchitis
B. Epididymitis
C. Testicular torsion
D. Appendiceal torsion

536. Which of the following hormones controls the embryologic testicular descent from the abdomen to the scrotum?

A. Testosterone
B. Follicle-stimulating hormone (FSH)
C. Human chorionic gonadotropin (hCG)
D. Androgen

537. What structure is the arrow pointing to in this image?

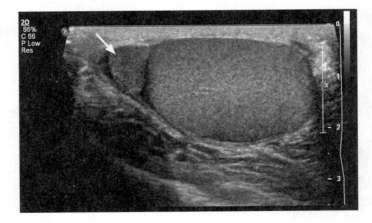

A. Epididymis
B. Mediastinum
C. Spermatic cord
D. Pampiniform plexus

AIT—Hotspot

538. This image was obtained from a neonatal patient. What is the most likely diagnosis for the pathology seen here (arrow)?

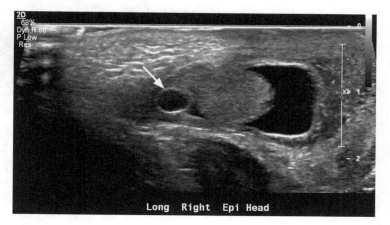

A. Epididymal cyst
B. Spermatocele
C. Epididymal cystadenoma
D. Lymphangioma

AIT—Hotspot

539. Which of the following conditions is associated with the bell-clapper deformity?
A. Extravaginal testicular torsion
B. Intravaginal testicular torsion
C. Neonatal testicular torsion
D. In utero testicular torsion

540. Which of the following maneuvers does NOT help with the diagnosis of the condition seen in this image?

See Color Plate 7 on page xxxvi.

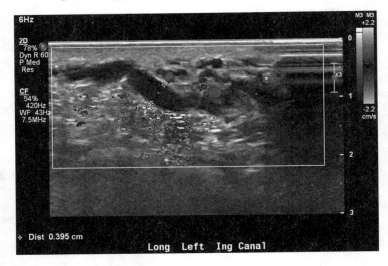

A. Standing position

B. Reverse Trendelenburg

C. Compression

D. Valsalva

541. Which of the following conditions is associated with ovotestis?

A. Hypospadias

B. True hermaphroditism

C. Cryptorchidism

D. Monorchidism

542. From which of the following vessels do the testicular arteries arise?

A. Vesicular arteries

B. External iliac arteries

C. Aorta

D. Internal iliac arteries

543. Which of the following is the most likely diagnosis of this benign testicular neoplasm?

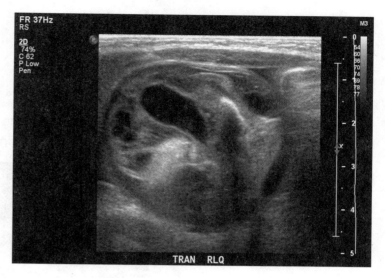

A. Endodermal sinus tumor

B. Seminoma

C. Epidermoid cyst

D. Teratoma

544. What structure is indicated by the arrow in this image?

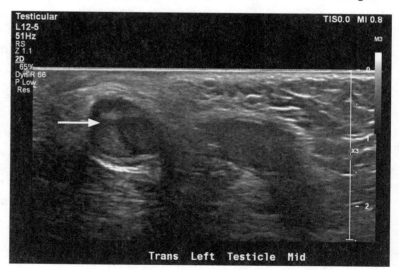

A. Penis

B. Right testis

C. Epididymis

D. Appendix testis

AIT—Hotspot

545. Which of the following measurements is considered a normal length of the prepubertal testis?

    A. 1.5 cm
    B. 2.5 cm
    C. 3.5 cm
    D. 4.5 cm

546. Which of the following syndromes is most likely to be associated with the findings seen in this image?

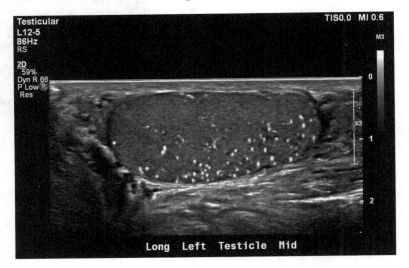

    A. Klinefelter syndrome
    B. Eagle-Barrett syndrome
    C. Prader-Willi syndrome
    D. Noonan syndrome

547. Which layer is disrupted when a testicular rupture occurs?

    A. External spermatic fascia
    B. Cremasteric fascia
    C. Tunica vaginalis
    D. Tunica albuginea

548. What layer of tissue forms the mediastinum testis?

    A. Cremasteric fascia
    B. Internal spermatic fascia
    C. Tunica vaginalis
    D. Tunica albuginea

549. What hormone induces and maintains male sexual secondary characteristics?
    A. Estrogen
    B. Luteinizing hormone (LH)
    C. Testosterone
    D. Inhibin

550. Bilateral agenesis of the testes is known as:
    A. Monorchidism
    B. Anorchidism
    C. Cryptorchidism
    D. Triorchidism

551. Which of the following is a rare pediatric testicular tumor associated with undescended testes?
    A. Seminoma
    B. Teratoma
    C. Embryonal carcinoma
    D. Endodermal sinus tumor

552. A teenage boy presents in the emergency room complaining of a sudden onset of left testicular pain. You perform an ultrasound exam and see the findings in this image. What is the likely diagnosis?

See Color Plate 8 on page xxxvi.

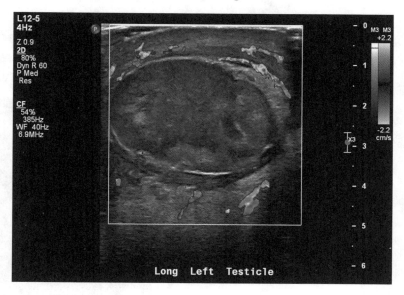

   A. Orchitis
   B. Testicular torsion
   C. Testicular hematoma
   D. Appendiceal torsion

553. This image supports the diagnosis of:

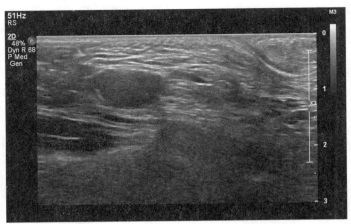

A. Herniated bowel

B. Herniated omentum

C. Cryptorchidism

D. Hydrocele

554. Which of the following abnormalities is associated with a blind-ending spermatic cord?

A. Anorchidism

B. Polyorchidism

C. Cryptorchidism

D. Monorchidism

555. This 15-year-old patient presented to the ultrasound department with orders for a scrotal ultrasound due to a painless palpable mass. Based on the imaging findings, what is the most likely diagnosis?

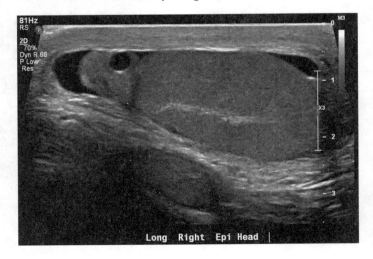

A. Epididymal cystadenoma

B. Spermatocele

C. Testicular cyst

D. Lymphangioma

556. The "blue dot sign" is associated with which of the following conditions?

    A. Testicular appendage torsion

    B. Testicular torsion

    C. Testicular infarction

    D. Testicular trauma

557. Which of the following masses is most commonly associated with the abnormal male karyotype?

    A. Teratoma

    B. Juvenile granulosa cell tumor

    C. Gonadoblastoma

    D. Sertoli cell tumor

PART 15
Soft Tissue

Normal ultrasound appearance

Use of the standoff pad

Imaging the contralateral side

Pathology

Note: The main topics of Part 15 are listed. For a complete study outline by topics and subtopics, see page xxxi of the table of contents. The clinical tasks on the ARDMS exam outline are cross-referenced to the entire text of this mock exam starting on page 607.

558. This structure was located in the sacrococcygeal region of a teenage male complaining of tenderness in the area. Based on the ultrasound findings and clinical symptoms, what is the most likely diagnosis?

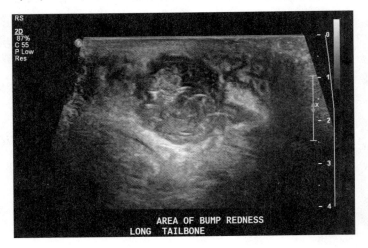

A. Sacrococcygeal teratoma

B. Synovial cyst

C. Meniscal cyst

D. Pilonidal cyst

559. The Achilles tendon connects which of the following muscles and bones?

A. Gastrocnemius and calcaneus

B. Subscapularis and humerus

C. Quadriceps and patella

D. Peroneal and fifth metatarsal

560. What type of hernia is represented in this image of a 1-year-old patient?

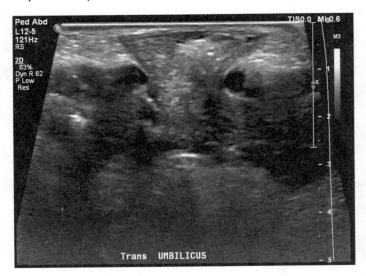

A. Umbilical hernia
B. Spigelian hernia
C. Linea alba hernia
D. Inguinal hernia

561. What is NOT a characteristic of a subcutaneous soft tissue lipoma?
    A. Compressibility
    B. Hypervascularity
    C. Mobility
    D. Painlessness

562. What is the most common vascular tumor of infancy?
    A. Hematoma
    B. Aneurysm
    C. Hemangioma
    D. Arteriovenous malformation

563. You are scanning a 17-year-old patient for a palpable mass in the wrist and you see the findings in this image. What is the most likely diagnosis?

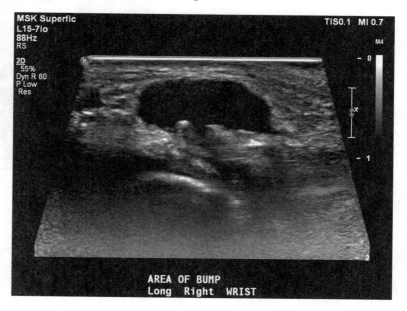

    A. Baker's cyst
    B. Meniscal cyst
    C. Ganglion cyst
    D. Sebaceous cyst

564. When evaluating a superficial structure, which of the following techniques would you use for better visualization in the near field?

   A. Compression with the transducer
   B. Panoramic imaging
   C. Harmonic imaging
   D. Standoff pad

565. Which term describes an infection of the subcutaneous soft tissue?

   A. Cellulitis
   B. Phlebitis
   C. Dermatitis
   D. Pyomyositis

566. Which number represents the hypodermis?

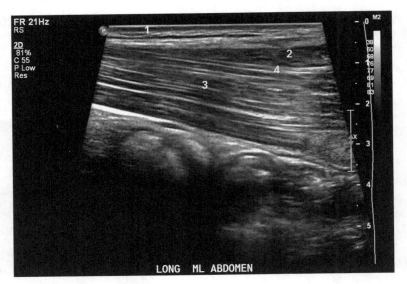

   A. 1
   B. 2
   C. 3
   D. 4

AIT—Hotspot

567. This image was obtained after a teenage boy was injured during a soccer game. What is the most likely diagnosis?

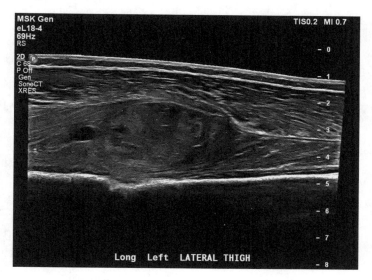

A. Hematoma
B. Seroma
C. Foreign body
D. Abscess

568. Which of the following soft-tissue foreign bodies cannot be seen with x-ray and may need to be evaluated with ultrasound?

A. Shard of glass
B. Pin
C. Nail
D. Splinter

569. What is the ultrasound appearance of the rectus abdominus muscle?

A. Hyperechoic
B. Anechoic
C. Hypoechoic
D. Isoechoic

570. Which structure connects bone to bone?

    A. Ligament

    B. Tendon

    C. Cartilage

    D. Epimysium

571. Which of these is one of the most common pediatric inflammatory masses of the neck?

    A. Fibromatosis colli

    B. Lymphadenopathy

    C. Thyroglossal duct cyst

    D. Hemangioma

572. Which type of imaging would be helpful when you are comparing a normal to an affected extremity?

    A. Panoramic

    B. 3D

    C. Split-screen

    D. Extended-field-of-view

573. Which of these is NOT one of the sonographic appearances of a torn tendon?

    A. Discontinuity of the tendon

    B. Hypoechoic in tear region

    C. Bell-clapper sign

    D. Color flow in tear region

574. A 14-year-old male presents for an ultrasound of a stab wound. Based on the sonographic appearance of the hematoma at the puncture site, what is the approximate length of time since the injury?

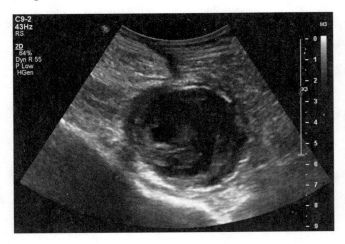

A. 2 hours

B. 1 day

C. 3 days

D. 2 weeks

575. The presence of gas within a complex collection of fluid in the subcutaneous soft tissue is most consistent with:

    A. Myositis

    B. Abscess

    C. Hematoma

    D. Seroma

576. This cystic structure, located in the gastrocnemius-semimembranosus bursa, represents a:

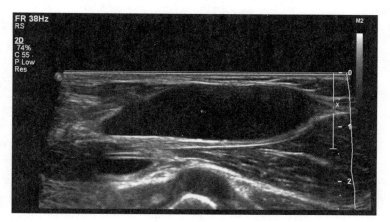

    A. Baker's cyst

    B. Meniscal cyst

    C. Ganglion cyst

    D. Sebaceous cyst

577. Which structure connects muscle to bone?

    A. Tendon

    B. Ligament

    C. Cartilage

    D. Nerve

PART 16
Vasculature of the Extremities

Normal anatomy

Pathology

Note: The main topics of Part 16 are listed. For a complete study outline by topics and subtopics, see page xxxi of the table of contents. The clinical tasks on the ARDMS exam outline are cross-referenced to the entire text of this mock exam starting on page 607.

578. Of the three layers that make up the walls of veins and arteries, which is the outer layer?

    A. Tunica media

    B. Tunica adventitia

    C. Tunica intima

    D. Tunica elastica

579. Which of these locations would NOT be chosen for insertion of a peripherally inserted central catheter (PICC) line?

    A. Femoral vein

    B. Subclavian vein

    C. Hepatic vein

    D. Internal jugular vein

580. What is the term for multiple abnormal vascular channels located between arteries and veins?

    A. Arteriovenous malformation

    B. Pseudoaneurysm

    C. Arteriovenous fistula

    D. Thrombus

581. With higher-grade arterial stenosis, you will see a tardus parvus waveform:

    A. At no time

    B. At the site of the stenosis

    C. Proximal to the stenosis

    D. Distal to the stenosis

582. Which maneuver is used to rule out thrombus and demonstrate vein patency?

    A. Pumping of the fists

    B. Valsalva

    C. Limb elevation

    D. Applying a blood pressure cuff

583. What vascular complication is commonly associated with a penetrating injury or a femoral artery catheterization?
    A. Deep venous thrombosis (DVT)
    B. Arteriovenous malformation (AVM)
    C. Pseudoaneurysm
    D. Nidus

584. Which artery gives rise to the radial and ulnar arteries?
    A. Axillary
    B. Brachial
    C. Basilic
    D. Subclavian

585. Which vein lies deep to the gastrocnemius muscle?
    A. Femoral
    B. Saphenous
    C. Popliteal
    D. Profunda femoris

586. Which vascular abnormality is associated with immobilization?
    A. Arteriovenous malformation (AVM)
    B. Arteriovenous fistula
    C. Pseudoaneurysm
    D. Deep venous thrombosis (DVT)

587. Atherosclerosis affects which part of the circulatory system?
    A. Arteries
    B. Veins
    C. Capillaries
    D. Lymphatic vessels

588. The confluence of the common iliac veins with the inferior vena cava occurs at which vertebral level?
   A. L2
   B. L3
   C. L4
   D. L5

589. A normal peripheral arterial waveform is:
   A. Triphasic and low-resistance
   B. Triphasic and high-resistance
   C. Biphasic and low-resistance
   D. Biphasic and high-resistance

590. Which of these arteries is NOT a direct branch off the aortic arch?
   A. Innominate
   B. Left common carotid
   C. Right subclavian
   D. Left subclavian

591. The deep and superficial veins of the thigh drain directly into which vessel?
   A. External iliac vein
   B. Popliteal vein
   C. Common iliac vein
   D. Common femoral vein

592. Which of these veins is the most medial vein of the upper leg?
   A. Common femoral
   B. Great saphenous
   C. Superficial femoral
   D. Deep femoral

PART 17
Physics and Instrumentation

Transducer selection

Image optimization

Harmonics

M-mode imaging

3D/4D imaging

Doppler imaging

Artifacts

Note: The main topics of Part 17 are listed. For a complete study outline by topics and subtopics, see page xxxii of the table of contents. The clinical tasks on the ARDMS exam outline are cross-referenced to the entire text of this mock exam starting on page 607.

593. Which of the following lesions in the liver most frequently causes a refraction artifact on ultrasound?

   A. Cyst

   B. Lipoma

   C. Hemangioma

   D. Hematoma

594. What type of imaging may help in visualizing the kidneys in a patient who is difficult to scan due to body habitus?

   A. High frequency

   B. Extended field of view

   C. 3D

   D. Harmonics

595. When scanning to rule out diaphragmatic paralysis, which of the following ultrasound techniques would you find helpful?

   A. M-mode

   B. B-mode

   C. A-mode

   D. D-mode

596. You are imaging an artery with color Doppler and note aliasing. Which of the following parameters could be causing this color artifact?

   A. Imaging at a shallow depth

   B. Transducer with a low Doppler frequency

   C. Increased Doppler frequency shift

   D. Low pulse repetition frequency (PRF)

AIT–SIC*

---

*Questions marked **AIT–SIC** are similar to ARDMS Advanced Item Type (AIT) questions called "Semi-Interactive Console" items. These require you to use your cursor to adjust controls on an onscreen console to correct a problem with the image presented. The console is "semi-interactive" because only some of the controls can be "adjusted." AIT–SIC items are currently limited to the Sonography Principles and Instrumentation (SPI) examination and as of this printing do not appear on the Pediatric Sonography exam, but as a bonus feature we have identified similar items in this mock exam.

597. Which of the following is an advantage of color Doppler imaging over pulsed Doppler imaging?
   A. The ability to measure velocities
   B. The fact that color Doppler is not angle-dependent
   C. The ability to display an entire vessel
   D. The ability to detect capillary flow

598. While scanning a rotator cuff you notice that the tendons appear hypoechoic. What artifact does this most likely represent?
   A. Posterior shadowing
   B. Anisotropy
   C. Reverberation
   D. Side-lobe artifact

599. In this image what artifact do the arrows indicate?

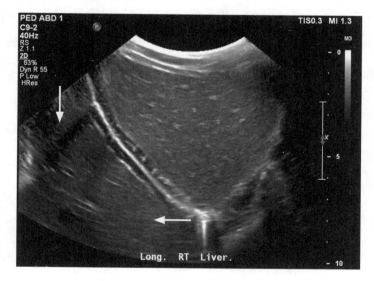

   A. Mirror-image
   B. Reverberation
   C. Refraction
   D. Ring-down

AIT—Hotspot

600. The purpose of using contrast agents in ultrasound is to:
   A. Detect the stiffness of tissues
   B. Enhance highly reflective structures
   C. Eliminate artifacts produced with gas
   D. Enhance blood flow signals

601. In which of the following structures would you most likely see a side-lobe artifact while scanning?
    A. Tendons
    B. Air
    C. Gallbladder
    D. Diaphragm

602. What is an advantage of power Doppler?
    A. Able to measure velocity
    B. Provides directional information
    C. Displays the strength of the signal
    D. Displays the Doppler frequency

603. What adjustment can be made to eliminate low frequency shifts?
    A. Increase the Doppler frequency.
    B. Increase the wall filter.
    C. Decrease the pulse repetition frequency (PRF).
    D. Decrease the packet size.

AIT—SIC

604. A three-dimensional (3D) scan allows you to obtain:
    A. Tissue stiffness
    B. Organ volume
    C. Blood flow velocity
    D. Time-motion display

605. The formation and oscillation of a gas bubble in a liquid are known as:
    A. Cavitation
    B. Thermal effect
    C. Infiltration
    D. Extravasation

606. Ring-down artifacts are likely to appear in the presence of:
    A. Fluid collections
    B. Large, smooth interfaces
    C. Gas bubbles
    D. Near-field highly reflective structures

607. In this image, what color artifact (arrow) is observed?

See Color Plate 9 on page xxxvi.

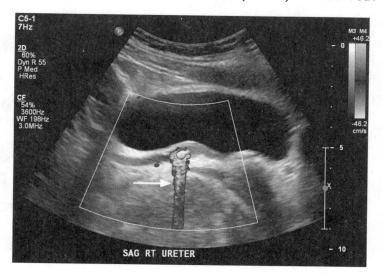

A. Aliasing

B. Ring-down

C. Doppler noise

D. Twinkle artifact

AIT—Hotspot

608. What type of artifact is represented by the arrows in this image?

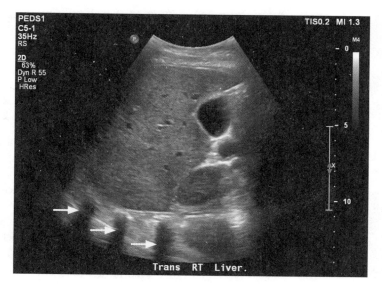

A. Shadowing

B. Enhancement

C. Side-lobe artifact

D. Reverberation

AIT—Hotspot

609. You are scanning a patient's bladder and see this artifact in the near field. What will eliminate the artifact?

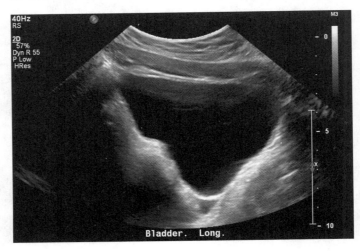

A. Increasing the power output

B. Decreasing the gain

C. Increasing the number of focal zones

D. Decreasing the dynamic range

AIT—SIC

610. When absolute velocities are to be measured, the beam/vessel angle should be:

A. 90 degrees or less

B. 80 degrees or less

C. 70 degrees or less

D. 60 degrees or less

611. To evaluate the liver for fibrosis, which of the following ultrasound techniques is helpful?

A. Elastography

B. Contrast-enhanced ultrasound

C. 3D imaging

D. B-mode ultrasound

612. When performing spectral Doppler, what should you do with the gate?

A. Open it as wide as possible.

B. Center it within the vessel.

C. Do not include angle correction.

D. Open the gate to a width of 25% of the vessel lumen.

AIT—SIC

PART 18

Patient Care and Management

Patient communication

Physician communication

Reporting and archiving

Sterile procedure

Infection control

Note: The main topics of Part 18 are listed. For a complete study outline by topics and subtopics, see page xxxii of the table of contents. The clinical tasks on the ARDMS exam outline are cross-referenced to the entire text of this mock exam starting on page 607.

613. Coagulation testing should be performed prior to procedures or surgery to assess:
    A. Family history of blood disorders
    B. Potential anesthesia complications
    C. Bleeding risk
    D. Healing time

614. The "time out" process verifies multiple components prior to surgery or interventional procedures. Which of the following is NOT one of these components?
    A. Correct site
    B. Correct patient
    C. Correct method
    D. Correct procedure

615. What is the easiest and most effective way of preventing the spread of infectious diseases?
    A. Wearing personal protective equipment (PPE)
    B. Using sterile precautions
    C. Not recapping needles
    D. Maintaining proper hand hygiene

616. What do the letters of the digital imaging system PACS stand for?
    A. Picture archiving and communication system
    B. Picture archive compression system
    C. Picture archive and completion system
    D. Picture archiving and computer system

617. While scanning a 2-year-old patient for abdominal pain after hours, you encounter these findings (arrow). What should you do?

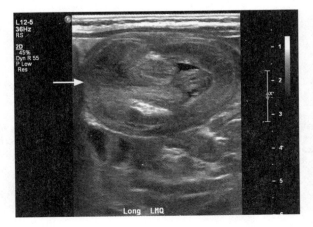

A. Tell the parent about the findings.
B. Leave the results to be read in the morning.
C. Communicate the findings to the radiologist.
D. Call the ordering physician with the results.

618. You are about to enter the room of a patient with known tuberculosis to perform a portable exam. What would be the most important personal protective equipment (PPE) you would need to put on?

A. Gown
B. N95 respirator
C. Protective eyewear
D. Gloves

619. While scanning a patient in the neonatal intensive care unit (NICU), you notice this echogenic intraluminal structure. What is the most likely cause?

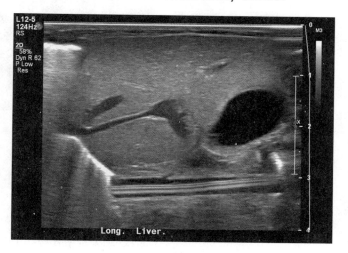

A. Umbilical artery catheter (UAC)
B. Transjugular intrahepatic portosystemic shunt (TIPS)
C. Umbilical vein catheter (UVC)
D. Ventriculoperitoneal shunt (VP shunt)

620. After performing an exam on a patient with *Clostridium difficile*, what is the correct method for cleaning your hands?

A. Alcohol foam
B. Hand washing with soap
C. Bleach and water
D. Betadine

621. While scanning a patient with a "fall risk" wristband, you are called out of the room. The patient does not appear to be in distress. Which of the following actions is appropriate patient care?

   A. Tell the patient you will be right back.
   B. Sit the patient up until you return.
   C. Leave the door to the exam room open.
   D. Put the bed rails up in your absence.

622. You are scanning a patient in the OR following an ultrasound-guided percutaneous renal biopsy and notice a thickening echogenic area (arrow) at the biopsy site. What should you do?

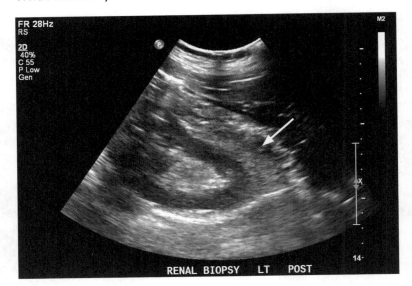

   A. Wait for the radiologist's dictation.
   B. Don't say anything.
   C. Discuss your findings with the performing physician.
   D. Tell your supervisor.

623. When you are scanning a patient under the age of 5, what is the best method to encourage cooperation for a successful exam?

   A. Use restraints.
   B. Engage with the patient and explain the procedure.
   C. Scold the patient on his or her behavior.
   D. Ignore the patient and proceed with the exam.

PART 19

Answers, Explanations, and References

Head

Spine

Neck and face

Chest

Liver

Gallbladder and biliary ducts

Pancreas

Spleen

Urinary tract

Adrenal glands

GI tract and mesentery

Pediatric hip

Female pelvis

Male pelvis, scrotum, and testes

Soft tissue

Vasculature of the extremities

Physics and instrumentation

Patient care and management

PART 1

Head

1. **C. Corpus callosum.**

    The cavum septi pellucidi (CSP) and the cavum vergae (when present) are bordered immediately cephalad by the corpus callosum. The cingulate sulcus appears as a bright echogenic line that also lies cephalad to the CSP and the corpus callosum. The third ventricle and the massa intermedia are both structures that lie caudate to the CSP.

    ▸ de Bruyn R (ed): *Pediatric Ultrasound: How, Why and When*, 2nd edition (e-book). Philadelphia, Churchill Livingstone/Elsevier, 2010, pp 252, 256–258.

    ▸ Rumack CM, Levine D (eds): *Diagnostic Ultrasound*, 5th edition. Philadelphia, Elsevier, 2018, p 1515.

    ▸ Siegel MJ (ed): *Pediatric Sonography*, 4th edition. Philadelphia, Lippincott Williams & Wilkins, 2011, pp 46–47.

2. **B. Congenital aqueductal stenosis.**

See Color Plate 10 on page xxxvii.

Ventricles of the Brain

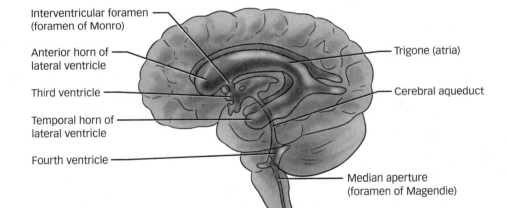

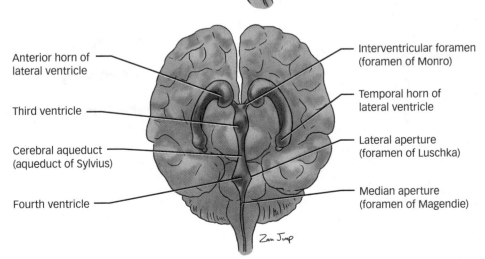

One of the most common causes of obstructive or noncommunicating hydrocephalus is congenital aqueductal stenosis. This should be suspected when there is dilatation of the lateral and third ventricles without dilatation of the fourth ventricle. With a vein of Galen aneurysm, dilatation of the ventricular system can be seen in conjunction with an abnormal midline cystic structure. In cases of hydrocephalus caused by a Chiari malformation, a downward displacement of brain tissue should also be seen. When there is failure of reabsorption of cerebrospinal fluid (CSF), or CSF malabsorption, the entire ventricular system appears abnormally dilated.

▸ de Bruyn R (ed): *Pediatric Ultrasound: How, Why and When*, 2nd edition (e-book). Philadelphia, Churchill Livingstone/Elsevier, 2010, p 275.

▸ Rumack CM, Levine D (eds): *Diagnostic Ultrasound*, 5th edition. Philadelphia, Elsevier, 2018, p 1538.

3. **D. Choroid plexus.**

The choroid plexus *is located mainly within the body and the trigones of the lateral ventricles. The choroid plexus extends midline through the foramen of Monro and into the roof of the third ventricle. The fourth ventricle also contains choroid plexus. The normal choroid plexus is never seen in the frontal or occipital horns of the lateral ventricles.* When there is a grade 2 intraventricular hemorrhage, *usually the blood clot lies in the dependent part of the lateral ventricles (the occipital horn).* Choroid plexus cysts *are anechoic structures seen within the echogenic choroid plexus.* Choroid plexus papillomas *commonly arise from the trigones of the lateral ventricles, but these neoplasms appear as large echogenic masses and are not seen in a normal head ultrasound.*

▸ de Bruyn R (ed): *Pediatric Ultrasound: How, Why and When*, 2nd edition (e-book). Philadelphia, Churchill Livingstone/Elsevier, 2010, pp 256–258, 260–261, 272.

▸ Rumack CM, Levine D (eds): *Diagnostic Ultrasound*, 5th edition. Philadelphia, Elsevier, 2018, pp 1522–1523.

▸ Siegel MJ (ed): *Pediatric Sonography*, 4th edition. Philadelphia, Lippincott Williams & Wilkins, 2011, pp 52–53.

ANSWERS

4. **A. Primitive prosencephalic vein.**

    A vein of Galen malformation or aneurysm is an arteriovenous malformation (AVM) that results from the shunting of multiple cerebral arteries into a dilated primitive prosencephalic vein. Although this malformation is referred to as a vein of Galen malformation, this abnormality occurs during embryonal development when the vein of Galen is not yet formed. The median prosencephalic vein of Markowski is the precursor to the vein of Galen and is the actual vessel that is affected in a vein of Galen malformation. This AVM appears as a midline cystic structure that can easily be differentiated from other cystic abnormalities with the use of color flow Doppler. Infants with a vein of Galen malformation can be treated with embolization of the feeding vessels. Magnetic resonance imaging (MRI) or conventional angiography is necessary before or during the procedure. The pericallosal artery is also a midline vessel, but it is located more anteriorly—formed from the anterior cerebral artery—and courses along the superior margin of the corpus callosum. The straight sinus is where the vein of Galen drains posteriorly and inferiorly.

    ▸ de Bruyn R (ed): *Pediatric Ultrasound: How, Why and When*, 2nd edition (e-book). Philadelphia, Churchill Livingstone/Elsevier, 2010, pp 252, 275–276.

    ▸ Rumack CM, Levine D (eds): *Diagnostic Ultrasound*, 5th edition. Philadelphia, Elsevier, 2018, p 1566.

    ▸ Siegel MJ (ed): *Pediatric Sonography*, 4th edition. Philadelphia, Lippincott Williams & Wilkins, 2011, pp 57, 81.

5. **A. Cytomegalovirus (CMV).**

    *TORCH is an acronym that refers to **t**oxoplasmosis, **o**ther (for other infections), **r**ubella, **c**ytomegalovirus, and the **h**erpes simplex virus. The most common of the congenital TORCH infections is cytomegalovirus (CMV), followed by toxoplasmosis. CMV can cause calcifications in the periventricular area. With toxoplasmosis and the herpes simplex virus (HSV) the calcifications are most likely to be in the cortex and basal ganglia area. Meningitis is not one of the TORCH infections and it is not associated with brain calcifications.*

    ▸ Rumack CM, Levine D (eds): *Diagnostic Ultrasound*, 5th edition. Philadelphia, Elsevier, 2018, pp 1557–1560.

    ▸ Siegel MJ (ed): *Pediatric Sonography*, 4th edition. Philadelphia, Lippincott Williams & Wilkins, 2011, pp 102–103.

6. **C. Holoprosencephaly.**

    Holoprosencephaly *results when there is failed or incomplete cleavage of the prosencephalon into the telencephalon and diencephalon. Three forms of holoprosencephaly have been described: alobar, semilobar, and lobar.* Alobar holoprosencephaly *is the most severe form and is commonly accompanied by midline facial anomalies like cyclopia and a proboscis. On ultrasound a monoventricle is seen.* Lobar holoprosencephaly *is the least severe form, with failure of cleavage frontally.* Lissencephaly *refers to the absence of gyri and sulci and is a migration disorder.* Hydranencephaly *is a condition in which there is almost complete destruction of the cerebral cortex.* Schizencephaly *is a migrational anomaly that leads to deep clefts of gray matter into the hemispheres.*

    ▶ de Bruyn R (ed): *Pediatric Ultrasound: How, Why and When*, 2nd edition (e-book). Philadelphia, Churchill Livingstone/Elsevier, 2010, p 271.

    ▶ Rumack CM, Levine D (eds): *Diagnostic Ultrasound*, 5th edition. Philadelphia, Elsevier, 2018, pp 1532, 1536–1537.

    ▶ Siegel MJ (ed): *Pediatric Sonography*, 4th edition. Philadelphia, Lippincott Williams & Wilkins, 2011, pp 92, 97, 100.

See Color Plate 10, "Ventricles of the Brain," on page xxxvii.

7. **B. The distance from the falx to the lateral wall of the frontal horn of the lateral ventricle.**

    The most universally accepted way to measure ventricular dilatation is to determine the ventricular index described by Malcolm I. Levene. This value is obtained by measuring the distance from the falx to the lateral wall of the anterior (frontal) horn of the lateral ventricle. This measurement should be taken in a coronal plane at the level of the third ventricle and the foramen of Monro. Another way to determine the ventricular index is to measure the distance between the frontal horns of the lateral ventricles and divide by 2. The margin of error with this measurement increases when there is a midline shift. When one is measuring ventricular dilatation, measurements from the medial wall of the lateral ventricles are not helpful and give no information about ventricular size.

    ▶ de Bruyn R (ed): *Pediatric Ultrasound: How, Why and When*, 2nd edition (e-book). Philadelphia, Churchill Livingstone/Elsevier, 2010, p 253.

    ▶ Levene MI: Measurement of the growth of the lateral ventricles in preterm infants with real-time ultrasound. Arch Dis Child 56:900–904, 1981.

8. **D. Connatal cysts.**

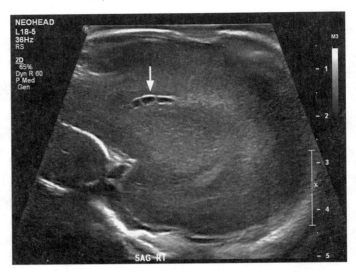

Connatal cysts *(arrow) are also known as* coarctation of the lateral ventricles, *and they are considered a normal variant. These cysts are located superolateral to the lateral ventricles near the frontal horns. It is important not to mistake connatal cysts for periventricular leukomalacia (PVL). In a coronal plane connatal cysts are located at 9 and 3 o'clock. PVL is typically located at 10–11 and 1–2 o'clock.* Subependymal cysts *are located in the subependymal lining of the ventricles and are most often associated with germinal matrix hemorrhage, ischemia, and TORCH infections (infections associated with toxoplasmosis, "other," rubella, cytomegalovirus, and herpes). An* arachnoid cyst *is not a common type of intracranial mass in childhood; when congenital, arachnoid cysts are most commonly located in the Sylvian fissures.* Choroid plexus cysts *are located within the choroid plexus.*

▸ de Bruyn R (ed): *Pediatric Ultrasound: How, Why and When*, 2nd edition (e-book). Philadelphia, Churchill Livingstone/Elsevier, 2010, pp 256, 259.
▸ Keller MS, DiPietro MA, Teele RL, et al: Periventricular cavitations in the first week of life. AJNR Am J Neuroradiol 8:291–295, 1987.
▸ Rumack CM, Levine D (eds): *Diagnostic Ultrasound*, 5th edition. Philadelphia, Elsevier, 2018, pp 1522, 1563–1566.
▸ Siegel MJ (ed): *Pediatric Sonography*, 4th edition. Philadelphia, Lippincott Williams & Wilkins, 2011, pp 52, 109–110.

9. **B. Group B streptococcus.**

In newborns, the two most common causes of central nervous system (CNS) infection are Escherichia coli *(E. coli) and group B streptococcus.* Enterococcus *can also cause meningitis but is less common.* Haemophilus influenzae *(H. influenzae) is a common cause of meningitis in older* children (between the ages of 3 months and 3 years), not in newborns. Cytomegalovirus (CMV) is not associated with infections of the central nervous system.

▶ Rumack CM, Levine D (eds): *Diagnostic Ultrasound*, 5th edition. Philadelphia, Elsevier, 2018, p 1560.

▶ Siegel MJ (ed): *Pediatric Sonography*, 4th edition. Philadelphia, Lippincott Williams & Wilkins, 2011, pp 103–104.

10. **C. Arachnoid cyst.**

An arachnoid cyst *is an intracranial cystic lesion that contains cerebrospinal fluid (CSF). These cysts are located between two layers of the arachnoid membranes and do not communicate with the ventricular system. Large arachnoid cysts can cause hydrocephalus due to compression of the foramen of Monro, third ventricle, or cerebral aqueduct; they can also cause a midline shift. A* Dandy-Walker cyst *is the enlargement of the cisterna magna and fourth ventricle in a Dandy-Walker malformation. The difference between an arachnoid cyst and a Dandy-Walker cyst is that the arachnoid cyst is separate from the fourth ventricle, whereas a Dandy-Walker cyst communicates with it. A* porencephalic cyst *usually connects with the lateral ventricles and is not between arachnoid membranes. A normal* cavum septi pellucidi *(CSP) is not located within the posterior fossa.*

▶ de Bruyn R (ed): *Pediatric Ultrasound: How, Why and When*, 2nd edition (e-book). Philadelphia, Churchill Livingstone/Elsevier, 2010, pp 25–26, 270–272.

▶ Rumack CM, Levine D (eds): *Diagnostic Ultrasound*, 5th edition. Philadelphia, Elsevier, 2018, pp 1529–1532, 1563–1565.

▶ Siegel MJ (ed): *Pediatric Sonography*, 4th edition. Philadelphia, Lippincott Williams & Wilkins, 2011, pp 87, 109.

11. **D. Arnold-Chiari malformation.**

Arnold-Chiari malformation, *also known as* Chiari malformation type 2, *is the most common of the different types of Chiari malformations. A* Chiari malformation *is a condition in which the brain tissue is inferiorly displaced into the spinal canal. The displaced vermis in an Arnold-Chiari malformation is often dysplastic, flat, and elongated. The vermis is seen extending through the foramen magnum and filling and obliterating the CSF space. With an Arnold-Chiari malformation there is also downward displacement of the cerebellar vermis, medulla, and fourth ventricle. An Arnold-Chiari malformation is almost always associated with a myelomeningocele. In a* Dandy-Walker complex, *the fourth ventricle appears dilated with an absent or dysplastic cerebellar vermis instead of displaced inferiorly as in a Chiari malformation.* Holoprosencephaly *and* colpocephaly *are conditions that normally do not alter the anatomy in the posterior fossa.*

▸ de Bruyn R (ed): *Pediatric Ultrasound: How, Why and When*, 2nd edition (e-book). Philadelphia, Churchill Livingstone/Elsevier, 2010, pp 270–272, 296–297.

▸ Rumack CM, Levine D (eds): *Diagnostic Ultrasound*, 5th edition. Philadelphia, Elsevier, 2018, pp 1526, 1529–1535.

▸ Siegel MJ (ed): *Pediatric Sonography*, 4th edition. Philadelphia, Lippincott Williams & Wilkins, 2011, pp 85–87.

12. D. Basal ganglia.

See also the answer to question 54.

The basal ganglia *comprise a group of structures located deep in the brain that include the caudate nucleus, putamen, globus pallidus, substantia nigra, and subthalamic nucleus. The thalamus and the caudate nucleus are separated by the caudothalamic groove. This junction is an area of concern for germinal matrix hemorrhage in early preterm infants. The* posterior fossa *is the space in the skull, located posterior and inferior in the head, that contains the brainstem and the cerebellum. The* brainstem *is the most inferior part of the brain and is composed of the midbrain, pons, and medulla. The* circle of Willis *is a group of cerebral arteries that supply blood to the brain.*

▸ de Bruyn R (ed): *Pediatric Ultrasound: How, Why and When*, 2nd edition (e-book). Philadelphia, Churchill Livingstone/Elsevier, 2010, p 260.

13. A. Porencephaly.

Porencephaly *(a porencephalic cyst) is the result of focal brain destruction after an ischemic, hemorrhagic, traumatic, or infectious event. These cysts are continuous with the ventricular system and normally do not extend to the surface of the brain.* Colpocephaly *refers to the enlargement and parallel orientation of the body and occipital horns of the lateral ventricles. This may be associated with agenesis of the corpus callosum, Chiari malformation, lissencephaly, and microcephaly. An* arachnoid cyst *is a cystic structure that contains cerebrospinal fluid (CSF) but does not communicate with the ventricular system.* Hydrocephalus *is an abnormal increased amount of CSF in the ventricular system and can be the result of obstruction, overproduction, or malabsorption.*

▸ de Bruyn R (ed): *Pediatric Ultrasound: How, Why and When*, 2nd edition (e-book). Philadelphia, Churchill Livingstone/Elsevier, 2010, p 270.

▸ Rumack CM, Levine D (eds): *Diagnostic Ultrasound*, 5th edition. Philadelphia, Elsevier, 2018, p 1528.

▸ Siegel MJ (ed): *Pediatric Sonography*, 4th edition. Philadelphia, Lippincott Williams & Wilkins, 2011, pp 91, 102, 107.

14. **D. Grade 4.**

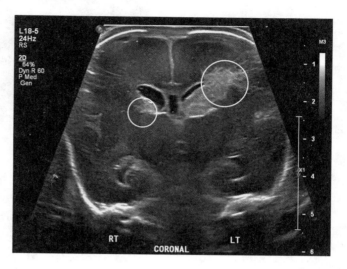

This image demonstrates intraparenchymal hemorrhages (circled), also referred to as grade 4 intraventricular hemorrhage (IVH). *This hemorrhage is an event that occurs primarily in premature infants with a gestational age of less than 30 weeks and a birth weight less than 1500 grams. Papile's grading system categorizes IVH in four grades. In a* grade 1 IVH, *the hemorrhage is confined to the subependymal (germinal matrix) region. In a* grade 2 IVH, *the bleeding extends into the ventricles without hydrocephalus. In a* grade 3 IVH *the blood fills and distends the ventricles, causing dilatation or hydrocephalus. In a* grade 4 IVH, *seen here, there is intraparenchymal hemorrhage.*

Types of intraventricular hemorrhage (IVH)— Papile's classification

Grade 1	Subependymal (germinal matrix) hemorrhage
Grade 2	Intraventricular hemorrhage
Grade 3	Intraventricular hemorrhage with hydrocephalus
Grade 4	Intraparenchymal hemorrhage

▸ de Bruyn R (ed): *Pediatric Ultrasound: How, Why and When*, 2nd edition (e-book). Philadelphia, Churchill Livingstone/Elsevier, 2010, pp 260–266.

▸ Rumack CM, Levine D (eds): *Diagnostic Ultrasound*, 5th edition. Philadelphia, Elsevier, 2018, p 1541.

▸ Siegel MJ (ed): *Pediatric Sonography*, 4th edition. Philadelphia, Lippincott Williams & Wilkins, 2011, pp 60–61.

15. **D. Thalamus.**

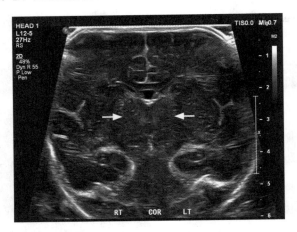

The thalamus *(arrows) is a paired paramedian structure located on each side of the third ventricle. Sonographically, the thalamus appears hypoechoic and is bordered inferiorly by the echogenic cerebral peduncles. The thalamus lies inferior to the choroid plexuses, located in the floor of the lateral ventricles. In alobar holoprosencephaly both sides of the thalamus are fused. The* massa intermedia *is a midline structure that connects the two thalami and lies within the third ventricle. The* corpus callosum *is also seen in the midline, superior to the cavum septi pellucidi (CSP). The pons is located within the posterior fossa anterior to the cerebellum.*

▶ de Bruyn R (ed): *Pediatric Ultrasound: How, Why and When*, 2nd edition (e-book). Philadelphia, Churchill Livingstone/Elsevier, 2010, p 260.

▶ Rumack CM, Levine D (eds): *Diagnostic Ultrasound*, 5th edition. Philadelphia, Elsevier, 2018, p 1514.

▶ Siegel MJ (ed): *Pediatric Sonography*, 4th edition. Philadelphia, Lippincott Williams & Wilkins, 2011, p 46.

16. **D. Nothing of clinical significance.**

Small, isolated choroid plexus cysts are common and have no clinical significance. When bilateral, multiple, and larger (>1 cm), choroid plexus cysts can be associated with chromosomal anomalies, such as trisomies 18 and 21 and Aicardi syndrome. Choroid plexus cysts can also develop after a choroid plexus hemorrhage, although this is uncommon. There is no association between choroid plexus cysts and ventriculomegaly.

▶ de Bruyn R (ed): *Pediatric Ultrasound: How, Why and When*, 2nd edition (e-book). Philadelphia, Churchill Livingstone/Elsevier, 2010, pp 24, 272.

▶ Rumack CM, Levine D (eds): *Diagnostic Ultrasound*, 5th edition. Philadelphia, Elsevier, 2018, p 1628.

▶ Siegel MJ (ed): *Pediatric Sonography*, 4th edition. Philadelphia, Lippincott Williams & Wilkins, 2011, p 110.

17. A. Hypoxic-ischemic injury.

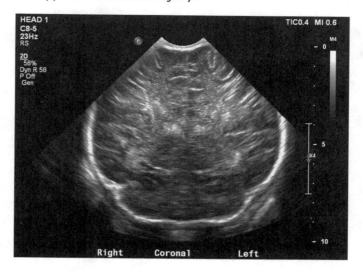

This image shows diffuse cerebral edema, which can be caused by hypoxic-ischemic injuries, *resulting in poor gyral-sulcal differentiation. In these cases, the ventricles may appear compressed (slit-like), although this is not specific for ischemia. The brain parenchyma may appear diffusely echogenic and eventually the condition can lead to cystic encephalomalacia. The newborn brain can be deprived of blood due to maternal and postpartum causes. Some maternal causes include maternal chronic cardiopulmonary disease and placenta-related problems. Postpartum causes include extracorporeal membrane oxygenation (ECMO), congenital heart disease (CHD), trauma, and meningitis. Cytomegalovirus (CMV) is not known to cause brain edema. A germinal matrix hemorrhage appears as a small echogenic mass in the caudothalamic groove area. When a hemorrhage extends to the brain parenchyma, it usually has the appearance of a focal, irregular hyperechoic mass that does not cause the diffuse echogenicity typical of poor gyral-sulcal differentiation.*

▶ de Bruyn R (ed): *Pediatric Ultrasound: How, Why and When*, 2nd edition (e-book). Philadelphia, Churchill Livingstone/Elsevier, 2010, pp 23, 267–268.

▶ Rumack CM, Levine D (eds): *Diagnostic Ultrasound*, 5th edition. Philadelphia, Elsevier, 2018, pp 1553–1555.

▶ Siegel MJ (ed): *Pediatric Sonography*, 4th edition. Philadelphia, Lippincott Williams & Wilkins, 2011, pp 61, 65, 72–76.

18. D. Cavum septi pellucidi (CSP).

The cavum septi pellucidi (CSP) is a cavity that separates the two frontal horns of the lateral ventricles and lies anterior to the foramen of Monro. The CSP contains cerebrospinal fluid (CSF) but does not communicate with the ventricular system. The CSP can have a posterior extension called the cavum vergae *that is located posterior to the foramen of Monro between the bodies of the lateral ventricles. The* third and fourth ventricles *do not separate the frontal horns of the lateral ventricles and lie inferior and posterior to the foramen of Monro.*

▶ de Bruyn R (ed): *Pediatric Ultrasound: How, Why and When*, 2nd edition (e-book). Philadelphia, Churchill Livingstone/Elsevier, 2010, p 256.

▶ Rumack CM, Levine D (eds): *Diagnostic Ultrasound*, 5th edition. Philadelphia, Elsevier, 2018, p 1521.

▶ Siegel MJ (ed): *Pediatric Sonography*, 4th edition. Philadelphia, Lippincott Williams & Wilkins, 2011, p 52.

19. **B. Lissencephaly.**

Lissencephaly *is a rare brain malformation secondary to a lack of development of the cerebral sulci and gyri. With this malformation the brain parenchyma appears smooth—without the folds and the grooves that characterize a normal brain. Patients with lissencephaly often have microcephaly, seizures, intellectual disabilities, and impaired motor functions.* Schizencephaly *is characterized by abnormal clefts or slits in the brain parenchyma and does not give the appearance of a smooth brain. An* intraparenchymal hemorrhage *is a more focal area that appears as an echogenic mass extending from the subependymal layer into the brain parenchyma.* Hydranencephaly *is a condition in which the brain is replaced by fluid.*

▶ Rumack CM, Levine D (eds): *Diagnostic Ultrasound*, 5th edition. Philadelphia, Elsevier, 2018, pp 1536–1538.

▶ Siegel MJ (ed): *Pediatric Sonography*, 4th edition. Philadelphia, Lippincott Williams & Wilkins, 2011, pp 65, 97–98.

20. **A. Agenesis of the corpus callosum.**

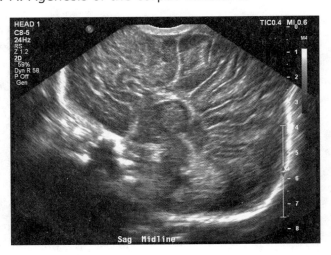

The corpus callosum is a midline structure that allows communication between the two cerebral hemispheres. The corpus callosum can be completely or partially absent. When the corpus callosum is absent on a coronal image, the lateral ventricles are widely separated, with a parallel orientation of the ventricular bodies and the occipital horns (colpocephaly). On a sagittal midline view, a "sunburst" sign can be seen due to the medial cerebral sulci and gyri radially arranged and extending perpendicular to the expected course of the corpus callosum (as seen in this image). Agyria *and* pachygyria *are abnormalities seen with lissencephaly and refer respectively to the complete and partial absence of gyri. In* holoprosencephaly, *the frontal horns of the lateral ventricles are fused in conjunction with the absence of the corpus callosum.*

▸ de Bruyn R (ed): *Pediatric Ultrasound: How, Why and When*, 2nd edition (e-book). Philadelphia, Churchill Livingstone/Elsevier, 2010, pp 24–25, 270, 272.

▸ Rumack CM, Levine D (eds): *Diagnostic Ultrasound*, 5th edition. Philadelphia, Elsevier, 2018, pp 1526–1528.

▸ Siegel MJ (ed): *Pediatric Sonography*, 4th edition. Philadelphia, Lippincott Williams & Wilkins, 2011, pp 90–92.

21. C. Subgaleal hematoma.

See Color Plate 11 on page xxxvii.

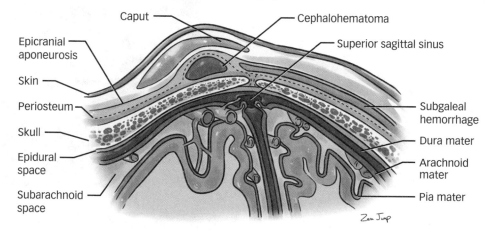

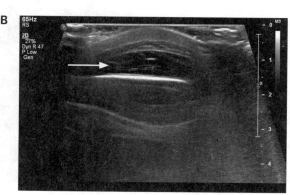

A Diagram showing intracranial and extracranial locations of hemorrhaging in the skull. *B* A subgaleal hemorrhage *is a serious injury in which there is bleeding between the skull's periosteum and the scalp galea or epicranial aponeurosis (arrow). The mirror artifact seen in this image should not be confused with an accompanying epidural hematoma. Since this bleed is located beneath the galeal layer, it can cross the midline. This type of bleed usually occurs after vacuum-assisted delivery. Infants can lose a large amount of blood in a small amount of time, which may lead to anemia, shock, coagulopathy, and even death. A* cephalohematoma *is located between the periosteum and the skull. A* caput succedaneum *is the swelling of the scalp. An* epidural hemorrhage *is an intracranial bleed between the dura mater and the skull.*

▸ Davis DJ: Neonatal subgaleal hemorrhage: diagnosis and management. CMAJ 164:1452–1453, 2001. Available at https:www.ncbi.nlm.nih.gov/pmc/articles/PMC81073/.

▸ Rumack CM, Levine D (eds): *Diagnostic Ultrasound*, 5th edition. Philadelphia, Elsevier, 2018, p 1557.

▸ Siegel MJ (ed): *Pediatric Sonography*, 4th edition. Philadelphia, Lippincott Williams & Wilkins, 2011, pp 45–49.

22. **C. Periventricular leukomalacia (PVL).**

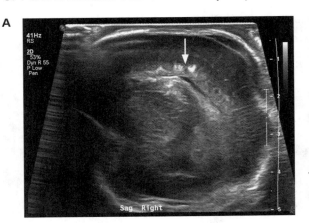

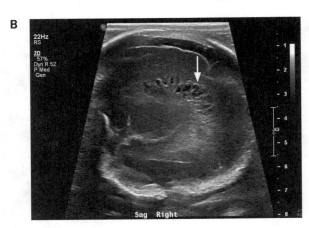

Periventricular leukomalacia *(PVL)* is a hypoxic-ischemic lesion affecting more premature infants than term infants. These infants are at a higher risk due to the lack of maturity of the cardiovascular system, resulting in episodes of hypotension. During these episodes the cerebral perfusion can be affected, causing a lack of oxygen or blood in the periventricular white matter. PVL is commonly related to prenatal events like placental abruption, perinatal asphyxia, cardiac arrest, and shock. **A** On ultrasound, during the first 2 weeks of the event, the periventricular white matter appears highly echogenic (arrow), more often anterior to the frontal horns and posterior to the occipital horns of the lateral ventricles. **B** Within 2 to 6 weeks the bright echogenic areas may start to become cystic (arrow), leading to cystic encephalomalacia (late phase).

Normal periventricular blush *can be differentiated from PVL because normal periventricular blush should never be more echogenic than the adjacent choroid plexus. In addition the blush disappears when looked at from the posterior fontanelle (demonstration of anisotropy), while echogenic PVL remains apparent. A* grade 4 intraventricular hemorrhage *(IVH) is usually asymmetric.* Meningitis *is not associated with prematurity or hypoxic events and usually has normal imaging findings.*

▶ de Bruyn R (ed): *Pediatric Ultrasound: How, Why and When*, 2nd edition (e-book). Philadelphia, Churchill Livingstone/Elsevier, 2010, pp 23, 267–268.

▶ Rumack CM, Levine D (eds): *Diagnostic Ultrasound*, 5th edition. Philadelphia, Elsevier, 2018, pp 1550, 1560.

▶ Siegel MJ (ed): *Pediatric Sonography*, 4th edition. Philadelphia, Lippincott Williams & Wilkins, 2011, pp 73–75.

23. **D. Mastoid fontanelle.**

The mastoid fontanelle *is used as an acoustic window to obtain axial images that best demonstrate the brainstem and posterior fossa. Most brain ultrasounds are done using mainly the* anterior fontanelle *with the mastoid fontanelle as a complement for a thorough examination of the posterior fossa. The* anterior fontanelle *is used to obtain sagittal and coronal images of the brain. The* posterior fontanelle *allows you to obtain axial scans of the trigones of the lateral ventricles and the posterior occipital horns. The* sphenoid fontanelle *is not used as an acoustic window for the evaluation of the brain.*

▶ de Bruyn R (ed): *Pediatric Ultrasound: How, Why and When*, 2nd edition (e-book). Philadelphia, Churchill Livingstone/Elsevier, 2010, pp 252, 255–256.

▶ Rumack CM, Levine D (eds): *Diagnostic Ultrasound*, 5th edition. Philadelphia, Elsevier, 2018, pp 1513–1517.

▶ Siegel MJ (ed): *Pediatric Sonography*, 4th edition. Philadelphia, Lippincott Williams & Wilkins, 2011, pp 45–49.

24. **A. Hydranencephaly.**

Hydranencephaly is an extreme form of porencephaly in which the cerebral hemispheres are absent to varying degrees and replaced by a cranial cavity filled with cerebrospinal fluid (CSF) due to destruction of the cerebral cortex. Hydranencephaly is believed to be caused by bilateral occlusion of the internal carotid arteries (ICAs) during fetal development. The presence of a falx cerebri, which is supplied by the external carotid artery (ECA), helps with the differentiation of this condition in comparison with holoprosencephaly. Cystic encephalomalacia shows areas of brain damage (focal or diffuse) that usually do not connect to the ventricular system. Arachnoid cysts are cystic structures that, when congenital, usually arise from the Sylvian fissures and retrocerebellar area, and the brain parenchyma is not replaced by the cyst.

▶ Rumack CM, Levine D (eds): *Diagnostic Ultrasound*, 5th edition. Philadelphia, Elsevier, 2018, p 1538.

▶ Siegel MJ (ed): *Pediatric Sonography*, 4th edition. Philadelphia, Lippincott Williams & Wilkins, 2011, p 100.

25. **B. Subdural hematoma.**

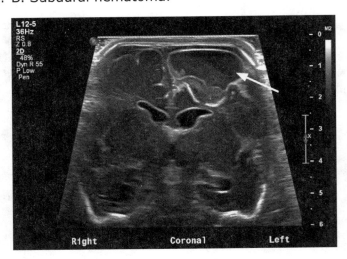

See Color Plate 11, "Locations of Hemorrhaging in the Skull," on page xxxvii.

Subdural hematomas are a type of brain injury commonly seen in full-term infants as a result of traumatic delivery. In a subdural hematoma, blood accumulates between the arachnoid and dura mater. When rapidly growing, a subdural hematoma can cause compression of the brain tissue, as seen in this image (arrow). This may result in brain injury that can lead to death. Subdural and epidural hemorrhages can be difficult to differentiate on ultrasound, and computed tomography (CT) or magnetic resonance imaging (MRI) may be the modality of choice for diagnosis. Cephalohematomas, caput succedaneum, and subgaleal hematomas are bleeding conditions that are seen extracranially (outside the skull).

▶ de Bruyn R (ed): *Pediatric Ultrasound: How, Why and When*, 2nd edition (e-book). Philadelphia, Churchill Livingstone/Elsevier, 2010, pp 260–261, 268, 274–275.

▶ Siegel MJ (ed): *Pediatric Sonography*, 4th edition. Philadelphia, Lippincott Williams & Wilkins, 2011, p 69.

26. **B. Teratoma.**

Teratomas, primitive neuroectodermal tumors, astrocytomas, and choroid plexus papillomas are the most common congenital brain neoplasms, frequently found within the first year of life. Ependymomas, germinomas, and gangliomas are rare. Teratomas are supratentorial in location and may arise in the suprasellar and pineal regions.

▶ Rumack CM, Levine D (eds): *Diagnostic Ultrasound*, 5th edition. Philadelphia, Elsevier, 2018, p 1562.

▶ Siegel MJ (ed): *Pediatric Sonography*, 4th edition. Philadelphia, Lippincott Williams & Wilkins, 2011, p 110.

27. **C. Lenticulostriate vasculopathy.**

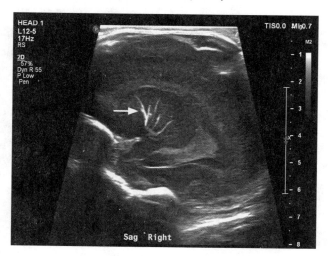

Although nonspecific for TORCH (toxoplasmosis, "other," rubella, cytomegalovirus, and herpes) infections, lenticulostriate vasculopathy *in the brain may be associated with cytomegalovirus (CMV). On ultrasound, calcifications or bright, linear, echogenic foci (arrow) are seen in the arteries of the thalamus and basal ganglia. These echogenic structures represent*

mineralized vessels. Abscesses, ventriculitis, and cerebral infarction are usually the result of an advanced acquired infection and not a congenital one like CMV.

▶ de Bruyn R (ed): *Pediatric Ultrasound: How, Why and When*, 2nd edition (e-book). Philadelphia, Churchill Livingstone/Elsevier, 2010, pp 272–273.
▶ Rumack CM, Levine D (eds): *Diagnostic Ultrasound*, 5th edition. Philadelphia, Elsevier, 2018, pp 1556–1557, 1560.
▶ Siegel MJ (ed): *Pediatric Sonography*, 4th edition. Philadelphia, Lippincott Williams & Wilkins, 2011, p 103.

28. **A. Extracorporeal membrane oxygenation (ECMO).**

    Extracorporeal membrane oxygenation (ECMO) is a technique used for the treatment of infants with acute, reversible respiratory failure. This technique helps to oxygenate the blood through a machine that performs the function of the heart and lungs. With ECMO the blood is bypassed from the right atrium of the heart to the aorta. Because infants on ECMO are on continuous heparinization, the risk of intracranial bleed and ischemia increases. Brain hemorrhages in infants on ECMO can appear hypoechoic due to the abnormal clotting of the blood. Therapeutic hypothermia and brain cooling are used to decrease the chances of severe brain damage in neonates suffering from hypoxic-ischemic encephalopathy. Dialysis is a treatment utilized on patients with renal failure and helps to perform the function of the kidneys by filtering the blood through a machine. A tracheostomy is a procedure that utilizes a neck incision as an alternative air passage when there is an obstruction of the airway. Therapeutic hypothermia and brain cooling, dialysis, and tracheostomy are not procedures used in children with acute respiratory failure because they do not help to oxygenate the blood.

    ▶ Rumack CM, Levine D (eds): *Diagnostic Ultrasound*, 5th edition. Philadelphia, Elsevier, 2018, pp 1578–1580.
    ▶ Siegel MJ (ed): *Pediatric Sonography*, 4th edition. Philadelphia, Lippincott Williams & Wilkins, 2011, pp 78–79.

29. **D. Choroid plexus papilloma.**

    Although brain tumors are very difficult to differentiate based on their sonographic appearance, the location of the neoplasm can help with the differential diagnosis. For example, choroid plexus papillomas are highly vascularized hyperechoic tumors that arise from the trigone of the lateral ventricle. Gliomas and ependymomas are usually infratentorial tumors that involve the brainstem. Teratomas are supratentorial in location, but, like any teratoma, their sonographic appearance typically includes calcifications and cystic areas of deterioration.

▶ Rumack CM, Levine D (eds): *Diagnostic Ultrasound*, 5th edition. Philadelphia, Elsevier, 2018, p 1562.

▶ Siegel MJ (ed): *Pediatric Sonography*, 4th edition. Philadelphia, Lippincott Williams & Wilkins, 2011, p 110.

30. C. Absent septum pellucidum.

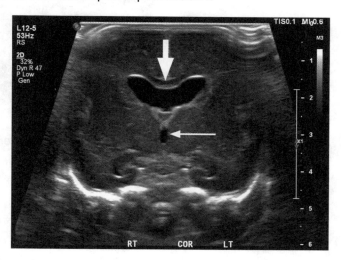

The cavum septi pellucidi (CSP) is fluid-filled space between the two leaves of the septum pellucidum, which is a usual finding in neonates. Some infants have a septum pellucidum without fluid and hence no cavum. The CSP is seen on ultrasound as a box-shaped structure that lies midline, superior to the roof of the third ventricle and between the lateral ventricles. When the CSP is partially or completely absent, continuous communication of the frontal horns of the lateral ventricles is seen. An absent septum pellucidum is often associated with septo-optic dysplasia, also known as de Morsier syndrome. In this coronal image, superior to the medial portion of the lateral ventricles, the corpus callosum is seen (thick arrow). In the midline, slightly inferior to the area of communication of the lateral ventricles, the thin third ventricle *appears normal (thin arrow). Although a large massa intermedia is often seen with Chiari 2 malformation, the massa intermedia is not seen in this image. It lies within the third ventricle and is easier to visualize when there is dilatation of the third ventricle.

▶ Rumack CM, Levine D (eds): *Diagnostic Ultrasound*, 5th edition. Philadelphia, Elsevier, 2018, pp 1521, 1535.

▶ Siegel MJ (ed): *Pediatric Sonography*, 4th edition. Philadelphia, Lippincott Williams & Wilkins, 2011, pp 52, 96–97.

31. C. Temporal lobe.

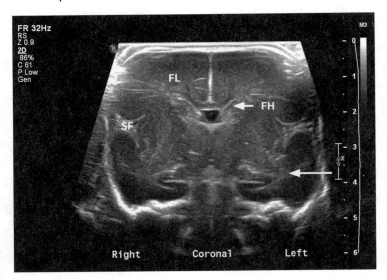

On a coronal plane, anterior to the frontal horns of the lateral ventricles, the frontal lobe (FL) of the brain is seen. Moving slightly posterior, at the level of the foramen of Monro (as seen in this image), the frontal horns (FH) of the lateral ventricles are visible, as well as the Sylvian fissures (SF) separating the frontal lobe from the temporal lobe (arrow). On a more posterior scan, at the level of the glomus of the choroid plexus, the parietal lobes are identified. In the most posterior aspect of the brain, past the occipital horns of the lateral ventricles and cerebellum, the occipital lobe is visualized.

▸ Rumack CM, Levine D (eds): *Diagnostic Ultrasound*, 5th edition. Philadelphia, Elsevier, 2018, pp 1514–1515.

▸ Siegel MJ (ed): *Pediatric Sonography*, 4th edition. Philadelphia, Lippincott Williams & Wilkins, 2011, p 45.

32. B. Hemorrhage.

Intracranial hemorrhages are asymptomatic 25%–50% of the time and are found during routine imaging. When symptoms are present, they can include an unexplained drop in hematocrit, apnea, or bradycardia. Symptomatic patients require "stat" head ultrasounds to rule out hemorrhage. On asymptomatic patients, head ultrasounds are usually performed within the first week of life. Most hemorrhages occur in the first three days after premature birth.

33. **D. Caput succedaneum.**

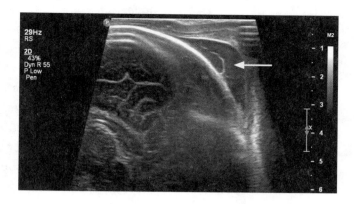

See Color Plate 11, "Locations of Hemorrhaging in the Skull" on page xxxvii.

A caput succedaneum is the swelling of an infant's scalp (arrow) due to the accumulation of blood in the presenting area of the head during delivery. This blood accumulation is the result of pressure during a prolonged, difficult labor. A caput succedaneum may cross the midline because the blood accumulation is in the scalp. It normally resolves within the first few days and usually does not cause any complications. This type of injury is usually diagnosed by physical exam only. Cerebral edema *occurs intracranially, not extracranially.* Subdural *and* epidural hematomas *are intracranial bleeds. When evaluating for extracranial lesions, incorporating the standoff pad in your exam helps to improve the visualization of the superficial layers.*

▸ Healthline: Caput succedaneum (swelling of the scalp during labor). Available at https://www.healthline.com/health/caput-succedaneum.

▸ Raines DA, Whitten RA: Cephalhematoma. In *StatPearls*, 2018. Available at https://www.ncbi.nlm.nih.gov/books/NBK470192.

▸ Siegel MJ (ed): *Pediatric Sonography*, 4th edition. Philadelphia, Lippincott Williams & Wilkins, 2011, p 105.

34. **D. Normal brain.**

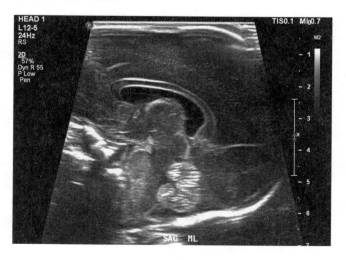

The parenchyma of a premature infant's brain has a different appearance when compared to a fully developed brain. A full-term brain shows the development of multiple sulci and gyri, since branching does not occur until after 33 weeks' gestation; prior to 33 weeks, the only sulci and gyri seen are the main ones. A 26-week premature brain that is undergoing normal brain development therefore has a smoother appearance, as seen in this image. The appearance is similar to that of lissencephaly, the abnormality characterized by the underdevelopment of sulci and gyri in the brain. The patient's gestational age at birth should, however, help differentiate lissencephaly from a normal premature brain. In addition, the parietal occipital fissure, usually present in the midline sagittal plane after 16 weeks' gestation, would be absent in lissencephaly. Cerebral ischemia and edema are most commonly seen in full-term infants and appear as poor gyral-sulcal differentiation with possible diffuse echogenic areas.

▶ Rumack CM, Levine D (eds): *Diagnostic Ultrasound*, 5th edition. Philadelphia, Elsevier, 2018, pp 1520–1521.

▶ Siegel MJ (ed): *Pediatric Sonography*, 4th edition. Philadelphia, Lippincott Williams & Wilkins, 2011, pp 49–51.

35. **B. Epidural hemorrhage.**

See Color Plate 11, "Locations of Hemorrhaging in the Skull," on page xxxvii.

An epidural hemorrhage *is a rare type of brain injury in which blood accumulates between the skull and the dura mater. This type of injury is commonly seen in full-term infants as a result of traumatic delivery. It is important not to mistake a mirror artifact of scalp fluid for an epidural fluid collection.* A subdural hemorrhage *is located between the dura and arachnoid mater. Ultrasound is not the best modality to differentiate a subdural from an epidural hemorrhage; computed tomography (CT) or magnetic resonance imaging (MRI) can best make the diagnosis.* A subgaleal hemorrhage *is located between the periosteum and the galea or epicranial aponeurosis.* A subarachnoid hemorrhage *is located within the subarachnoid space.*

▶ Davis DJ: Neonatal subgaleal hemorrhage: diagnosis and management. CMAJ 164:1452–1453, 2001. Available at https:www.ncbi.nlm.nih.gov/pmc/articles/PMC81073/.

▶ de Bruyn R (ed): *Pediatric Ultrasound: How, Why and When*, 2nd edition (e-book). Philadelphia, Churchill Livingstone/Elsevier, 2010, pp 261–262.

▶ Rumack CM, Levine D (eds): *Diagnostic Ultrasound*, 5th edition. Philadelphia, Elsevier, 2018, p 1557.

▶ Siegel MJ (ed): *Pediatric Sonography*, 4th edition. Philadelphia, Lippincott Williams & Wilkins, 2011, pp 69–71.

36. **C. Supratentorial.**

   Most brain tumors in infancy arise from the supratentorial region. By contrast, in older children brain tumors are infratentorial. Although brain tumors are difficult to differentiate on ultrasound, their location helps to reduce the list of differential diagnoses. In most cases, additional imaging modalities, such as magnetic resonance imaging (MRI), are utilized for better evaluation and localization of the lesion. The sella turcica is used as a landmark specifically for pituitary tumors.

   ▶ Rumack CM, Levine D (eds): *Diagnostic Ultrasound*, 5th edition. Philadelphia, Elsevier, 2018, p 1562.

   ▶ Siegel MJ (ed): *Pediatric Sonography*, 4th edition. Philadelphia, Lippincott Williams & Wilkins, 2011, p 110.

37. **A. Grade 1.**

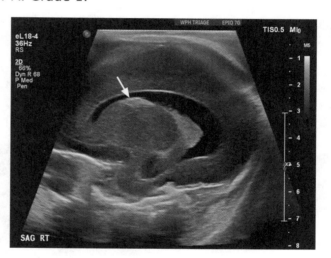

   In a grade 1 or germinal matrix (subependymal) intraventricular hemorrhage (IVH), the bleed is confined to the subependymal region (germinal matrix). The sonographic appearance of a grade 1 IVH is of a small hyperechoic, irregular structure (arrow) in the caudothalamic groove. Subependymal hemorrhages are more common in early premature infants because the germinal matrix, a highly vascular structure located mainly in the subependymal region, starts regressing after 34 weeks' gestation and by 36 weeks has nearly disappeared. Due to the nature of the germinal matrix, the infant's gestational age is directly related to the incidence of hemorrhage. Premature infants who are less than 30 weeks old or have a birth weight less than 1500 grams are at higher risk for hemorrhage.

   ▶ de Bruyn R (ed): *Pediatric Ultrasound: How, Why and When*, 2nd edition (e-book). Philadelphia, Churchill Livingstone/Elsevier, 2010, pp 260, 264.

▸ Rumack CM, Levine D (eds): *Diagnostic Ultrasound*, 5th edition. Philadelphia, Elsevier, 2018, pp 1541–1544.

▸ Siegel MJ (ed): *Pediatric Sonography*, 4th edition. Philadelphia, Lippincott Williams & Wilkins, 2011, pp 61–62.

38. **C. Occipital lobe.**

    The most posterior lobe of the brain is the occipital lobe. *The occipital lobe is located superior to the cerebellum and posterior to the* parietal *and* temporal lobes. *When scanning through the anterior fontanelle coronally, you can image the occipital lobe by angling toward the most posterior aspect of the head, superior and posterior to the cerebellum. In this view the lateral ventricles are not visualized. The midline posterior interhemispheric fissure is seen, and on each side increased echogenicity of the white matter is normally visualized.*

    ▸ Rumack CM, Levine D (eds): *Diagnostic Ultrasound*, 5th edition. Philadelphia, Elsevier, 2018, p 1515.

    ▸ Siegel MJ (ed): *Pediatric Sonography*, 4th edition. Philadelphia, Lippincott Williams & Wilkins, 2011, p 46.

39. **B. Dandy-Walker malformation.**

    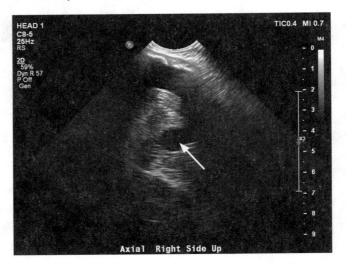

    Dandy-Walker complex *is a group of congenital brain malformations that include the Dandy-Walker malformation and the Dandy-Walker variant. The Dandy-Walker malformation is characterized by a dilated fourth ventricle (arrow) in communication with the cisterna magna. There is elevation of the tentorium cerebelli, and the cerebellar vermis can be absent or hypoplastic and displaced laterally by the enlarged fourth ventricle. Differential diagnoses for Dandy-Walker malformation*

include mega cisterna magna *and posterior* subarachnoid cyst. *To differentiate these two abnormalities from Dandy-Walker malformation it is important to know that a mega cisterna magna is not commonly associated with hydrocephalus and a posterior subarachnoid cyst does not communicate with the fourth ventricle. With a* Chiari malformation, *the cisterna magna and fourth ventricle are obliterated, not enlarged.*

▶ de Bruyn R (ed): *Pediatric Ultrasound: How, Why and When*, 2nd edition (e-book). Philadelphia, Churchill Livingstone/Elsevier, 2010, pp 270–271.

▶ Siegel MJ (ed): *Pediatric Sonography*, 4th edition. Philadelphia, Lippincott Williams & Wilkins, 2011, pp 87–90.

40. **D. Temporal bone.**

For the evaluation and Doppler interrogation of the middle cerebral artery (MCA), the temporal bone is the best approach or window. Due to the angle and location of the MCA, the MCA's blood flow is toward the transducer and the angle of insonation is close to zero when you are scanning through the transtemporal window. The opposite happens when you scan through the anterior fontanelle. The perpendicular relationship between the MCA and the sound beam gives an angle of insonation that is close to 90 degrees. The temporal bone approach is also helpful to evaluate most of the main branches of the circle of Willis.

▶ Rumack CM, Levine D (eds): *Diagnostic Ultrasound*, 5th edition. Philadelphia, Elsevier, 2018, p 1574.

▶ Siegel MJ (ed): *Pediatric Sonography*, 4th edition. Philadelphia, Lippincott Williams & Wilkins, 2011, p 58.

41. **A. Cephalohematoma.**

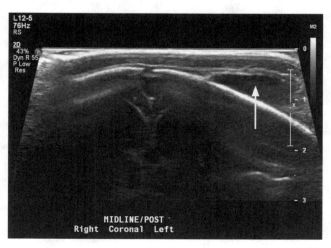

See Color Plate 11, "Locations of Hemorrhaging in the Skull," on page xxxvii.

A cephalohematoma *(arrow) is a hemorrhage between the skull (the echogenic line beneath the hemorrhage) and the membrane underneath the skin or periosteum. The periosteum keeps the bleeding contained and unable to cross the midline. Therefore, the key point in differentiating a cephalohematoma from a* caput succedaneum *and a* subgaleal hemorrhage *is the ability of the hemorrhage to cross the midline suture line. A* subarachnoid hemorrhage *is a bleed deeper within the skull, between the pia and the arachnoid mater. When evaluating for extracranial lesions, incorporating the standoff pad in your exam helps to improve the visualization of the superficial layers.*

▶ Davis DJ: Neonatal subgaleal hemorrhage: diagnosis and management. CMAJ 15:1452–1453, 2001. Available at https:www.ncbi.nlm.nih.gov/pmc/articles/PMC81073/.

▶ Healthline: Caput succedaneum (swelling of the scalp during labor). Available at https://www.healthline.com/health/caput-succedaneum.

▶ Raines DA, Whitten RA: Cephalhematoma. In *StatPearls*, 2018. Available at https://www.ncbi.nlm.nih.gov/books/NBK470192.

42. **D. Schizencephaly.**

Schizencephaly *is a cortical neuronal migration malformation in utero that causes abnormal clefts or slits in the brain parenchyma. These clefts are lined with gray matter and extend from the ependyma of the lateral ventricles to the pia mater. The clefts can be unilateral or bilateral, and in 70% of cases there is also absence of the septum pellucidum.* **Lissencephaly** *is a malformation characterized by the smooth appearance of the brain.* **Hydranencephaly** *results when the cerebral hemispheres are replaced by a cranial cavity filled with cerebrospinal fluid (CSF) due to destruction of the cerebral cortex.* **Porencephaly**, *unlike schizencephaly, involves cysts (not clefts) that do not extend to the surface cortex of the brain.*

▶ Rumack CM, Levine D (eds): *Diagnostic Ultrasound*, 5th edition. Philadelphia, Elsevier, 2018, pp 1536–1538.

▶ Siegel MJ (ed): *Pediatric Sonography*, 4th edition. Philadelphia, Lippincott Williams & Wilkins, 2011, p 98.

43. **B. Grade 2.**

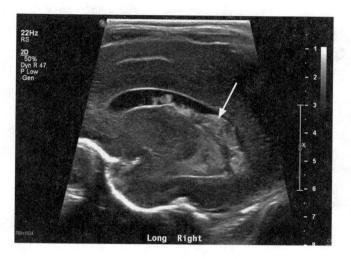

See also the answer to question 14.

In a grade 2 intraventricular hemorrhage (IVH), the bleeding extends from the subependymal region into the ventricles. On ultrasound, echogenic material (arrow) is seen within the ventricles or attached to the choroid plexus. Grade 2 IVHs can be difficult to diagnose because on occasion the blood products are small and located in the occipital horn of the lateral ventricle. Scanning through the mastoid fontanelle increases the level of detection of these small bleeds.

▶ de Bruyn R (ed): *Pediatric Ultrasound: How, Why and When*, 2nd edition (e-book). Philadelphia, Churchill Livingstone/Elsevier, 2010, p 264.
▶ Rumack CM, Levine D (eds): *Diagnostic Ultrasound*, 5th edition. Philadelphia, Elsevier, 2018, pp 1544–1545.
▶ Siegel MJ (ed): *Pediatric Sonography*, 4th edition. Philadelphia, Lippincott Williams & Wilkins, 2011, pp 62–64.

44. **B. Cerebellar hemorrhage.**

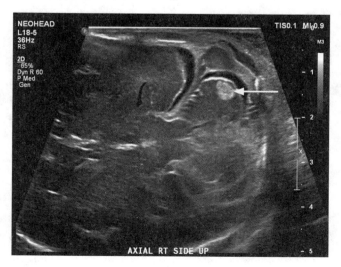

The sonographic appearance of a cerebellar hemorrhage *is a hyperechoic mass (arrow) within the cerebellum. Cerebellar hemorrhages can be unilateral or bilateral and can occur in preterm or full-term infants. In premature infants, a cerebellar hemorrhage can be related to an extension of an intraventricular hemorrhage (IVH) or subarachnoid hemorrhage. In full-term infants, it can be secondary to traumatic birth and has also been associated with tight-fitting facemasks for ventilation. The lesion demonstrated in this image of the cerebellum would less likely represent a* hemangioblastoma, *an* astrocytoma, *or a* liponeurocytoma *because these are uncommon tumors and are not usually associated with IVH. Only the liponeurocytoma is a cerebellar tumor; the others occur in the brain or spinal cord.*

▶ de Bruyn R (ed): *Pediatric Ultrasound: How, Why and When*, 2nd edition (e-book). Philadelphia, Churchill Livingstone/Elsevier, 2010, pp 261–263.

▶ Rumack CM, Levine D (eds): *Diagnostic Ultrasound*, 5th edition. Philadelphia, Elsevier, 2018, pp 1548–1550.

▶ Siegel MJ (ed): *Pediatric Sonography*, 4th edition. Philadelphia, Lippincott Williams & Wilkins, 2011, pp 72–73.

45. **A. Cystic encephalomalacia.**

    Cystic encephalomalacia *is the result of damage to brain parenchyma, usually caused by cerebral ischemia, infection, hemorrhage, trauma, or other insults. In diffuse brain damage, large areas of cystic encephalomalacia may be seen. These cystic lesions normally do not connect with the ventricular system.* Ventriculitis *can occur when a meningeal infection progresses and affects the ventricles.* Hydrocephalus *can be the result of ventricular obstruction, malabsorption of cerebrospinal fluid (CSF), or overproduction.* Schizencephaly *does not result from brain damage during the neonatal period; it is a neuronal migration malformation that occurs in utero.*

    ▶ Rumack CM, Levine D (eds): *Diagnostic Ultrasound*, 5th edition. Philadelphia, Elsevier, 2018, p 1538.

    ▶ Siegel MJ (ed): *Pediatric Sonography*, 4th edition. Philadelphia, Lippincott Williams & Wilkins, 2011, p 102.

46. **C. Colpocephaly.**

    Colpocephaly *is the enlargement and parallel orientation of the occipital horns of the lateral ventricles and is associated with absence of the corpus callosum. In colpocephaly the frontal horns appear widely separated and often smaller than the occipital horns. Other brain anomalies that are associated with* an absent corpus callosum include Dandy-Walker complex, holoprosencephaly, septo-optic dysplasia, lipomas, and Aicardia syndrome.

▶ de Bruyn R (ed): *Pediatric Ultrasound: How, Why and When*, 2nd edition (e-book). Philadelphia, Churchill Livingstone/Elsevier, 2010, p 272.
▶ Rumack CM, Levine D (eds): *Diagnostic Ultrasound*, 5th edition. Philadelphia, Elsevier, 2018, pp 1526–1528.
▶ Siegel MJ (ed): *Pediatric Sonography*, 4th edition. Philadelphia, Lippincott Williams & Wilkins, 2011, pp 90–91.

47. C. Grade 3.

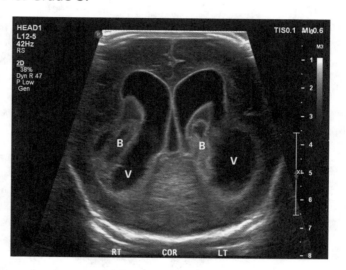

See also the answer to question 14.

A grade 3 intraventricular hemorrhage (IVH) occurs when there is intraventricular bleed associated with hydrocephalus. As seen in this image, the ventricles (V) become dilated due to a block in the ventricular system caused by a clot. A grade 3 IVH is usually easier to diagnose, because the dilated ventricles provide better visualization of the blood (B) within the ventricles. Grade 3 hemorrhages usually resolve or improve after five to six weeks, because the obstructing clot starts to dissolve and allows cerebrospinal fluid (CSF) to flow normally within the ventricular system. As indicated by the clots' echotexture, this is not an acute hemorrhage and demonstrates the change in appearance as a clot dissolves. The echogenic ventricular walls are due to posthemorrhagic ventriculitis.

▶ de Bruyn R (ed): *Pediatric Ultrasound: How, Why and When*, 2nd edition (e-book). Philadelphia, Churchill Livingstone/Elsevier, 2010, p 264.
▶ Rumack CM, Levine D (eds): *Diagnostic Ultrasound*, 5th edition. Philadelphia, Elsevier, 2018, pp 1545–1547.
▶ Siegel MJ (ed): *Pediatric Sonography*, 4th edition. Philadelphia, Lippincott Williams & Wilkins, 2011, pp 64–65.

48. **B. Prosencephalon.**

During early development of the central nervous system (CNS), there are three primary vesicles of the brain: the prosencephalon (forebrain), the mesencephalon (midbrain), and the rhombencephalon (hindbrain). The prosencephalon *divides into the telencephalon and the diencephalon. Eventually the telencephalon becomes the cerebral hemispheres and the basal ganglia, and the diencephalon becomes the thalamus and hypothalamus. The* mesencephalon *forms the cerebral peduncles, cerebral aqueduct, and corpora quadrigemina. The* rhombencephalon *divides into the metencephalon and myelencephalon to eventually form the cerebellum, pons, and medulla oblongata.*

▶ Rumack CM, Levine D (eds): *Diagnostic Ultrasound*, 5th edition. Philadelphia, Elsevier, 2018, p 1167.

49. **C. Parietal lobe.**

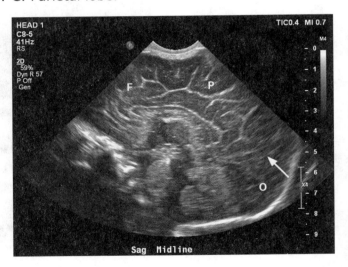

There are two parietal lobes *(P), and they are located superior to the* temporal lobes, *anterior to the* occipital lobe *(O), and posterior to the* frontal lobes *(F). On a midline parasagittal view (as in this image), the* parieto-occipital fissure *(arrow) is seen separating the parietal lobe from the occipital lobe. Laterally, on a sagittal plane, the* Sylvian fissure *(not visualized in this image) is seen separating the parietal lobe from the temporal lobe inferiorly. The central sulcus separates the parietal lobe from the frontal lobe but is difficult to visualize on ultrasound.*

▶ Rumack CM, Levine D (eds): *Diagnostic Ultrasound*, 5th edition. Philadelphia, Elsevier, 2018, p 1516.

50. **A. 8.5 MHz.**

When selecting your transducer frequency, you should consider both resolution and penetration. For a preterm infant, a transducer with the highest frequency possible is better because it provides the best resolution. For a full-term infant, a lower frequency provides the needed penetration for the larger head. The most adequate transducer for a full-term infant with macrocephaly is one with a lower frequency.

▸ de Bruyn R (ed): *Pediatric Ultrasound: How, Why and When*, 2nd edition (e-book). Philadelphia, Churchill Livingstone/Elsevier, 2010, p 252.
▸ Rumack CM, Levine D (eds): *Diagnostic Ultrasound*, 5th edition. Philadelphia, Elsevier, 2018, p 1512.
▸ Siegel MJ (ed): *Pediatric Sonography*, 4th edition. Philadelphia, Lippincott Williams & Wilkins, 2011, p 44.

51. **B. Fourth ventricle.**

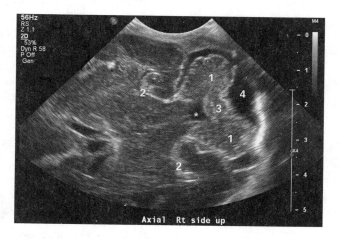

The posterior fossa *is a space in the skull located posterior and inferior in the calvaria, and it contains the brainstem and the cerebellum. The* brainstem *is composed of the midbrain, pons, and medulla and is continuous with the spinal cord. The* cerebellum *(numbered 1 in this image) is an echogenic peanut- or dumbbell-shaped structure located below the* tentorium cerebelli *(2) and behind the top portion of the brainstem. The echogenic structure seen connecting the two sides of the cerebellum is the* cerebellar vermis *(3). Also contained in the posterior fossa, the* fourth ventricle *(asterisk) is located within the pons, the dorsal roof being formed by the cerebellum. The* cisterna magna *(4) is the space filled with cerebrospinal fluid (CSF) located inferior to the cerebellar vermis, which is continuous with the fourth ventricle. The* third ventricle *is not located within the posterior fossa.*

▸ Rumack CM, Levine D (eds): *Diagnostic Ultrasound*, 5th edition. Philadelphia, Elsevier, 2018, p 1524.

See also the answer to question 14.

52. **D. Ventricular distention.**

The difference between a grade 2 and a grade 3 intraventricular hemorrhage (IVH) is the presence of hydrocephalus or ventricular enlargement. When a blood clot causes an obstruction within the ventricular system, cerebrospinal fluid (CSF) starts to accumulate, causing enlargement of the ventricles. Blood products within the ventricles are seen in both a grade 2 and a grade 3 IVH. However, in a grade 3 IVH there must be ventricular distension/hydrocephalus accompanying the blood products within the ventricles. When there is extension of the bleed into the brain parenchyma, it is considered a grade 4 IVH. With a grade 3 IVH, the lateral and third ventricles are usually affected because the aqueduct of Sylvius is a common location for clot obstruction. In most cases, the blockage resolves on its own; a ventriculoperitoneal (VP) shunt is required in only a small percentage of patients.

▶ de Bruyn R (ed): *Pediatric Ultrasound: How, Why and When*, 2nd edition (e-book). Philadelphia, Churchill Livingstone/Elsevier, 2010, p 264.
▶ Rumack CM, Levine D (eds): *Diagnostic Ultrasound*, 5th edition. Philadelphia, Elsevier, 2018, pp 1545–1547.
▶ Siegel MJ (ed): *Pediatric Sonography*, 4th edition. Philadelphia, Lippincott Williams & Wilkins, 2011, pp 64–65.

53. **A. Rhombencephalon.**

The rhombencephalon, or hindbrain, is one of the primary vesicles that develops in the early embryo. During the early stages of development, the rhombencephalon subdivides into the metencephalon and myelencephalon. The metencephalon eventually becomes the pons and cerebellum. The medulla oblongata develops from the most posterior part of the rhombencephalon, the myelencephalon. The mesencephalon is the primary vesicle that develops into the cerebral peduncles, the corpora quadrigemina, and the cerebral aqueduct. The prosencephalon is another primary vesicle, which subdivides into the telencephalon and diencephalon, and they become the cerebrum, the thalamus, and the hypothalamus.

▶ Rumack CM, Levine D (eds): *Diagnostic Ultrasound*, 5th edition. Philadelphia, Elsevier, 2018, p 1167.

54. B. Caudate nucleus.

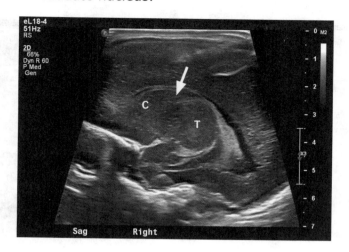

The caudate nucleus (labeled C in the image) is a bilateral C-shaped structure that forms part of the basal ganglia. The caudate nucleus is located lateral to and below the floor of the frontal horns of the lateral ventricles. The caudate nucleus is separated inferiorly from the thalamus (T) by the echogenic caudothalamic groove (arrow). This area is an important landmark for the evaluation of intracranial bleeds because germinal matrix hemorrhages occur in this region.

▶ de Bruyn R (ed): *Pediatric Ultrasound: How, Why and When*, 2nd edition (e-book). Philadelphia, Churchill Livingstone/Elsevier, 2010, p 258.
▶ Rumack CM, Levine D (eds): *Diagnostic Ultrasound*, 5th edition. Philadelphia, Elsevier, 2018, p 1524.

55. B. To produce cerebrospinal fluid (CSF).

The main function of the choroid plexus is the production of cerebrospinal fluid (CSF). The largest portion of the choroid plexus (glomus) is located within the trigone of the lateral ventricle bilaterally. Within the lateral ventricles, the normal choroid plexus never extends into the frontal or occipital horns. The choroid plexus is also located in the roof of the third and fourth ventricles. Some pathologies involving the choroid plexus, such as choroid plexus hypertrophy, tumors, and neural tube defects, can cause overproduction of CSF, leading to hydrocephalus.

▶ de Bruyn R (ed): *Pediatric Ultrasound: How, Why and When*, 2nd edition (e-book). Philadelphia, Churchill Livingstone/Elsevier, 2010, p 275.
▶ Rumack CM, Levine D (eds): *Diagnostic Ultrasound*, 5th edition. Philadelphia, Elsevier, 2018, pp 1522–1523.
▶ Siegel MJ (ed): *Pediatric Sonography*, 4th edition. Philadelphia, Lippincott Williams & Wilkins, 2011, pp 52–53.

56. C. Corpus callosum.

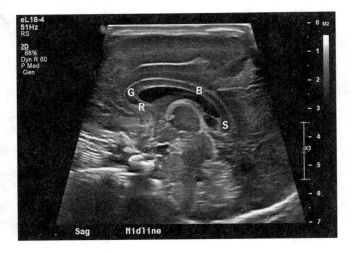

The corpus callosum *is a white-matter midline structure that connects both sides of the brain. On a midline sagittal view, the corpus callosum appears as a C-shaped structure that borders the* cavum septi pellucidi *(CSP) anteriorly and superiorly. The most anterior section of the corpus callosum is called the* genu *(G) and borders the CSP anteriorly. From the anterior aspect of the genu, the inferior and backward extension is called the* rostrum *(R). The* body *(B) of the corpus callosum is the largest section and connects the posterior aspect of the genu with the* splenium *(S). When there is partial agenesis of the corpus callosum, the portion of the corpus callosum that is usually present is the genu.*

▶ de Bruyn R (ed): *Pediatric Ultrasound: How, Why and When*, 2nd edition (e-book). Philadelphia, Churchill Livingstone/Elsevier, 2010, pp 256, 258.
▶ Rumack CM, Levine D (eds): *Diagnostic Ultrasound*, 5th edition. Philadelphia, Elsevier, 2018, p 1526.
▶ Siegel MJ (ed): *Pediatric Sonography*, 4th edition. Philadelphia, Lippincott Williams & Wilkins, 2011, pp 90, 92.

57. A. Cavum septi pellucidi (CSP).

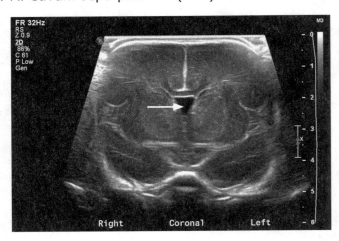

The cavum septi pellucidi *(CSP; see arrow) is a box-shaped midline cavity that is filled with cerebrospinal fluid (CSF). The CSP is located between the anterior horns of the lateral ventricles and anterior to the foramen of Monro. Early in gestation (usually before 24 weeks), the CSP can have a posterior extension called the* cavum vergae. *The* cavum veli interpositi *is a possible extension of the cavum vergae that appears below the columns of the fornices and anteroinferior to the splenium of the corpus callosum. This cystic structure can appear separated from the cavum vergae by a thin septation, and, although it is considered a normal variant, observation may be needed to ensure the right diagnosis. On ultrasound the* corpus callosum *appears hypoechoic with echogenic borders, not anechoic.*

▶ de Bruyn R (ed): *Pediatric Ultrasound: How, Why and When*, 2nd edition (e-book). Philadelphia, Churchill Livingstone/Elsevier, 2010, pp 256, 265.
▶ Rumack CM, Levine D (eds): *Diagnostic Ultrasound*, 5th edition. Philadelphia, Elsevier, 2018, pp 1521–1522.
▶ Siegel MJ (ed): *Pediatric Sonography*, 4th edition. Philadelphia, Lippincott Williams & Wilkins, 2011, p 52.

58. **D. Frontal and parietal.**

The skull bones are separated from one another by fontanelles and sutures. The anterior fontanelle *is a diamond-shaped space located centrally between the two frontal and parietal bones. It is the space formed when the coronal, metopic, and sagittal sutures meet. The* frontal *or* metopic suture *separates both frontal lobes medially. The* coronal suture *separates the frontal bones from the parietal bones. The* sagittal suture, *located in the midline, separates both parietal bones.*

▶ Rumack CM, Levine D (eds): *Diagnostic Ultrasound*, 5th edition. Philadelphia, Elsevier, 2018, p 44.

59. **C. Holoprosencephaly.**

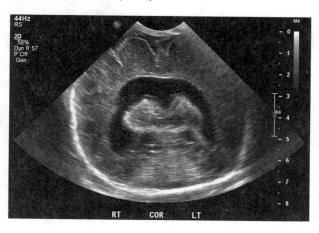

Holoprosencephaly *is a congenital malformation, occurring during the organogenesis period, in which the cerebral hemispheres fail to divide. On ultrasound, all forms of holoprosencephaly can be identified. Holoprosencephaly is often diagnosed prenatally, and magnetic resonance imaging (MRI) is usually best for the final diagnosis. Holoprosencephaly consists of multiple midline defects that can include a central common ventricle (monoventricle) and partial or complete fusion of the thalami, depending on the severity. Absence of the cavum septi pellucidi (CSP) is seen in all forms of holoprosencephaly.* Porencephaly *is seen as cystic areas of focal tissue destruction that communicate with the ventricular system.* Colpocephaly *refers to the parallel orientation of the lateral ventricles.* Schizencephaly *appears as clefts in the brain parenchyma that may extend throughout the brain hemisphere.*

▶ de Bruyn R (ed): *Pediatric Ultrasound: How, Why and When*, 2nd edition (e-book). Philadelphia, Churchill Livingstone/Elsevier, 2010, p 271.

▶ Rumack CM, Levine D (eds): *Diagnostic Ultrasound*, 5th edition. Philadelphia, Elsevier, 2018, pp 1525, 1532.

▶ Siegel MJ (ed): *Pediatric Sonography*, 4th edition. Philadelphia, Lippincott Williams & Wilkins, 2011, p 92.

60. C. 3

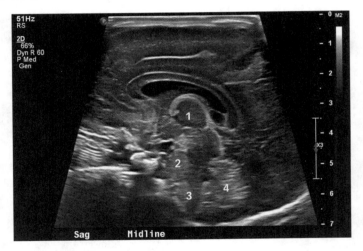

On a midline sagittal plane the pons (2) appears superior and anterior to the medulla oblongata (3). These structures are seen anterior to the fourth ventricle and appear slightly echogenic. Posterior to the fourth ventricle, the hyperechoic cerebellar vermis (4) is seen. The massa intermedia (1) is seen within the thin third ventricle superiorly.

▶ Rumack CM, Levine D (eds): *Diagnostic Ultrasound*, 5th edition. Philadelphia, Elsevier, 2018, p 1516.

▶ Siegel MJ (ed): *Pediatric Sonography*, 4th edition. Philadelphia, Lippincott Williams & Wilkins, 2011, p 45.

See Color Plate 1 on page xxxiii.

61. **A. Subarachnoid space.**

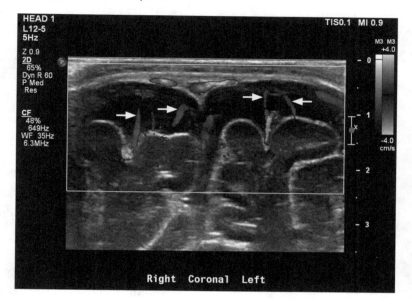

See Color Plate 11 "Locations of Hemorrhaging in the Skull," on page xxxvii.

Extra-axial fluid collections can be seen within the subarachnoid, subdural, and epidural spaces. Although they are difficult to differentiate on ultrasound, the use of color Doppler can help with the diagnosis. The presence of the cortical vessels crossing the fluid (arrows) is indicative of a subarachnoid *fluid collection. In a* subdural *fluid collection, the vessels are pushed toward the brain surface and are not seen crossing the fluid. The* subgaleal space *is located outside the skull. Epidural hemorrhages are located between the skull and the dura mater, and they cause a mass effect in the adjacent parenchyma. High-frequency transducers are best for imaging this superficial area.*

▶ de Bruyn R (ed): *Pediatric Ultrasound: How, Why and When*, 2nd edition (e-book). Philadelphia, Churchill Livingstone/Elsevier, 2010, pp 41, 252, 254–255, 261–263.

▶ Rumack CM, Levine D (eds): *Diagnostic Ultrasound*, 5th edition. Philadelphia, Elsevier, 2018, pp 1557–1558.

▶ Siegel MJ (ed): *Pediatric Sonography*, 4th edition. Philadelphia, Lippincott Williams & Wilkins, 2011, p 71.

62. **B. 12 months.**

Intracranial ultrasound exams are usually performed between the ages of newborn and 12 months old. At about 9 months old, the anterior fontanelle starts to close, and closure is usually complete by 24 months. Because the anterior fontanelle is the main acoustic window used for neonatal brain ultrasound, the earlier the exam is performed, the better its quality will be. Limited visualization of the brain can occur when there are overlapping sutures. If ultrasound appears suboptimal, other imaging modalities may be indicated.

▸ Rumack CM, Levine D (eds): *Diagnostic Ultrasound*, 5th edition. Philadelphia, Elsevier, 2018, p 1513.

▸ Siegel MJ (ed): *Pediatric Sonography*, 4th edition. Philadelphia, Lippincott Williams & Wilkins, 2011, p 43.

63. C. 5.

There are 5 main sutures in the skull. These sutures are the frontal (metopic) suture, coronal suture, sagittal suture, lambdoid suture, and squamous suture. The frontal suture *is located between the two frontal bones. The* sagittal suture *separates the two parietal bones. The* coronal suture *lies between the frontal and parietal bones. The* lambdoid suture *separates the parietal bones from the occipital bone posteriorly. The* squamous suture, *located on each side, divides the parietal bone from the temporal bone.*

▸ Radiology Masterclass: CT brain anatomy: skull bones and sutures. Available at https://www.radiologymasterclass.co.uk/tutorials/ct/ct_brain_anatomy/ct_brain_anatomy_skull.

▸ Rumack CM, Levine D (eds): *Diagnostic Ultrasound*, 5th edition. Philadelphia, Elsevier, 2018, p 44.

64. D. Papile's.

The most popular grading system for intraventricular hemorrhage (IVH) is Papile's classification. The Papile system is divided into four grades of IVH. A grade 1 IVH *occurs when there is subependymal (germinal matrix) hemorrhage only.* A grade 2 IVH *includes extension of the hemorrhage into the normal-sized ventricles.* A grade 3 IVH *includes hemorrhage into the ventricles with ventricular dilatation or hydrocephalus.* A grade 4 IVH *occurs when there is intraparenchymal extension of the hemorrhage. The Levene grading system is also accepted but is more complicated than Papile's system.*

▸ de Bruyn R (ed): *Pediatric Ultrasound: How, Why and When*, 2nd edition (e-book). Philadelphia, Churchill Livingstone/Elsevier, 2010, pp 263–266.

▸ Siegel MJ (ed): *Pediatric Sonography*, 4th edition. Philadelphia, Lippincott Williams & Wilkins, 2011, p 61.

65. **A. Congenital neoplasms.**

Congenital brain malformations can be classified based on the stage of brain development during which the alteration occurs. The stages of brain development are cytogenesis, histogenesis, and organogenesis. Cytogenesis *refers to the formation of cells from molecules. Congenital neoplasms are an example of alterations during this stage. Because cytogenesis disorders are microscopic, they cannot be identified on ultrasound.* Histogenesis *refers to the formation of tissues from cells. Examples of malformations occurring during this stage are tuberous sclerosis and congenital vascular malformations (vein of Galen malformation). Disorders of histogenesis can be recognized by ultrasound.* Organogenesis *refers to the formation of organs from tissues. Disorders of organogenesis can be subdivided into more stages. Disorders of neural tube closure, disorders of diverticulation and cleavage, and disorders of sulcation and cellular migration are some of them. Disorders of neural tube closure include Chiari malformation, agenesis of the corpus callosum, Dandy-Walker malformation, and posterior fossa arachnoid cyst. Septo-optic dysplasia and holoprosencephaly are disorders occurring during brain diverticulation and cleavage. Lissencephaly, schizencephaly, polymicrogyria, and pachymicrogyria are some examples of disorders occurring during sulcation and cellular migration.*

▶ Rumack CM, Levine D (eds): *Diagnostic Ultrasound*, 5th edition. Philadelphia, Elsevier, 2018, pp 1524–1525.

▶ Siegel MJ (ed): *Pediatric Sonography*, 4th edition. Philadelphia, Lippincott Williams & Wilkins, 2011, p 81.

66. **A. Deep in the brain.**

The white matter is located deep in the brain. The white matter allows fast communication between both sides of the brain. The corpus callosum is one of the largest white-matter structures in the brain. The gray matter is more superficial and is composed of neurons. The basal ganglia and brainstem are examples of gray matter deep in the brain.

▶ Fields DR: Change in the brain's white matter: the role of the brain's white matter in active learning and memory may be underestimated. Science 330:768–769, 2010. Available at https://www.ncbi.nlm.nih.gov/pmc/articles/PMC3201847/.

67. B. Tentorium cerebelli.

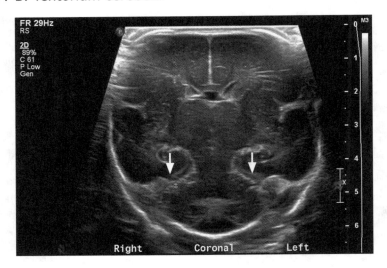

The tentorium cerebelli (arrows) is the structure that separates the cerebrum from the cerebellum. The tentorium is an extension or infolding of the dura mater. On ultrasound, the tentorium appears as an echogenic lining that borders the cerebellum superiorly. The tentorium is an important landmark, because neoplasms and some pathologies can be classified as supratentorial or infratentorial depending on their location.

▶ Murphy A, Maingard J, et al: Tentorium cerebelli. Available from Radiopaedia at https://radiopaedia.org/articles/tentorium-cerebelli.

68. D. Sylvian fissure.

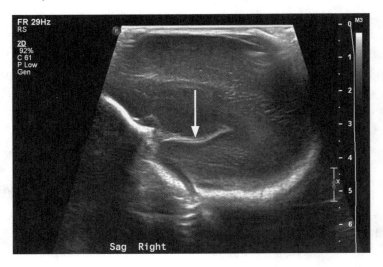

The Sylvian fissure (arrow) is located laterally, separating the frontal and temporal lobes of the brain. In the sagittal plane the Sylvian fissure appears as an echogenic line angling toward the most lateral aspect of each side of the brain.

The cingulate sulcus *and* cingulate gyrus *are both located midline in the brain superior and parallel to the course of the corpus callosum. The* interhemispheric fissure *is midline and separates both brain hemispheres.*

▸ Rumack CM, Levine D (eds): *Diagnostic Ultrasound*, 5th edition. Philadelphia, Elsevier, 2018, pp 1514–1515, 1521.

▸ Siegel MJ (ed): *Pediatric Sonography*, 4th edition. Philadelphia, Lippincott Williams & Wilkins, 2011, pp 46–47.

69. **D. Septo-optic dysplasia.**

    Absence of the septum pellucidum can be an isolated finding or it can be associated with other brain anomalies. Septo-optic dysplasia *is an anomaly associated with absence of the septum pellucidum. Other brain anomalies associated with absence of the septum pellucidum include holoprosencephaly, Chiari II malformation, schizencephaly, and hydranencephaly. On ultrasound, the frontal horns of the lateral ventricles communicate and have a square-shape appearance. Absence of the septum pellucidum does not always indicate absence of the corpus callosum.*

    ▸ Rumack CM, Levine D (eds): *Diagnostic Ultrasound*, 5th edition. Philadelphia, Elsevier, 2018, pp 1532–1534.

    ▸ Siegel MJ (ed): *Pediatric Sonography*, 4th edition. Philadelphia, Lippincott Williams & Wilkins, 2011, pp 96–97.

70. **C. Ependyma.**

    The ependyma *is the lining that borders the ventricles and the spinal cord. The ependyma helps in the production of cerebrospinal fluid (CSF), although CSF is produced mainly by the choroid plexus. When a germinal matrix hemorrhage occurs in the caudothalamic groove area, the rupture of the ependyma allows the bleed to extend into the ventricles (grade 2 intraventricular hemorrhage). Inflammation of the ependyma is also referred to as* ventriculitis. *The* germinal matrix *is a vascular area of the brain that is located in the caudothalamic groove region. The* pia mater *is the most internal meningeal layer and recovers the brain. The* tentorium cerebelli *is an infolding of dura mater and separates the cerebrum and the cerebellum.*

    ▸ Rumack CM, Levine D (eds): *Diagnostic Ultrasound*, 5th edition. Philadelphia, Elsevier, 2018, p 1538.

71. **B. Aqueduct of Sylvius.**

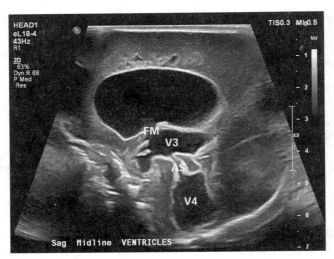

See Color Plate 10, "Ventricles of the Brain," on page xxxvii.

In the normal ventricular circulation, the cerebrospinal fluid (CSF) is produced by the choroid plexus, accumulates within the lateral ventricles, and then courses through the foramen of Monro (FM) into the third ventricle (V3). From the third ventricle, the CSF passes through the aqueduct of Sylvius (AS) into the fourth ventricle. From the fourth ventricle (V4), the CSF goes laterally through the foramen of Lushka and medially through the foramen of Magendie (not visualized). After passing through the foramen of Lushka on either side, the CSF goes around the brain into the subarachnoid space, where fluid is reabsorbed. The CSF that passes through the foramen of Magendie travels downward into the subarachnoid cisterns and into the spinal space.

▶ de Bruyn R (ed): *Pediatric Ultrasound: How, Why and When*, 2nd edition (e-book). Philadelphia, Churchill Livingstone/Elsevier, 2010, p 256.

▶ Rumack CM, Levine D (eds): *Diagnostic Ultrasound*, 5th edition. Philadelphia, Elsevier, 2018, p 1538.

72. **A. Massa intermedia.**

The massa intermedia *is a gray-matter structure that connects both sides of the thalamus. The massa intermedia lies across the third ventricle and is easily seen when there is dilatation of the third ventricle. Enlargement of the massa intermedia can be seen with Chiari II malformation. The* third ventricle *separates the two thalami, and the* tentorium cerebelli *separates the brain from the cerebellum. The* quadrigeminal cistern *is located inferior to the thalamus and is an extension of the third ventricle.*

▶ de Bruyn R (ed): *Pediatric Ultrasound: How, Why and When*, 2nd edition (e-book). Philadelphia, Churchill Livingstone/Elsevier, 2010, pp 259, 260.

▶ Rumack CM, Levine D (eds): *Diagnostic Ultrasound*, 5th edition. Philadelphia, Elsevier, 2018, p 1526.

▶ Siegel MJ (ed): *Pediatric Sonography*, 4th edition. Philadelphia, Lippincott Williams & Wilkins, 2011, pp 47–48.

73. **B. Internal carotid artery (ICA).**

The middle cerebral artery *(MCA) is a branch from the internal carotid artery (ICA) that is located laterally within the Sylvian fissure. The MCA suppies blood to part of the frontal, temporal, and parietal lobes of the brain. The* external carotid artery *(ECA) bifurcates into the superficial, temporal, and maxillary arteries, supplying blood to the face and neck. The* anterior cerebral artery *(ACA), as well as the MCA, is a branch of the ICA. The* posterior cerebral artery *(PCA) forms from the bifurcation of the basilar artery (BA) and posterior communicating artery (PCoA).*

▶ Rumack CM, Levine D (eds): *Diagnostic Ultrasound*, 5th edition. Philadelphia, Elsevier, 2018, p 1514.

74. **B. 2.**

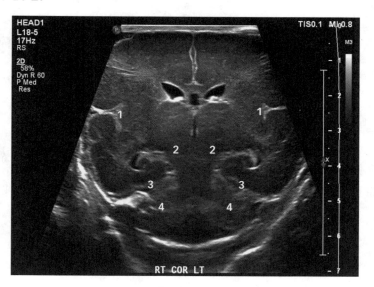

In a coronal plane, the cerebral peduncles *(2) are seen as heart-shaped hypoechoic structures that connect the cerebral hemispheres with the brainstem. The number 1 represents the echogenic* Sylvian fissures *bilaterally. The* tentorium cerebelli *(3) is seen separating the* cerebellum *(4) from the cerebrum.*

▶ Rumack CM, Levine D (eds): *Diagnostic Ultrasound*, 5th edition. Philadelphia, Elsevier, 2018, pp 1514–1515.

▶ Siegel MJ (ed): *Pediatric Sonography*, 4th edition. Philadelphia, Lippincott Williams & Wilkins, 2011, p 46.

75. A. Middle cerebral artery (MCA).

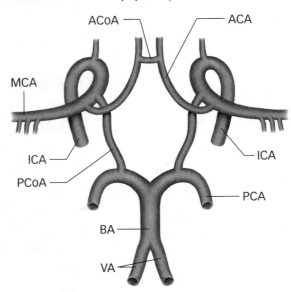

The middle cerebral artery (MCA)—although it supplies blood to the brain—is not a part of the circle of Willis. The circle of Willis is composed by the right and left anterior cerebral arteries (ACAs), the anterior communicating artery (ACoA), the right and left internal carotid arteries (ICAs), the right and left posterior cerebral arteries (PCAs), and the right and left posterior communicating arteries (PoCAs). The circle of Willis supplies blood to the brain hemispheres and receives its blood from the ICAs and vertebral arteries. (BA = basilar artery, VA = vertebral arteries.)

▶ Rumack CM, Levine D (eds): *Diagnostic Ultrasound*, 5th edition. Philadelphia, Elsevier, 2018, pp 1592–1593.

PART 2

Spine

76. **C. Neurulation.**

   Neurulation *is the formation of the neural tube in vertebrates. Failure of neurulation or incomplete neurulation results in spinal dysraphisms—a spectrum of disorders including open and closed neural tube defects. The brain and spinal cord originate from the neural tube. Within the first month of the gestation period, the ectoderm thickens to form a neural plate and neural folds. The neural folds bend dorsally to meet in the midline. When the folds fuse together, the neural tube closes. The ectoderm separates from the neural tissue, fusing to the midline and covering the neural structures. The majority of the neural tube is formed during primary neurulation. Canalization and retrogressive differentiation take place during secondary neurulation of the caudal cell mass in the distal spine.* Gastrulation *is the transition from a blastula into a multilayered (endoderm, mesoderm, and ectoderm) organism.* Invagination *and* ingression *occur during the gastrulation process.*

   ▶ Kenyon College Biology Department: Gastrulation and neurulation. Available at http://biology.kenyon.edu/courses/biol114/Chap14/Chapter_14.html.

   ▶ Rothman TP: Ectoderm: neurulation, neural tube, neural crest. Available at http://www.columbia.edu/itc/hs/medical/humandev/2004/Chapt4-Ectoderm.pdf.

   ▶ Rumack CM, Levine D (eds): *Diagnostic Ultrasound*, 5th edition. Philadelphia, Elsevier, 2018, pp 1672–1673.

   ▶ Siegel MJ (ed): *Pediatric Sonography*, 4th edition. Philadelphia, Lippincott Williams & Wilkins, 2011, pp 647–649.

77. **A. Sacral dimple.**

   Dorsal cutaneous stigma *refers to skin lesions located on the back. Other stigmata include skin tags, hair tufts, discolorations, asymmetric gluteal folds, and hemangiomas. These skin signs are common indications for the infant to have a spine ultrasound exam before the infant is released from the hospital. The simple* sacral dimple *(also called a* sacral pit*) is the most common and least likely to be associated with spinal dysraphism. Often "sacral" dimple is listed as the indication for the exam, but the dimple is actually located in the coccyx region. The term* coccygeal dimple *is not typically used. An open sacral dimple, known as a* pinpoint ostium, *is associated with a* dorsal dermal sinus *(DDS). A DDS is* a fistula connecting the skin to the neural components of the spine, and it is commonly located in the lumbosacral region. Sonographically, a DDS will appear as an anechoic or hypoechoic tract leading from the skin through the soft tissues into the spinal canal. A tethered cord may or may not be present.

▶ Ben-Sira L, Ponger P, Miller E, et al: Low-risk lumbar skin stigmata in infants: the role of ultrasound screening. J Pediatrics 155:864–869, 2009. Available at https://pedclerk.uchicago.edu/sites/pedclerk.uchicago.edu/files/uploads/low%20risk.pdf.

▶ de Bruyn R (ed): *Pediatric Ultrasound: How, Why and When*, 2nd edition (e-book). Philadelphia, Churchill Livingstone/Elsevier, 2010, pp 294–295.

▶ Siegel MJ (ed): *Pediatric Sonography*, 4th edition. Philadelphia, Lippincott Williams & Wilkins, 2011, pp 656, 661–662.

78. **B. Changing the patient's position.**

    Nerve roots that clump together to cause the appearance of a mass in the decubitus position are collectively termed a "pseudomass." When the patient is returned to the prone position, the nerves will resume their normal position and the mass will disappear. Adjusting the transducer or machine parameters will not aid in ruling out a pseudomass.

    ▶ Siegel MJ (ed): *Pediatric Sonography*, 4th edition. Philadelphia, Lippincott Williams & Wilkins, 2011, pp 654–655.

79. **D. Pilonidal abscess.**

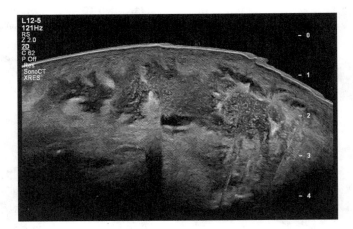

    A pilonidal sinus is a channel or tract leading from the subcutaneous tissue to the coccyx region. The opening of the sinus appears as a small pit in the skin. These sinuses do not communicate with the neural space. When the sinus becomes dilated, a pilonidal cyst may form and even contain hair or debris. If the cyst becomes infected, an abscess can form. An abscess would most likely be expected given the findings

in this image, which demonstrates a hypoechoic collection of echogenic fluid with poorly defined, hyperechoic borders. Peripheral hyperemia around the abscess is usually noted with color Doppler. A pilonidal cyst would appear smaller, rounder, and with a well-defined border. A simple meningocele *occurs when cerebrospinal fluid–filled meninges herniate through a posterior bony defect, producing a cystic mass underneath the subcutaneous tissues. Simple meningoceles typically occur in the lumbosacral region. Sacrococcygeal teratomas share the location and vascularity characteristics of a pilonidal abscess, but vascularity would additionally be seen within the mass. Teratomas are usually diagnosed prenatally.*

▶ Siegel MJ (ed): *Pediatric Sonography*, 4th edition. Philadelphia, Lippincott Williams & Wilkins, 2011, pp 658–659, 662.

80. **A. At or below L3.**

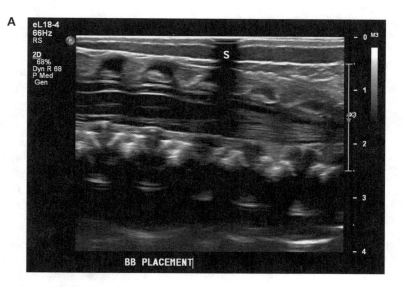

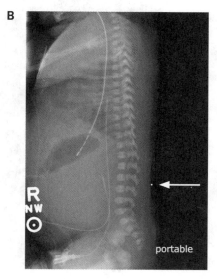

The conus medullaris is the tapered caudal end of the spinal cord that blends into the filum terminale without interruption. The normal termination of the conus medullaris should be at the level of the L2-L3 disk space or higher, although usually it terminates within the L1-L2 disk space. If the conus reaches the superior end plate of L3 or extends past L3, it is considered abnormal or tethered. However, a conus medullaris located at the level of L3 is normal 1% of the time. An extended-field-of-view or panoramic ultrasound image can provide a more global view of the lower spine. **A** *If the conus extends beyond the L2-L3 disk space, a BB, which will create a shadow (S), should be placed by the sonographer at the level of the conus termination.* **B** *A radiograph will be taken with a radiopaque BB in place (arrow), so that the radiologist can verify the true level of termination. Occasionally an infant may be missing a sacral bone or rib, which can cause the sonographer's count to be off. This can be verified on the radiograph as well.*

▶ DiPietro MA: The conus medullaris: normal US findings throughout childhood. Radiology 188:149–153, 1993.

▶ Rumack CM, Levine D (eds): *Diagnostic Ultrasound*, 5th edition. Philadelphia, Elsevier, 2018, pp 1216–1217, 1678.

▶ Siegel MJ (ed): *Pediatric Sonography*, 4th edition. Philadelphia, Lippincott Williams & Wilkins, 2011, pp 652–653, 662.

▶ Unsinn KM, Geley T, Freund MC, et al: US of the spinal cord in newborns: spectrum of normal findings, variants, congenital anomalies, and acquired diseases. RadioGraphics 20:923–938, 2000. Available at https://pubs.rsna.org/doi/full/10.1148/radiographics.20.4.g00jl06923.

81. **B. Syrinx.**

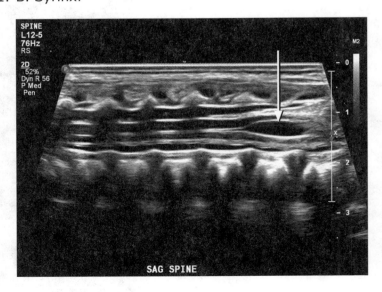

A syrinx, also known as syringomyelia, is an enclosed fluid-filled cystic sac located within the spinal cord. This image demonstrates a syrinx (arrow) arising from the central complex of the spinal cord. A syrinx can grow over time and compress the cord from the inside outward. If a syrinx is found in conjunction with hydromyelia (the central portion of the cord dilated by cerebrospinal fluid or CSF), it is termed syringohydromyelia. Syringomyelia and hydromyelia are difficult to differentiate with ultrasound. A filar cyst would be present caudal to the conus, where the filum would originate. More recent higher-resolution probes show that the presence of a filar cyst is very common. The thecal sac is filled with CSF and serves as the protective covering of the spinal cord and nerve roots. A myelocystocele is a type of occult spinal dysraphism where a dilated (hydromyelic) spinal cord herniates through a dorsal bony spinal defect.

▶ Rumack CM, Levine D (eds): *Diagnostic Ultrasound*, 5th edition. Philadelphia, Elsevier, 2018, pp 1674–1675, 1678, 1681, 1683–1684.

▶ Siegel MJ (ed): *Pediatric Sonography*, 4th edition. Philadelphia, Lippincott Williams & Wilkins, 2011, pp 654, 659–660.

▶ Unsinn KM, Geley T, Freund MC, et al: US of the spinal cord in newborns: spectrum of normal findings, variants, congenital anomalies, and acquired diseases. RadioGraphics 20:923–938, 2000. Available at https://pubs.rsna.org/doi/full/10.1148/radiographics.20.4.g00jl06923.

82. **C. Lipoma.**

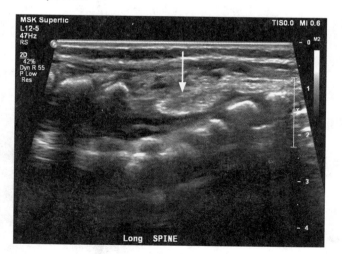

Spinal lipomas (arrow) are echogenic fatty masses that communicate with the spinal cord. There are four categories of sacral lipoma: lipomyelocele, lipomyelomeningocele, intradural lipomas, and fibrolipomas of the filum terminale. Lipomyeloceles and lipomyelomeningoceles make up 50% of occult spinal dysraphisms. On ultrasound, an echogenic spinal

spinal mass will extend through a posterior spinal defect into the canal and communicate with a tethered cord. Lipomas run along the subcutaneous tissues. A lipoma has a flat plane with the skin of the back. With a lipomyelomeningocele, the cord and neural placode are raised above the skin surface by an enlarged subarachnoid space. An intradural lipoma is located within the spine but beneath the pia mater. There is a clear differentiation between an intradural lipoma and the subcutaneous tissues on ultrasound. A fibrolipoma of the filum terminale, also called a filar lipoma, will appear as a thickened echogenic filum with no distinct mass. Small fibrolipomas are asymptomatic, but larger ones are associated with tethered cord.

The coccyx usually appears in early infancy as a hypoechoic cartilaginous structure without ossification. The cauda equina is an echogenic nerve root bundle seen lying in the dependent portion of the thecal sac. The notochord is an embryologic cartilaginous rod that acts as support until the vertebral column is formed.

▶ de Bruyn R (ed): *Pediatric Ultrasound: How, Why and When*, 2nd edition (e-book). Philadelphia, Churchill Livingstone/Elsevier, 2010, pp 295–296.

▶ Rumack CM, Levine D (eds): *Diagnostic Ultrasound*, 5th edition. Philadelphia, Elsevier, 2018, pp 1216–1217, 1686–1689.

▶ Siegel MJ (ed): *Pediatric Sonography*, 4th edition. Philadelphia, Lippincott Williams & Wilkins, 2011, pp 652–653, 658, 663–664.

▶ Unsinn KM, Geley T, Freund MC, et al: US of the spinal cord in newborns: spectrum of normal findings, variants, congenital anomalies, and acquired diseases. RadioGraphics 20:923–938, 2000. Available at https://pubs.rsna.org/doi/full/10.1148/radiographics.20.4.g00jl06923.

83. **A. Filum terminale.**

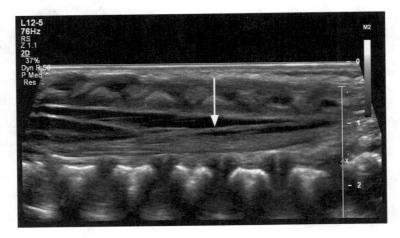

The filum terminale *(arrow)* is the terminal portion of the spinal cord extending from the conus medullaris. The most caudal aspect of the filum, the filum terminale externum, attaches to the back of the coccyx. On ultrasound, a normal filum will appear as an echogenic, string-like projection extending from the conus and mobile with pulsations, breathing, or crying. Normal measurements of the filum terminale should not exceed 2 mm in diameter.

The cauda equina *(Latin for "horse's tail")* is the thicker, echogenic bundle of nerve roots seen on either side of the spinal cord and filum. The cauda equina will also display movement in a normal spinal cord. Meninges consist of the external dura mater, the middle arachnoid mater, and the innermost pia mater, which together enclose the brain and spine. On ultrasound, the dura mater is seen as an echogenic lining of the spinal canal. The term leptomeninges refers to the inner two meningeal layers (arachnoid and pia mater).

▶ Cramer GD, Ro C-S: The sacrum, sacroiliac joint, and coccyx. In Cramer GD, Darby SA (eds): *Clinical Anatomy of the Spine, Spinal Cord, and ANS*, 3rd edition. Philadelphia, Mosby, 2014. Available at www.sciencedirect.com/topics/neuroscience/coccygeal-nerve.

▶ de Bruyn R (ed): *Pediatric Ultrasound: How, Why and When*, 2nd edition (e-book). Philadelphia, Churchill Livingstone/Elsevier, 2010, p 296.

▶ Hacking V, Trajcevska E, et al: Filum terminale. Available from Radiopaedia at https://radiopaedia.org/articles/filum-terminale.

▶ Rumack CM, Levine D (eds): *Diagnostic Ultrasound*, 5th edition. Philadelphia, Elsevier, 2018, pp 1673–1675.

▶ Unsinn KM, Geley T, Freund MC, et al: US of the spinal cord in newborns: spectrum of normal findings, variants, congenital anomalies, and acquired diseases. RadioGraphics 20:923–938, 2000. Available at https://pubs.rsna.org/doi/full/10.1148/radiographics.20.4.g00jl06923.

84. **D. 12 MHz linear array.**

The optimal transducer for neonatal spine ultrasound would be a 12 MHz linear transducer. You should always use the highest-frequency transducer that allows adequate penetration and visualization of the body part you are examining. In neonatal spine cases, even an 18 MHz transducer has proved sufficient. Although magnetic resonance imaging (MRI) is felt to be the preferred examination in older infants, spine ultrasounds are cost-effective and allow screening for an early diagnosis and characterization of defects. Sonography is ideal for infants until the age of 4–6 months because the spine is a superficial structure and the cartilaginous spinal arches provide an acoustic window. Infants are typically placed prone with a rolled towel under the lower abdomen to create a slight kyphosis, separating the spinous processes. Longitudinal and transverse images are obtained, along with a panoramic or extended-field-of-view image, which allows a more global interpretation.

▶ de Bruyn R (ed): *Pediatric Ultrasound: How, Why and When*, 2nd edition (e-book). Philadelphia, Churchill Livingstone/Elsevier, 2010, p 291.
▶ Rumack CM, Levine D (eds): *Diagnostic Ultrasound*, 5th edition. Philadelphia, Elsevier, 2018, p 1674.
▶ Siegel MJ (ed): *Pediatric Sonography*, 4th edition. Philadelphia, Lippincott Williams & Wilkins, 2011, pp 647, 650.

85. **B. Alpha-fetoprotein (AFP).**

   An elevated level of alpha-fetoprotein *(AFP) is associated with an increased risk of neural tube defect. AFP is a protein produced by the fetal liver. It passes through the placenta into the mother's blood, which is tested during the second trimester screening. AFP is also a tumor marker for liver cancers and some germ cell cancers. A dietary deficiency of folic acid has also been linked with spinal dysraphisms.* Human chorionic gonadotropin *(hCG) is a hormone produced within the placenta.* Inhibin-A *is a protein produced by the placenta and the ovaries. Low levels of AFP combined with abnormal levels of hCG and inhibin-A could indicate a chromosomal abnormality.*

   ▶ Keough J: *Nursing Laboratory and Diagnostic Tests Demystified*, 2nd edition. New York, McGraw-Hill, 2017, pp 258–262, 264–267.

86. **C. Sacrococcygeal teratoma.**

   Sacrococcygeal teratomas *are not associated with bony vertebral defects and usually do not involve the spinal canal. Sacrococcygeal teratomas comprise 40% of fetal and neonatal germ cell tumors, and 10% of sacrococcygeal teratomas are malignant. Sacrococcygeal teratomas occur more often in girls. There are four types, and they are classified by the location of the teratoma. Type 1 comprises 50%; these are external with a small presacral component. Type 2 is external with a large intrapelvic component. Type 3 is predominantly internal with a small external component. Type 4 is entirely* *presacral without any external component. On ultrasound, sacrococcygeal teratomas appear heterogeneous, having soft tissue and cystic components. The benign teratomas tend to appear more cystic. Other spinal tumors can be intramedullary or extramedullary. Cord enlargement, displacement, or decreased pulsatility may occur with spinal tumors. Meningocele, lipomeningocele,* and *myelocystocele are all associated with bony vertebral defects.*

▶ Rumack CM, Levine D (eds): *Diagnostic Ultrasound*, 5th edition. Philadelphia, Elsevier, 2018, pp 1238–1239, 1691.

▶ Siegel MJ (ed): *Pediatric Sonography*, 4th edition. Philadelphia, Lippincott Williams & Wilkins, 2011, pp 657–660, 664–668.

87. **C. Myelomeningocele.**

Myelomeningoceles are involved in 99% of spina bifida aperta cases and are the most common congenital malformation of the spine. The other 1% are myeloceles. When the neural plate does not fold during neurulation, it is left exposed and will eventually appear as a reddish tissue mass on the back. The majority of myelomeningoceles are lumbosacral. Depending on the level of defect, patients with spina bifida aperta experience neurological deficits and bowel or bladder dysfunction. Myelomeningoceles contain nerve roots and are lifted up above the skin surface by a dilated subarachnoid space. Sonography is usually not performed due to the risk of infection or injury. If necessary, sterile precautions should be taken. Myelomeningoceles are associated with tethered cord, hydromyelia or syringomyelia, diastematomyelia, Chiari II malformation, hydrocephalus, agenesis of the corpus callosum, and Dandy-Walker malformation. Lipomyeloceles, myelocystoceles, and *sacrococcygeal teratomas are all skin-covered defects.*

▶ de Bruyn R (ed): *Pediatric Ultrasound: How, Why and When*, 2nd edition (e-book). Philadelphia, Churchill Livingstone/Elsevier, 2010, p 296.

▶ Rumack CM, Levine D (eds): *Diagnostic Ultrasound*, 5th edition. Philadelphia, Elsevier, 2018, pp 1681–1683.

▶ Siegel MJ (ed): *Pediatric Sonography*, 4th edition. Philadelphia, Lippincott Williams & Wilkins, 2011, pp 657–660.

▶ Unsinn KM, Geley T, Freund MC, et al: US of the spinal cord in newborns: spectrum of normal findings, variants, congenital anomalies, and acquired diseases. RadioGraphics 20:923–938, 2000. Available at https://pubs.rsna.org/doi/full/10.1148/radiographics.20.4.g00jl06923.

88. **B. T12.**

   The last rib is normally located at the 12th thoracic vertebra, T12. Spine ultrasounds are performed to locate the vertebral level where the conus medullaris terminates and to evaluate for spinal dysraphisms. To determine the level of the conus, you can count down from the 12th rib, located at T12, up from the L5-S1 junction or up from the most distal sacral vertebra. In rare situations, there may be an absent sacral bone or rib. Placement of a radiopaque BB at the conus and obtaining an x-ray will assist in the determination of the level of the conus.

   ▶ Rumack CM, Levine D (eds): *Diagnostic Ultrasound*, 5th edition. Philadelphia, Elsevier, 2018, p 1677.

   ▶ Siegel MJ (ed): *Pediatric Sonography*, 4th edition. Philadelphia, Lippincott Williams & Wilkins, 2011, p 653.

89. **B. Occult spina bifida.**

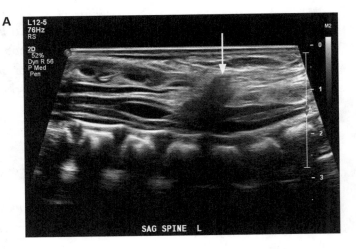

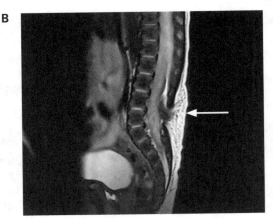

   *This **A** ultrasound image and **B** corresponding magnetic resonance image (MRI) demonstrate an occult spina bifida or closed neural tube defect (NTD). Each imaging modality shows a communicating defect between the spinal canal and subcutaneous tissues. Also present is a syrinx within the*

central spinal cord. Spina bifida aperta *is defined as an* open *NTD, where you would see a defect communicating to an open surface of the skin.* Diastematomyelia *is defined as two hemicords, each with its own central complex, resulting from a cleft in the middle of the spinal cord. Two cords are not seen in this image. Because the sacral bones are visible in this image,* caudal regression syndrome *would not be a correct choice, since this syndrome includes sacral agenesis.*

▸ de Bruyn R (ed): *Pediatric Ultrasound: How, Why and When*, 2nd edition (e-book). Philadelphia, Churchill Livingstone/Elsevier, 2010, pp 291, 294–297.

▸ Rumack CM, Levine D (eds): *Diagnostic Ultrasound*, 5th edition. Philadelphia, Elsevier, 2018, pp 1682–1686.

▸ Siegel MJ (ed): *Pediatric Sonography*, 4th edition. Philadelphia, Lippincott Williams & Wilkins, 2011, pp 657–660, 664.

▸ Unsinn KM, Geley T, Freund MC, et al: US of the spinal cord in newborns: spectrum of normal findings, variants, congenital anomalies, and acquired diseases. RadioGraphics 20:923–938, 2000. Available at https://pubs.rsna.org/doi/full/10.1148/radiographics.20.4.g00jl06923.

90. **D. Skin covering.**

The main difference between spina bifida aperta and occult spina bifida is the presence of skin covering. Spina bifida aperta *includes the open spinal defects myelocele (1%) and myelomeningocele (99%). The majority are found in the lumbosacral region. Patients with spina bifida aperta show neurological deficits such as paresis or paralysis, depending on the level of the defect, and may also demonstrate bowel or bladder dysfunction. Chiari II malformation accompanies almost all of spina bifida aperta cases. Open neural tube defects are associated with other congenital anomalies, hydrocephalus, agenesis of the corpus callosum, and Dandy-Walker malformation.* Occult spina bifida *includes any skin-covered posterior bony defect where various combinations of neural structures may protrude through. The presence of meninges, a bony defect, and a tethered cord can be found in both spina bifida aperta and occult spina bifida. Ultrasound would not usually be performed in cases of spina bifida aperta due to risk of injury or infection of the open defect. If ultrasound is requested, special care should be taken to perform the exam with a sterile transducer cover and sterile gel.*

▸ de Bruyn R (ed): *Pediatric Ultrasound: How, Why and When*, 2nd edition (e-book). Philadelphia, Churchill Livingstone/Elsevier, 2010, p 294.

▸ Rumack CM, Levine D (eds): *Diagnostic Ultrasound*, 5th edition. Philadelphia, Elsevier, 2018, pp 1681–1682.

▶ Siegel MJ (ed): *Pediatric Sonography*, 4th edition. Philadelphia, Lippincott Williams & Wilkins, 2011, pp 658–661.

▶ Unsinn KM, Geley T, Freund MC, et al: US of the spinal cord in newborns: spectrum of normal findings, variants, congenital anomalies, and acquired diseases. RadioGraphics 20:923–938, 2000. Available at https://pubs.rsna.org/doi/full/10.1148/radiographics.20.4.g00jl06923.

91. **D. Caudal regression syndrome.**

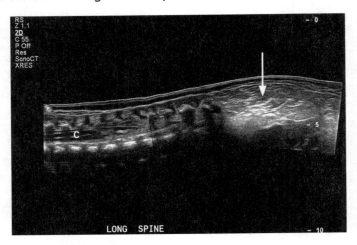

Caudal regression syndrome *is a spectrum of congenital anomalies of varying degrees. The lower spine, extremities, anus, rectum, and genitourinary tract are commonly affected. Caudal regression is associated with infants of diabetic mothers. Clinical signs may include sacral agenesis (arrow), imperforate anus, malformed genitalia, sirenomelia, renal aplasia, and pulmonary hypoplasia. On ultrasound, the spinal cord (C) is often hypoplastic and tethered, and it may have a thickened filum or echogenic lipoma. If the cord is not tethered, it usually terminates above L1 and instead of tapering into a conical shape will appear blunted and squared off.* Spina bifida aperta *would not show a skin covering, as seen in this image.* Tight filum syndrome *refers to neurological deficits, orthopedic deformities, and pain when the spine is stretched during growth spurts or exercise.* Diastematomyelia *refers to a midline cleft within the spinal cord, resulting in two symmetric hemicords.*

▶ de Bruyn R (ed): *Pediatric Ultrasound: How, Why and When*, 2nd edition (e-book). Philadelphia, Churchill Livingstone/Elsevier, 2010, p 297.

▶ Rumack CM, Levine D (eds): *Diagnostic Ultrasound*, 5th edition. Philadelphia, Elsevier, 2018, pp 1218, 1237–1238.

▶ Siegel MJ (ed): *Pediatric Sonography*, 4th edition. Philadelphia, Lippincott Williams & Wilkins, 2011, pp 657–658, 660–661, 662–664.

▶ Unsinn KM, Geley T, Freund MC, et al: US of the spinal cord in newborns: spectrum of normal findings, variants, congenital anomalies, and acquired diseases. RadioGraphics 20:923–938, 2000. Available at https://pubs.rsna.org/doi/full/10.1148/radiographics.20.4.g00jl06923.

92. A. Lumbar puncture.

A lumbar puncture or spinal tap is a minimally invasive procedure performed to diagnose disorders of the brain and spinal cord. Lumbar punctures are routinely done for febrile neonates or when there is a suspicion of a central nervous system (CNS) infection or neoplasm. Under sterile conditions, a spinal tap withdraws cerebrospinal fluid (CSF) from the spinal canal to be sent for testing. Lumbar punctures are usually performed without ultrasound guidance, but ultrasound can be helpful in guiding the needle through the spinous processes and into the thecal sac. Complications include laceration of the dura mater or other meninges, causing a CSF leak or hematoma. An epidural is a way of administering medication into the epidural space within the spinal cord. A laminotomy is an invasive surgical procedure that removes the lamina of the vertebrae in an effort to relieve pressure within the spinal canal. A quad screen is a blood test done in the second trimester to screen for neural tube defects and chromosomal abnormalities in the fetus.

▶ Rumack CM, Levine D (eds): *Diagnostic Ultrasound*, 5th edition. Philadelphia, Elsevier, 2018, p 1695.

▶ Siegel MJ (ed): *Pediatric Sonography*, 4th edition. Philadelphia, Lippincott Williams & Wilkins, 2011, pp 669, 697.

93. C. L2-L3.

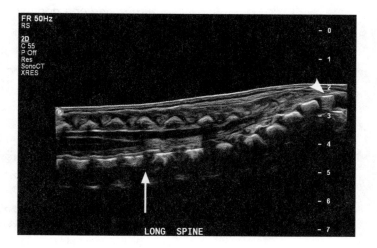

In this image, the conus terminates at the L2-L3 disk space (arrow). The last vertebra seen in the image is S5 (arrowhead), so counting upward, the conus is seen ending prior to L3. The level of the conus is important, to rule out tethering of the spinal cord. As the spine grows and elongates, mechanical stretching of the cord occurs. Tethering, which occurs when the conus extends past the L3 vertebra, can

impair the blood flow to the cord, causing ischemia and neural dysfunction. Surgery is necessary to clip the filum and release the tethering. The earlier the diagnosis and repair are made, the better the outcome is. A tethered cord can occur as an isolated finding, but most often tethered cords are found in conjunction with spinal dysraphisms.

▶ Rumack CM, Levine D (eds): *Diagnostic Ultrasound*, 5th edition. Philadelphia, Elsevier, 2018, p 1678.

▶ Siegel MJ (ed): *Pediatric Sonography*, 4th edition. Philadelphia, Lippincott Williams & Wilkins, 2011, p 657.

▶ Unsinn KM, Geley T, Freund MC, et al: US of the spinal cord in newborns: spectrum of normal findings, variants, congenital anomalies, and acquired diseases. RadioGraphics 20:923–938, 2000. Available at https://pubs.rsna.org/doi/full/10.1148/radiographics.20.4.g00jl06923.

94. **B. Diastematomyelia.**

The congenital fissure of the spinal cord is a split cord malformation known as diastematomyelia. *This midline cleft results in two symmetric hemicords, each having a central canal and each surrounded by pia. Diastematomyelia most commonly occurs in the thoracic or lumbar region and affects girls more often than boys. Half of patients will demonstrate cutaneous stigmata and symptoms related to a tethered cord. A large majority of patients have another vertebral abnormality along with diastematomyelia. On ultrasound, two cords with an echogenic central complex can be visualized on either side of a bony spur or cartilage that separates them. Typically, the two cords will reunite distal to the dividing spur or cartilage. The* notochord *is the embryologic skeletal support before the vertebrae are formed.* Dysraphism *refers to any disorder resulting from abnormal neurulation.* Bicordism *is not a medical term.*

▶ de Bruyn R (ed): *Pediatric Ultrasound: How, Why and When*, 2nd edition (e-book). Philadelphia, Churchill Livingstone/Elsevier, 2010, p 295.

▶ Rumack CM, Levine D (eds): *Diagnostic Ultrasound*, 5th edition. Philadelphia, Elsevier, 2018, p 1688.

▶ Siegel MJ (ed): *Pediatric Sonography*, 4th edition. Philadelphia, Lippincott Williams & Wilkins, 2011, pp 655, 660–661.

▶ Unsinn KM, Geley T, Freund MC, et al: US of the spinal cord in newborns: spectrum of normal findings, variants, congenital anomalies, and acquired diseases. RadioGraphics 20:923–938, 2000. Available at https://pubs.rsna.org/doi/full/10.1148/radiographics.20.4.g00jl06923.

95. D. Spinal cord.

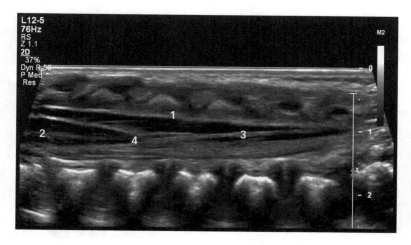

The cylindrical spinal cord (2) extends from the medulla oblongata to the conus medullaris (4). It is composed of gray and white matter (nervous tissue) and surrounded by cerebrospinal fluid (CSF). The cord is narrowest in the mid thoracic region. A normal spinal cord tapers to a conical point known as the conus medullaris (4) prior to the L3 vertebral body. The central canal is the echogenic linear structure seen within the center of the cord. The cord is surrounded by the anterior and posterior subarachnoid spaces and housed by vertebrae. There are 33 vertebrae in the spinal column: 7 cervical, 12 thoracic, 5 lumbar, 5 sacral, and 4 fused coccygeal bones. The dura mater (1) and the filum terminale (3) are not hypoechoic but are hyperechoic linear structures on ultrasound.

▶ de Bruyn R (ed): *Pediatric Ultrasound: How, Why and When*, 2nd edition (e-book). Philadelphia, Churchill Livingstone/Elsevier, 2010, pp 291–294.

▶ Rumack CM, Levine D (eds): *Diagnostic Ultrasound*, 5th edition. Philadelphia, Elsevier, 2018, pp 1674–1677.

▶ Siegel MJ (ed): *Pediatric Sonography*, 4th edition. Philadelphia, Lippincott Williams & Wilkins, 2011, p 651.

▶ Unsinn KM, Geley T, Freund MC, et al: US of the spinal cord in newborns: spectrum of normal findings, variants, congenital anomalies, and acquired diseases. RadioGraphics 20:923–938, 2000. Available at https://pubs.rsna.org/doi/full/10.1148/radiographics.20.4.g00jl06923.

96. A. Hydromyelia.

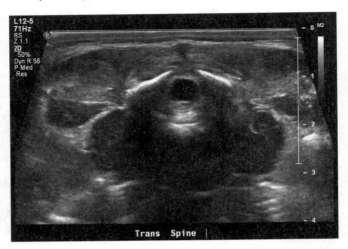

Hydromyelia *describes an area of increased fluid or dilatation of the central canal within the spinal cord that is not enclosed, but open to communicate with the fourth ventricle. In this transverse image, the central portion of the spinal cord has been replaced with fluid, leaving the cord difficult to visualize. Hydromyelia in newborns is associated with myelomeningocele and Chiari II malformation. Clinical symptoms of hydromyelia in older children and adults include weakness, spastic paraparesis, and sensory disturbances. A dilated or enlarged thecal sac would compress the cord. A* filar cyst *is a small, fusiform-shaped cystic structure located at the origin of the filum where it meets the conus. A* meningocele *is a congenital herniation of a cerebrospinal fluid–filled sac through a defect in the spine or skull.*

▶ Rumack CM, Levine D (eds): *Diagnostic Ultrasound*, 5th edition. Philadelphia, Elsevier, 2018, p 1688.
▶ Siegel MJ (ed): *Pediatric Sonography*, 4th edition. Philadelphia, Lippincott Williams & Wilkins, 2011, pp 654, 658–659, 668.
▶ Unsinn KM, Geley T, Freund MC, et al: US of the spinal cord in newborns: spectrum of normal findings, variants, congenital anomalies, and acquired diseases. RadioGraphics 20:923–938, 2000. Available at https://pubs.rsna.org/doi/full/10.1148/radiographics.20.4.g00jl06923.

97. B. Trauma.

Spinal cord compression *is often the result of trauma. Although it can happen during delivery, spinal cord trauma is rare in children under 15, because it is most often the result of motor vehicle or sports accidents. Spinal cord compression or displacement can occur if there is an epidural or subdural hematoma present. On ultrasound, the spinal cord may appear echogenic secondary to edema or an acute hemorrhage. Other causes of spinal cord compression include spondylosis, tumors, disk abnormalities, and abscess.* Sacrococcygeal teratomas *and* pilonidal sinus *do not communicate with the spinal canal.* Caudal regression syndrome *results in a high or tethered cord but is not associated with cord compression.*

▸ de Bruyn R (ed): *Pediatric Ultrasound: How, Why and When*, 2nd edition (e-book). Philadelphia, Churchill Livingstone/Elsevier, 2010, pp 297–298.

▸ Rumack CM, Levine D (eds): *Diagnostic Ultrasound*, 5th edition. Philadelphia, Elsevier, 2018, p 1695.

▸ Siegel MJ (ed): *Pediatric Sonography*, 4th edition. Philadelphia, Lippincott Williams & Wilkins, 2011, pp 664–668.

▸ Unsinn KM, Geley T, Freund MC, et al: US of the spinal cord in newborns: spectrum of normal findings, variants, congenital anomalies, and acquired diseases. RadioGraphics 20:923–938, 2000. Available at https://pubs.rsna.org/doi/full/10.1148/radiographics.20.4.g00jl06923.

98. **B. Ventriculus terminalis.**

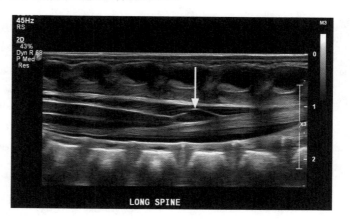

The terms ventriculus terminalis *and* filar cyst *(arrow) are used interchangeably to describe an oval cystic structure located at the caudal end of the conus medullaris and the proximal end of the filum terminale. A ventriculus terminalis is an ependyma-lined structure that is an asymptomatic normal variant, and it will typically decrease in size within the first month of life. A* syrinx *(syringomyelia) is a fluid-filled oval-shaped cavity located within the spinal cord, not caudal to it.* Hydromyelia *is the dilatation or widening of the spinal cord where spinal fluid accumulates.* Tight filum syndrome *results in a short, thick filum and a low conus but is not associated with a cystic structure or fluid accumulation.*

▸ de Bruyn R (ed): *Pediatric Ultrasound: How, Why and When*, 2nd edition (e-book). Philadelphia, Churchill Livingstone/Elsevier, 2010, pp 293–294.

▸ Siegel MJ (ed): *Pediatric Sonography*, 4th edition. Philadelphia, Lippincott Williams & Wilkins, 2011, pp 654, 662–663, 668.

▸ Unsinn KM, Geley T, Freund MC, et al: US of the spinal cord in newborns: spectrum of normal findings, variants, congenital anomalies, and acquired diseases. RadioGraphics 20:923–938, 2000. Available at https://pubs.rsna.org/doi/full/10.1148/radiographics.20.4.g00jl06923.

99. A. Nerve root.

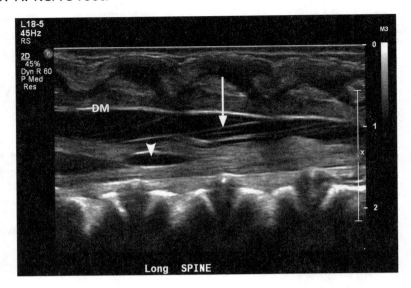

The structure indicated by the arrow is a nerve root. Nerve roots, *as seen in this image, appear as wispy echogenic linear structures within the posterior subarachnoid space. The* filum *is a thicker linear echogenic structure extending from the conus. A* filar cyst *or* ventriculus terminalis, *appearing as a hypoechoic ovoid structure (arrowhead), is also noted in this image but is not indicated by the arrow. The dura mater (DM) is the bold echogenic lining of the spinal canal.*

▶ de Bruyn R (ed): *Pediatric Ultrasound: How, Why and When*, 2nd edition (e-book). Philadelphia, Churchill Livingstone/Elsevier, 2010, pp 291–294.

▶ Rumack CM, Levine D (eds): *Diagnostic Ultrasound*, 5th edition. Philadelphia, Elsevier, 2018, p 1676.

▶ Siegel MJ (ed): *Pediatric Sonography*, 4th edition. Philadelphia, Lippincott Williams & Wilkins, 2011, p 651.

▶ Unsinn KM, Geley T, Freund MC, et al: US of the spinal cord in newborns: spectrum of normal findings, variants, congenital anomalies, and acquired diseases. RadioGraphics 20:923–938, 2000. Available at https://pubs.rsna.org/doi/full/10.1148/radiographics.20.4.g00jl06923.

100. C. Dorsal dermal sinus.

A dorsal dermal sinus is an epithelium-lined sinus or tract connecting the skin to the neural components (spinal cord, cauda equina, or arachnoid) of the spine. Most often, dorsal dermal sinuses are located within the lumbosacral area. They are commonly accompanied by dorsal subcutaneous stigmata such as a sacral dimple *or* pinpoint ostium, *but the presence of a dimple or ostium is seen in many infants and children with normal spines. Sonographically, a hypoechoic or anechoic tract from the skin through the soft tissues and into the spinal canal is seen. A tethered cord may be present. If there is an accompanying intraspinal lipoma or tumor, it may be adherent to the spinal cord and nerves. A pilonidal sinus or sacrococcygeal teratoma does not communicate with the spinal neural components.*

▶ de Bruyn R (ed): *Pediatric Ultrasound: How, Why and When*, 2nd edition (e-book). Philadelphia, Churchill Livingstone/Elsevier, 2010, p 295.

▶ Rumack CM, Levine D (eds): *Diagnostic Ultrasound*, 5th edition. Philadelphia, Elsevier, 2018, p 1686.

▶ Siegel MJ (ed): *Pediatric Sonography*, 4th edition. Philadelphia, Lippincott Williams & Wilkins, 2011, pp 649, 656, 661–662, 664–666.

▶ Unsinn KM, Geley T, Freund MC, et al: US of the spinal cord in newborns: spectrum of normal findings, variants, congenital anomalies, and acquired diseases. RadioGraphics 20:923–938, 2000. Available at https://pubs.rsna.org/doi/full/10.1148/radiographics.20.4.g00jl06923.

PART 3

Neck and Face

101. **A. Thyroglossal duct cyst.**

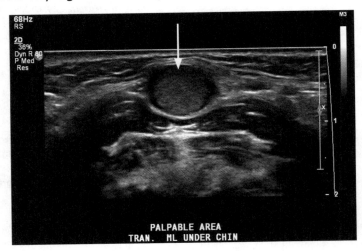

Thyroglossal duct cysts *(arrow) are cystic structures located anteriorly below the hyoid bone at or slightly off midline. They present as a soft, painless lump characterized by movement with swallowing. The* thyroglossal duct *is an embryologic channel between the base of the tongue and the normal position of the thyroid that serves as a path for the thyroid to descend during fetal development. Usually the thyroglossal duct then disappears, but sometimes a remnant remains as a pocket, a thyroglossal duct cyst. These cysts are present at birth and are often seen in children; they are commonly diagnosed after an infection of the upper respiratory tract causes them to enlarge and become painful. Branchial cleft* cysts *and* ranulas *normally are not located in this midline area. They, as well as* thyroid cysts, *do not move with swallowing.*

▶ de Bruyn R (ed): *Pediatric Ultrasound: How, Why and When*, 2nd edition (e-book). Philadelphia, Churchill Livingstone/Elsevier, 2010, pp 281–283.
▶ Rumack CM, Levine D (eds): *Diagnostic Ultrasound*, 5th edition. Philadelphia, Elsevier, 2018, pp 1639, 1643.
▶ Siegel MJ (ed): *Pediatric Sonography*, 4th edition. Philadelphia, Lippincott Williams & Wilkins, 2011, p 132.

102. **D. 4.**

There are usually 4 parathyroid glands. The superior parathyroid glands are located near the superior lobe of the thyroid and the inferior glands are adjacent to the lower poles of the thyroid. The main function of the parathyroid glands is to maintain calcium and phosphate homeostasis. Normal parathyroid glands are difficult to visualize with ultrasound due their small size (<5 mm) and their similar echogenicity and proximity to the normal thyroid gland.

▶ de Bruyn R (ed): *Pediatric Ultrasound: How, Why and When*, 2nd edition (e-book). Philadelphia, Churchill Livingstone/Elsevier, 2010, pp 280–281.

▶ Rumack CM, Levine D (eds): *Diagnostic Ultrasound*, 5th edition. Philadelphia, Elsevier, 2018, p 1650.

▶ Siegel MJ (ed): *Pediatric Sonography*, 4th edition. Philadelphia, Lippincott Williams & Wilkins, 2011, p 158.

103. C. Parotid gland.

See Color Plate 12 on page xxxviii.

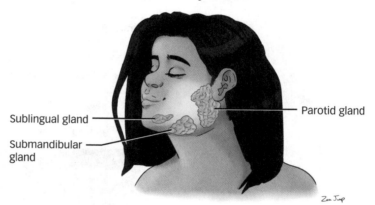

The Salivary Glands

Locations of the salivary glands are illustrated above. Hemangiomas are the most common neoplasms of the salivary glands in children. Hemangiomas are most commonly encountered in the parotid gland and present at birth or during the neonatal period. The patient may have a nontender palpable mass in the mandibular area and occasionally show a skin discoloration. Most infantile hemangiomas have a rapid neonatal growth and normally regress later in childhood. In general, neoplasms involving the salivary glands are located within the parotid gland 90% to 95% of the time. The remainder occur in the submandibular and sublingual glands. The parathyroid glands are not salivary glands.

▶ de Bruyn R (ed): *Pediatric Ultrasound: How, Why and When*, 2nd edition (e-book). Philadelphia, Churchill Livingstone/Elsevier, 2010, pp 288–289.

▶ Rumack CM, Levine D (eds): *Diagnostic Ultrasound*, 5th edition. Philadelphia, Elsevier, 2018, p 1636.

▶ Siegel MJ (ed): *Pediatric Sonography*, 4th edition. Philadelphia, Lippincott Williams & Wilkins, 2011, p 121.

104. **D. Parathyroid hormone (PTH).**

The hormones associated with the thyroid gland are triiodothyronine (T3), thyroxine (T4), and thyroid-stimulating hormone (TSH). T3 and T4 are the hormones secreted by the thyroid gland, and their production and release are controlled by TSH. The anterior lobe of the pituitary gland controls the release of TSH and is dependent on the serum levels of T3 and T4. When there are high levels of the T3 and T4 the TSH levels decrease, whereas with low levels of thyroid hormones, TSH levels increase. Thyrotropin-releasing hormone (TRH) is a hormone released by the hypothalamus and regulates the TSH. Parathyroid hormone is the hormone secreted by the parathyroid glands and is not associated with the thyroid.

▸ Brady B: Thyroid gland: overview. Available at https://www.endocrineweb.com/conditions/thyroid-nodules/thyroid-gland-controls-bodys-metabolism-how-it-works-symptoms-hyperthyroid.

▸ Siegel MJ (ed): *Pediatric Sonography*, 4th edition. Philadelphia, Lippincott Williams & Wilkins, 2011, p 147.

105. **B. Parotid gland.**

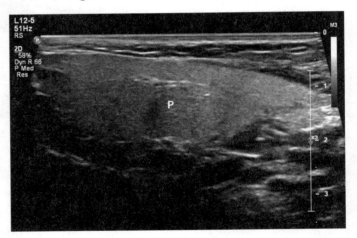

See Color Plate 12, "The Salivary Glands," on page xxxviii.

The parotid gland (P) is the largest of the three main salivary glands and is located anterior and slightly inferior to the ear lobe. Most of the parotid gland tissue lies superficial to the masseter muscle and has an elliptical shape. The parotid gland appears homogeneous and hyperechoic when compared to the adjacent muscle, and small lymph nodes can be visualized within the gland. The submandibular gland *lies under the mandible and can often be visualized by placing the transducer below the jaw on each side of the midline. The* sublingual gland *may be visualized by placing the transducer in the submental space (under the chin). Lymph nodes usually appear more hypoechoic on ultrasound and demonstrate a central hilum.*

▶ de Bruyn R (ed): *Pediatric Ultrasound: How, Why and When*, 2nd edition (e-book). Philadelphia, Churchill Livingstone/Elsevier, 2010, pp 286–289.
▶ Rumack CM, Levine D (eds): *Diagnostic Ultrasound*, 5th edition. Philadelphia, Elsevier, 2018, p 1630.
▶ Siegel MJ (ed): *Pediatric Sonography*, 4th edition. Philadelphia, Lippincott Williams & Wilkins, 2011, pp 118–120.

106. A. Fibromatosis colli.

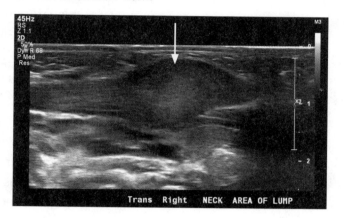

Fibromatosis colli is the most common cause of neonatal torticollis and is usually related to traumatic birth or uterine malpresentation. Fibromatosis colli occurs when the sternocleidomastoid muscle contracts and becomes fibrotic and short, causing an ipsilateral tilt of the head. Sonographically, fibromatosis colli appears as a focal thickening of the sternocleidomastoid muscle (arrow), especially when compared to the unaffected side. Some patients with fibromatosis colli can have associated musculoskeletal anomalies like hip dysplasia and tibial torsion. Aggressive fibromatosis is a lesion in which there is aggressive fibrous tissue proliferation and occurs most commonly after puberty. Aggressive fibromatosis will appear as a poorly circumscribed mass on ultrasound. Nodular fasciitis and inflammatory myofibroblastic tumor are uncommon fibrous lesions of the neck that have a nonspecific sonographic appearance, and additional imaging and biopsy are needed for their diagnosis.

▶ de Bruyn R (ed): *Pediatric Ultrasound: How, Why and When*, 2nd edition (e-book). Philadelphia, Churchill Livingstone/Elsevier, 2010, pp 284–285.
▶ Rumack CM, Levine D (eds): *Diagnostic Ultrasound*, 5th edition. Philadelphia, Elsevier, 2018, pp 1663–1664.
▶ Siegel MJ (ed): *Pediatric Sonography*, 4th edition. Philadelphia, Lippincott Williams & Wilkins, 2011, pp 137–138.

107. C. Papillary carcinoma.

In general, thyroid carcinomas are rare in children. The most common type is the papillary thyroid carcinoma, *accounting for 70% to 90% of all thyroid cancers. There is a higher incidence in females between the ages of 15 and 19 years. Following papillary carcinomas,* follicular carcinomas *account for 10% to 20% of thyroid cancers.* Medullary carcinomas *and* acinar cell carcinomas *are very rare in children, and medullary carcinoma is linked to a strong family history of the disease.*

▶ de Bruyn R (ed): *Pediatric Ultrasound: How, Why and When*, 2nd edition (e-book). Philadelphia, Churchill Livingstone/Elsevier, 2010, p 279.
▶ Rumack CM, Levine D (eds): *Diagnostic Ultrasound*, 5th edition. Philadelphia, Elsevier, 2018, p 1648.
▶ Siegel MJ (ed): *Pediatric Sonography*, 4th edition. Philadelphia, Lippincott Williams & Wilkins, 2011, p 152.

108. C. Masseter muscles.

The thyroid gland is bordered anterolaterally by the sternocleidomastoid *and* strap muscles. *Posterolateral to the thyroid lobes, the* longus colli muscles *border the gland. The* masseter muscles *are located in the face, connecting the mandible to the cheek bone on each side; these muscles do not border the thyroid gland.*

▶ Rumack CM, Levine D (eds): *Diagnostic Ultrasound*, 5th edition. Philadelphia, Elsevier, 2018, p 1630.
▶ Siegel MJ (ed): *Pediatric Sonography*, 4th edition. Philadelphia, Lippincott Williams & Wilkins, 2011, p 119.

109. D. Parathyroid adenoma.

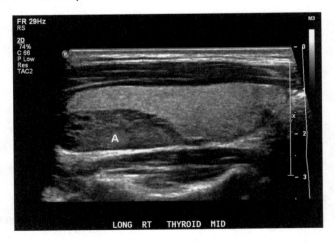

Hypercalcemia, pruritus, and bone pain are symptoms associated with hyperparathyroidism. Parathyroid adenoma *(A) is the most common cause of primary hyperparathyroidism and on ultrasound will appear as a hypoechoic, oval structure*

located posterior to the thyroid gland. The normal parathyroid glands are difficult to differentiate from the thyroid. A functioning parathyroid carcinoma can also cause primary hyperparathyroidism but is less likely to be the cause. Thyroid neoplasms like adenoma and carcinoma will not cause hypercalcemia.

▶ Mayo Clinic: Hyperparathyroidism. Available at https://www.mayoclinic.org/diseases conditions/hyperparathyroidism/symptoms causes/syc-20356194.

▶ Siegel MJ (ed): *Pediatric Sonography*, 4th edition. Philadelphia, Lippincott Williams & Wilkins, 2011, p 159.

110. **B. Sublingual duct.**

A ranula is a cyst composed of retained mucus beneath the tongue and may be caused by obstruction of the sublingual gland or ducts. Ranulas are located in the sublingual space (where the sublingual ducts drain). When restricted to this area, they are known as simple ranulas. On ultrasound, simple ranulas appear as well-defined simple cysts under the tongue. When ranulas extend below the mylohyoid muscle (under the chin) they are termed as plunging ranulas. The Stensen duct drains the parotid gland and is on each side of the face, crossing the masseter muscle. The Wharton duct is the main duct of the submandibular gland and drains in the anterior portion of the mouth floor. The Wirsung duct, also known as the pancreatic duct, is not located in the mouth.

▶ Rumack CM, Levine D (eds): *Diagnostic Ultrasound*, 5th edition. Philadelphia, Elsevier, 2018, pp 1639–1640.

▶ Siegel MJ (ed): *Pediatric Sonography*, 4th edition. Philadelphia, Lippincott Williams & Wilkins, 2011, pp 118–121, 123–124.

111. **D. Internal jugular vein.**

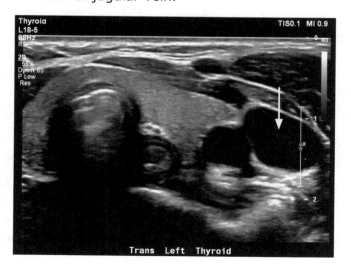

At the level of the thyroid in a transverse scan, the common carotid artery and the internal jugular vein (arrow) can be seen along the posterolateral margin of the gland. The common carotid artery is more medial and posterior than the internal jugular vein. The echogenic wall of the common carotid artery helps to differentiate the vessels. A normal variant of the internal jugular vein is the asymmetry of both veins. It is a common finding for the right internal jugular vein to be larger in diameter than the left. The common carotid artery bifurcates superiorly at the level of the angle of the mandible into the internal and external carotid arteries. The external jugular vein is more lateral and superficial than the internal jugular vein and is not commonly seen during ultrasound of the thyroid gland.

▸ Rumack CM, Levine D (eds): *Diagnostic Ultrasound*, 5th edition. Philadelphia, Elsevier, 2018, p 1642.

▸ Siegel MJ (ed): *Pediatric Sonography*, 4th edition. Philadelphia, Lippincott Williams & Wilkins, 2011, pp 143–144.

112. B. Parotid.

See Color Plate 12, "The Salivary Glands," on page xxxviii.

The parotid gland *is the largest of the three main salivary glands and is located anterior and slightly inferior to the ear lobe. Most of the parotid gland tissue lies superficial to the masseter muscle, and the gland has an elliptical shape. The* sublingual gland *is the smallest of the major salivary glands. It is located on each side of the floor of the mouth. The* submandibular gland *is smaller than the parotid but larger than the sublingual gland and is located along the border of the mandible on each side. The thyroid gland is not a salivary gland.*

▸ de Bruyn R (ed): *Pediatric Ultrasound: How, Why and When*, 2nd edition (e-book). Philadelphia, Churchill Livingstone/Elsevier, 2010, pp 286–288.

▸ Rumack CM, Levine D (eds): *Diagnostic Ultrasound*, 5th edition. Philadelphia, Elsevier, 2018, pp 1629–1631.

▸ Siegel MJ (ed): *Pediatric Sonography*, 4th edition. Philadelphia, Lippincott Williams & Wilkins, 2011, pp 118–121.

113. A. Hyperechoic and homogeneous.

The normal thyroid gland echogenicity is slightly hyperechoic and homogeneous compared to the adjacent muscle. In a transverse scan, the thyroid gland appears as a bilobed structure connected by an isthmus anterior to the trachea. Each thyroid lobe is bordered posterolaterally by the longus colli muscle, which appears as a triangular and hypoechoic structure in transverse imaging. In sagittal imaging, the lobes of the thyroid have an elliptical shape. About 50% of patients have a superior extension of the isthmus called the pyramidal lobe. Commonly in the left lobe of the thyroid, the esophagus can be seen lying medial and posterior to the gland as a hypoechoic rounded structure that may contain air within it. The normal thyroid may have colloid follicles, which appear as small cystic structures within the thyroid parenchyma. The size of the thyroid changes with age and body height.

▶ Rumack CM, Levine D (eds): *Diagnostic Ultrasound*, 5th edition. Philadelphia, Elsevier, 2018, pp 1640–1642.

▶ Siegel MJ (ed): *Pediatric Sonography*, 4th edition. Philadelphia, Lippincott Williams & Wilkins, 2011, pp 147–148.

114. **A. Kidneys.**

The kidneys and the liver are target organs of parathyroid hormone (PTH). PTH is secreted by the parathyroid glands and is responsible for the regulation of the calcium and phosphate levels in the body. When the parathyroid glands secrete elevated amounts of PTH, regardless of the calcium levels in the body, this condition is known as hyperparathyroidism. The spleen, pancreas, and gallbladder are not target organs of PTH.

▶ Sargis RM: An overview of the parathyroid: the calcium regulating gland that helps keep bones healthy. Available at https://www.endocrineweb.com/endocrinology/overview-parathyroid.

▶ Siegel MJ (ed): *Pediatric Sonography*, 4th edition. Philadelphia, Lippincott Williams & Wilkins, 2011, p 158.

115. **B. Trachea.**

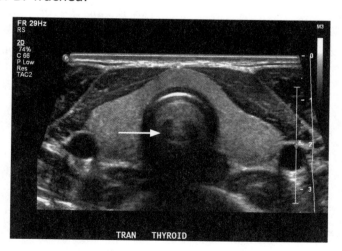

The trachea (arrow), also known as the windpipe, is a long tubular structure with cartilaginous rings. The trachea connects the larynx to the bronchial tubes and is located posterior to the thyroid isthmus. Because the trachea is a hollow tube and is filled with air, it is difficult to evaluate with ultrasound. The anterior echogenic curved margin posterior to the thyroid isthmus represents the air-mucosal interface followed by the reverberation artifact posterior to it (bullet sign). The esophagus is seen posterior to and left of the trachea and appears as a hypoechoic structure. The hyoid bone and cervical spine are not normally seen in a thyroid ultrasound.

▶ Rumack CM, Levine D (eds): *Diagnostic Ultrasound*, 5th edition. Philadelphia, Elsevier, 2018, p 1642.

▶ Siegel MJ (ed): *Pediatric Sonography*, 4th edition. Philadelphia, Lippincott Williams & Wilkins, 2011, p 147.

116. A. Branchial cleft cyst.

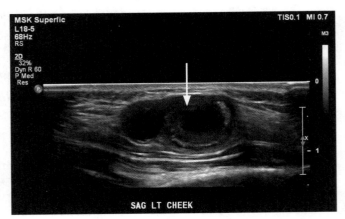

A painless cystic structure located posterior to and below the ear is most likely a branchial cleft cyst. Branchial cleft cysts (arrow) are the most common abnormality of the "branchial apparatus," which is the embryologic structure that develops into the neck tissues. There are four types of branchial cleft cysts—designated type I (around the ear lobe or under the jaw), type II (lower-neck sinus tract cysts), type III (near the thyroid gland—rare), and type IV (below the neck—also rare). Type II branchial cleft cysts are the most common. Sonographically, branchial cleft cysts appear as anechoic, well-defined structures with posterior enhancement; if infected or hemorrhagic they may appear hypoechoic. Thyroglossal duct cysts are located in the midline of the neck or slightly to the left adjacent to the hyoid bone. Cystadenomas of the salivary glands are uncommon tumors. Ranulas are sublingual cystic structures caused by obstruction of the sublingual ducts.

▶ de Bruyn R (ed): *Pediatric Ultrasound: How, Why and When*, 2nd edition (e-book). Philadelphia, Churchill Livingstone/Elsevier, 2010, pp 281–283.

▶ Rumack CM, Levine D (eds): *Diagnostic Ultrasound*, 5th edition. Philadelphia, Elsevier, 2018, pp 1640, 1643, 1651.

▶ Siegel MJ (ed): *Pediatric Sonography*, 4th edition. Philadelphia, Lippincott Williams & Wilkins, 2011, pp 121–123, 132–134.

117. **A. Microcalcifications.**

Differentiation between benign and malignant thyroid nodules is difficult with ultrasound, and a final diagnosis is obtained only by biopsy. Some of the sonographic characteristics that can suggest a malignant thyroid nodule are microcalcifications, nodule size greater than 1 cm, irregular margins, absence of peripheral halo, lesion with more height than width, and abnormal adjacent lymph nodes. With the presence of adjacent lymphadenopathy, the concern for metastatic disease increases. Comet-tail artifact, nodule size less than 1 cm, and large eggshell calcifications are all characteristics suggesting benign thyroid nodules.

▶ de Bruyn R (ed): *Pediatric Ultrasound: How, Why and When*, 2nd edition (e-book). Philadelphia, Churchill Livingstone/Elsevier, 2010, p 279.

▶ Rumack CM, Levine D (eds): *Diagnostic Ultrasound*, 5th edition. Philadelphia, Elsevier, 2018, p 1648.

▶ Siegel MJ (ed): *Pediatric Sonography*, 4th edition. Philadelphia, Lippincott Williams & Wilkins, 2011, p 154.

118. **D. Viral parotitis.**

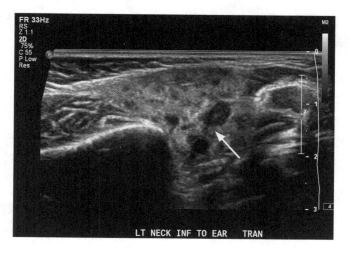

Inflammation of the salivary glands caused by viral infections is more common than bacterial infections of the salivary glands. Viral parotitis *is commonly caused by mononucleosis, cytomegalovirus (CMV), human immunodeficiency virus (HIV), and mumps. Sonographically, acute nonsuppurative viral parotitis appears as an enlarged and heterogeneous parotid gland (arrow) with a hypoechoic multinodular*

appearance. Bacterial infections of the salivary gland are uncommon but can be caused by Staphylococcus aureus *and* Streptococcus. *On ultrasound,* bacterial parotitis *may also appear multinodular and may include the presence of an abscess, because with bacterial parotitis abscess development can occur.* Sialadenitis *is a chronic inflammation of the parotid gland that is associated with cystic fibrosis. On ultrasound, recurrent sialadenitis appears as a normal or small sized heterogeneous parotid gland.* Sialolithiasis *is the formation of calculi in the salivary glands and most commonly occurs in the submandibular gland. Sialolithiasis is uncommon in children and appears as echogenic foci with posterior shadowing.*

▶ Rumack CM, Levine D (eds): *Diagnostic Ultrasound*, 5th edition. Philadelphia, Elsevier, 2018, p 1634.

▶ Siegel MJ (ed): *Pediatric Sonography*, 4th edition. Philadelphia, Lippincott Williams & Wilkins, 2011, pp 124–126.

119. **A. Under the tongue.**

The term sublingual *refers to the area under the tongue. In this area, there is a pair of salivary glands known as the* sublingual glands. *The area under the mandible is known as the* submandibular area. *The area under the nose is known as the* subnasal area. *The area below the ear is known as the* subauricular area.

▶ Siegel MJ (ed): *Pediatric Sonography*, 4th edition. Philadelphia, Lippincott Williams & Wilkins, 2011, p 119.

120. **B. Thyroid dysgenesis.**

Congenital hypothyroidism is relatively common, affecting approximately 1 in 4000 infants. Thyroid dysgenesis *(a defect of the gland) is the most common cause of congenital hypothyroidism and is related to mental retardation and delayed bone development.* Maternal thyrotoxicosis *(hyperthyroidism),* dyshormonogenesis *(abnormal synthesis and secretion of the hormones), and* pituitary/hypothalamic hypothyroidism *are other, less common causes of congenital hypothyroidism.*

▶ de Bruyn R (ed): *Pediatric Ultrasound: How, Why and When*, 2nd edition (e-book). Philadelphia, Churchill Livingstone/Elsevier, 2010, p 277.

▶ Rumack CM, Levine D (eds): *Diagnostic Ultrasound*, 5th edition. Philadelphia, Elsevier, 2018, p 1642.

▶ Siegel MJ (ed): *Pediatric Sonography*, 4th edition. Philadelphia, Lippincott Williams & Wilkins, 2011, pp 148–149.

121. **D. Mandible.**

    The angle of the jaw bone is formed by the **mandible**, *the most inferior bone of the face. The* **maxilla** *forms the upper jaw bone and together with the mandible forms the mouth structure. The* **zygoma** *forms the cheekbone lateral and inferior to the orbits. The* **vomer** *is a midline bone that separates the nasal cavities.*

    ▸ Jahan-Parwar B: Facial bone anatomy. Available at https://emedicine.medscape.com/article/835401-overview.

122. **C. Parallel and lateral to the horizontal portion of the mandible.**

    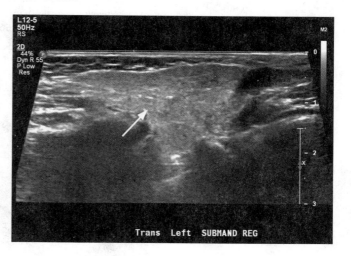

    See Color Plate 12, "The Salivary Glands," on page xxxviii.

    This image of the submandibular gland (arrow) can be obtained by placing the transducer parallel to the mandible and slightly lateral under the jaw on each side of the midline. The submandibular gland is one of the three main salivary glands and has an oval or triangular shape. The submandibular gland appears homogeneous and hyperechoic when compared to adjacent structures. If you scanned parallel and anterior to the ear, you would be imaging the parotid gland, which is the largest of the major salivary glands. Placing the transducer sagittal and midline under the chin will allow you to visualize the sublingual salivary gland, the smallest of the three major salivary glands. Perpendicular and anterior to the trachea, the thyroid gland can be imaged.

    ▸ de Bruyn R (ed): *Pediatric Ultrasound: How, Why and When*, 2nd edition (e-book). Philadelphia, Churchill Livingstone/Elsevier, 2010, pp 285, 288.

    ▸ Rumack CM, Levine D (eds): *Diagnostic Ultrasound*, 5th edition. Philadelphia, Elsevier, 2018, p 1630.

    ▸ Siegel MJ (ed): *Pediatric Sonography*, 4th edition. Philadelphia, Lippincott Williams & Wilkins, 2011, pp 118–121.

123. A. Generalized parathyroid hyperplasia.

Secondary hyperparathyroidism *occurs when there is an excessive production of parathyroid hormone (PTH) caused initially by decreased levels of calcium from another disease.* Generalized parathyroid hyperplasia *occurs as a response to this lack of calcium, increasing the amount of PTH in the body. Chronic renal disease and intestinal malabsorption are common causes of secondary hyperparathyroidism. Functional* parathyroid adenomas, carcinomas, *and* cysts *are all causes of primary hyperparathyroidism, with adenomas being the most common.*

▸ Mayo Clinic: Hyperparathyroidism: symptoms and causes. Available at https://www.mayoclinic.org/diseases conditions/hyperparathyroidism/symptoms causes/syc 20356194.

▸ Siegel MJ (ed): *Pediatric Sonography*, 4th edition. Philadelphia, Lippincott Williams & Wilkins, 2011, p 159.

124. C. Goiter.

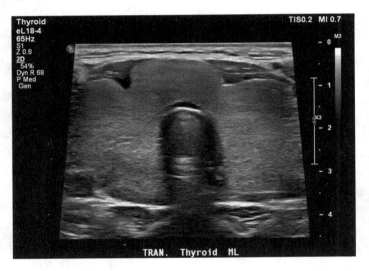

Goiter *is a general term that refers to the diffuse enlargement of the thyroid gland. Goiter can be caused by inflammatory or autoimmune conditions like Hashimoto's thyroiditis, also known as lymphocytic thyroiditis, and Graves' disease. The term* thyroid inferno *refers to the markedly increased vascularity that the thyroid presents on ultrasound with Graves' disease.* Multinodular goiter *refers to the nodular enlargement to the thyroid gland caused by adenomatous tissue. Multinodular goiter is also known as* adenomatous goiter *or* nodular hyperplasia *and may be associated with renal disease and polydactyly.*

▸ de Bruyn R (ed): *Pediatric Ultrasound: How, Why and When*, 2nd edition (e-book). Philadelphia, Churchill Livingstone/Elsevier, 2010, p 279.

▸ Rumack CM, Levine D (eds): *Diagnostic Ultrasound*, 5th edition. Philadelphia, Elsevier, 2018, p 1648.

▸ Siegel MJ (ed): *Pediatric Sonography*, 4th edition. Philadelphia, Lippincott Williams & Wilkins, 2011, pp 154, 157.

125. **D. Adenoma.**

Thyroid adenomas are the most common benign neoplasm of the gland. Sonographic characteristics of a thyroid adenoma include hyperechogenicity, hypoechoic rim, peripheral curvilinear calcifications ("eggshell"), peripheral vascularity, cystic changes corresponding to internal hemorrhage, and comet-tail artifact produced by colloid crystals. Thyroid adenomas may be associated with hyperthyroidism. Papillary *and* medullary carcinomas *are malignant lesions; the sonographic characteristics described in the question are of a benign nodule.* Colloid cysts *are mostly anechoic structures.*

▸ Rumack CM, Levine D (eds): *Diagnostic Ultrasound*, 5th edition. Philadelphia, Elsevier, 2018, pp 1646, 1648.

▸ Siegel MJ (ed): *Pediatric Sonography*, 4th edition. Philadelphia, Lippincott Williams & Wilkins, 2011, pp 150–151, 154.

126. **C. Lateral cervical lymph nodes.**

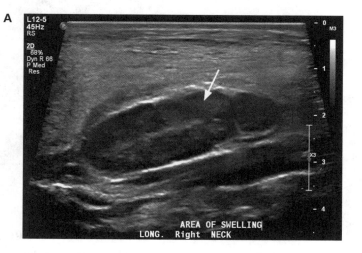

See Color Plate 15 on page xxxix.

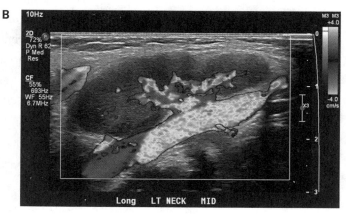

Lymph nodes *in the neck and face, as seen in image* **A** *(arrow), are divided into a superficial and a deep group. The* superficial group *includes parotid, submandibular, facial, and occipital nodes. The* deep group *includes the sublingual, retropharyngeal, and lateral cervical nodes. The lateral cervical nodes can be subdivided into superficial and deep, the deep group being the most involved in disease processes. Normal lymph nodes in children typically measure 5 mm or less in the short axis. With color Doppler a vascular hilum is seen (image* **B***).*

▶ de Bruyn R (ed): *Pediatric Ultrasound: How, Why and When*, 2nd edition (e-book). Philadelphia, Churchill Livingstone/Elsevier, 2010, pp 284–286.
▶ Rumack CM, Levine D (eds): *Diagnostic Ultrasound*, 5th edition. Philadelphia, Elsevier, 2018, p 1658.
▶ Siegel MJ (ed): *Pediatric Sonography*, 4th edition. Philadelphia, Lippincott Williams & Wilkins, 2011, p 128.

127. A. Isthmus.

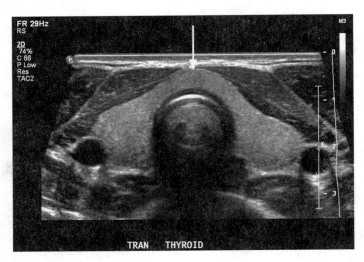

The midline structure that connects both lobes of the thyroid is known as the isthmus. *The isthmus is a narrow strip of thyroid tissue that runs along the anterior border of the trachea. The thyroid is a butterfly-shaped organ, with the isthmus mimicking the butterfly's "body" and the lobes being the "wings." The* pyramidal lobe *of the thyroid is a superior extension of the isthmus that can be seen in normal patients.* Thyroid arch *and* accessory lobe *are not terms used in reference to thyroid anatomy.*

▶ Rumack CM, Levine D (eds): *Diagnostic Ultrasound*, 5th edition. Philadelphia, Elsevier, 2018, p 1642.
▶ Siegel MJ (ed): *Pediatric Sonography*, 4th edition. Philadelphia, Lippincott Williams & Wilkins, 2011, p 147.

128. **A. Lymphangioma.**

Lymphangiomas are benign congenital malformations of dilated lymphatic channels that are also known as cystic hygromas. This congenital malformation is usually found by the first year of life and presents as an asymptomatic mass. Lymphangiomas are the second most common vascular lesion of the parotid gland, following hemangiomas. Hemangiomas are also congenital masses, but they comprise multiple hypoechoic tubular vessels. Pleomorphic adenomas are usually homogeneous hypoechoic masses and, along with cystadenomas, are not congenital and are rare in childhood.

▸ de Bruyn R (ed): *Pediatric Ultrasound: How, Why and When*, 2nd edition (e-book). Philadelphia, Churchill Livingstone/Elsevier, 2010, pp 283–284, 290.

▸ Rumack CM, Levine D (eds): *Diagnostic Ultrasound*, 5th edition. Philadelphia, Elsevier, 2018, p 1636.

▸ Siegel MJ (ed): *Pediatric Sonography*, 4th edition. Philadelphia, Lippincott Williams & Wilkins, 2011, pp 121–122.

129. **B. Hashimoto's thyroiditis.**

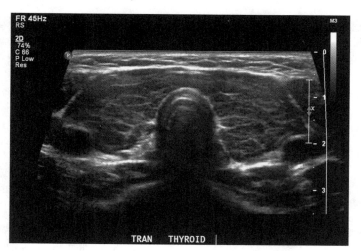

Hashimoto's thyroiditis, also known as chronic lymphocytic thyroiditis, is the most common cause of hypothyroidism and thyroiditis in children and adolescents. Hashimoto's thyroiditis is a chronic autoimmune disease in which lymphocytes infiltrate the gland. Patients with Hashimoto's thyroiditis present with a painless enlarged thyroid. Sonographically, the thyroid gland appears enlarged and heterogeneous with a hypoechoic multinodular appearance, as seen in this image. With color Doppler, hyperemia is commonly seen. Graves' disease is an autoimmune disorder and is the most common

cause of hyperthyroidism (not hypothyroidism) in children. Focal thyroiditis, also known as subacute (de Quervain) thyroiditis, and acute suppurative thyroiditis are inflammatory, not autoimmune, diseases and are uncommon.

▸ de Bruyn R (ed): *Pediatric Ultrasound: How, Why and When*, 2nd edition (e-book). Philadelphia, Churchill Livingstone/Elsevier, 2010, pp 278–280.
▸ Rumack CM, Levine D (eds): *Diagnostic Ultrasound*, 5th edition. Philadelphia, Elsevier, 2018, pp 1645–1646.
▸ Siegel MJ (ed): *Pediatric Sonography*, 4th edition. Philadelphia, Lippincott Williams & Wilkins, 2011, pp 154–157.

130. D. Sialolithiasis.

Sialolithiasis *refers to the presence of calculi in a submandibular gland.* Sialolithiasis *most commonly affects the submandibular gland due to its alkaline nature.* Sialolithiasis *may be an isolated finding, but it has also been associated with cystic fibrosis.* Ranulas *are cystic structures caused by obstruction of the sublingual ducts.* Mumps *affects the parotid gland and is the most common cause of parotiditis. The majority of the salivary gland* hemangiomas *occur in the parotid gland.*

▸ de Bruyn R (ed): *Pediatric Ultrasound: How, Why and When*, 2nd edition (e-book). Philadelphia, Churchill Livingstone/Elsevier, 2010, p 288.
▸ Rumack CM, Levine D (eds): *Diagnostic Ultrasound*, 5th edition. Philadelphia, Elsevier, 2018, pp 1632, 1635–1636.
▸ Siegel MJ (ed): *Pediatric Sonography*, 4th edition. Philadelphia, Lippincott Williams & Wilkins, 2011, pp 121, 123–124.

131. A. Carotid bifurcation mass.

Fine needle biopsy *(FNB) of the neck is a procedure in which a fine needle is inserted into the neck with the purpose of aspirating fluid or tissue from a suspicious lesion for diagnosis. FNB may be indicated in cases of enlarged lymph nodes, thyroid gland lesions, cystic neck lesions, and parathyroid neoplasms. Although FNB may be used for any neck masses, carotid body tumors are neoplasms near the carotid bifurcation; therefore, due to the known risks of complications, FNB should be avoided in this area. FNB as well as percutaneous drainage should always be performed using sterile technique. Ultrasound guidance may be employed to localize the lesion to be biopsied or drained.*

▸ Boone J: Biopsy, fine needle, neck mass. Available at https://emedicine.medscape.com/article/1520111-overview#a7.
▸ Siegel MJ (ed): *Pediatric Sonography*, 4th edition. Philadelphia, Lippincott Williams & Wilkins, 2011, p 685.

132. **B. Nodular formation.**

Graves' disease and Hashimoto's thyroiditis are autoimmune disorders and sonographically have very similar appearances. Both conditions can be visualized on ultrasound as an enlarged hypervascular thyroid with possible lobulated contours. Nodular formation is not a feature of Graves' disease, but it is seen with Hashimoto's thyroiditis. The term thyroid inferno *is used to describe the marked hypervascularity of the gland with Graves' disease. Patients with Graves' disease present with weight loss, nervousness, palpitations, and heat intolerance (symptoms of hyperthyroidism). With Graves' disease there is an increase in thyroxine (T4) and triiodothyronine (T3) hormones, and thyroid-stimulating hormone (TSH) is decreased.*

▶ de Bruyn R (ed): *Pediatric Ultrasound: How, Why and When*, 2nd edition (e-book). Philadelphia, Churchill Livingstone/Elsevier, 2010, pp 278–280.

▶ Rumack CM, Levine D (eds): *Diagnostic Ultrasound*, 5th edition. Philadelphia, Elsevier, 2018, pp 1645–1646.

▶ Siegel MJ (ed): *Pediatric Sonography*, 4th edition. Philadelphia, Lippincott Williams & Wilkins, 2011, pp 155–157.

133. **C. Parathyroid adenoma.**

The most common cause of primary hyperparathyroidism is parathyroid adenoma. *Hyperparathyroidism occurs when there is an excessive production of parathyroid hormone (PTH), regardless of the calcium levels. Patients with hyperparathyroidism are diagnosed when the PTH is increased and there is hypercalcemia. Treatment for primary hyperparathyroidism is removal of the adenomatous gland.* Multiple endocrine neoplasia (MEN) type I *and* parathyroid carcinoma *are rarely the cause of primary hyperparathyroidism. Generalized parathyroid hyperplasia causes secondary hyperparathyroidism.*

▶ Mayo Clinic: Hyperparathyroidism. Available at https://www.mayoclinic.org/diseases conditions/hyperparathyroidism/symptoms causes/syc-20356194.

▶ Siegel MJ (ed): *Pediatric Sonography*, 4th edition. Philadelphia, Lippincott Williams & Wilkins, 2011, p 159.

134. D. Esophagus.

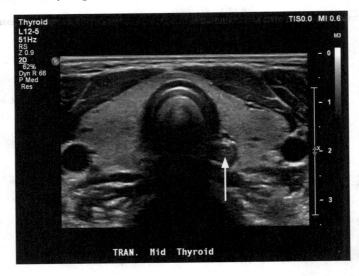

In the normal thyroid, the esophagus (arrow) appears as a hypoechoic rounded structure posterior and medial to the left lobe of the thyroid. The esophagus has a hypoechoic muscular wall and may contain air within it. Normal parathyroid glands are very difficult to visualize with ultrasound due to their small size and echogenicity similar to the thyroid. Lymph nodes appear as oval structures with an echogenic vascular hilum. Thyroid adenomas appear as hyperechoic neoplasms with a hypoechoic fibrous capsule.

▶ de Bruyn R (ed): *Pediatric Ultrasound: How, Why and When,* 2nd edition (e-book). Philadelphia, Churchill Livingstone/Elsevier, 2010, p 277.

▶ Siegel MJ (ed): *Pediatric Sonography,* 4th edition. Philadelphia, Lippincott Williams & Wilkins, 2011, p 150.

135. C. Sublingual.

See Color Plate 12, "The Salivary Glands," on page xxxviii.

The sublingual gland *is the smallest of the major salivary glands. One of these glands is located on each side of the floor of the mouth. The* parotid gland *is the largest of the major salivary glands and is located mainly anterior and inferior to the ear. The* submandibular gland *is smaller than the parotid but larger than the sublingual gland and is located along the border of the mandible on each side. The* thyroid gland *is not a salivary gland.*

▶ Rumack CM, Levine D (eds): *Diagnostic Ultrasound,* 5th edition. Philadelphia, Elsevier, 2018, pp 1630–1631.

▶ Siegel MJ (ed): *Pediatric Sonography,* 4th edition. Philadelphia, Lippincott Williams & Wilkins, 2011, pp 118–121.

PART 4

Chest

136. **B. 12.5 MHz linear transducer.**

A 12.5 MHz linear transducer is best when evaluating the pleural cavity of an infant. This transducer allows sufficient resolution and penetration in smaller patients, and the larger footprint assists in a better evaluation of the near-field structures. The selection of transducers and frequency for chest ultrasounds should be based on the patient's age, size, and clinical question. An 8.5 MHz sector transducer with a small footprint can be helpful when scanning through the suprasternal, intercostal, and subxiphoid spaces due to easy access, but because near-field resolution is not as optimal, this is not the best choice for evaluating fluid collections. A 5.0 MHz transducer is best when penetration is needed in larger children and adolescents. A 17.5 MHz transducer provides high resolution with very little penetration and generally is not optimal for the evaluation of the pleural space.

▶ de Bruyn R (ed): *Pediatric Ultrasound: How, Why and When*, 2nd edition (e-book). Philadelphia, Churchill Livingstone/Elsevier, 2010, pp 342, 348–350.

▶ Rumack CM, Levine D (eds): *Diagnostic Ultrasound*, 5th edition. Philadelphia, Elsevier, 2018, pp 1701–1702.

▶ Siegel MJ (ed): *Pediatric Sonography*, 4th edition. Philadelphia, Lippincott Williams & Wilkins, 2011, p 164.

137. **A. Atelectasis.**

Atelectasis occurs when the alveoli are collapsed and not filled with air. The term "hepatization" of the lung is used when the bronchi are not filled with air, thus allowing transmission of the ultrasound beam and giving an appearance similar to the liver. Hepatization of the lung can be seen in atelectasis and lung consolidation. Congenital pulmonary airway malformation (CPAM, formerly known as congenital cystic adenomatoid malformation of the lung or CCAML) is a benign condition of abnormal lung tissue comprising cysts. Empyema *refers to a complex fluid collection with internal debris and septations.* Pneumothorax *is the term for air within the pleural cavity. Pneumothorax does not allow transmission of the ultrasound beam.*

▶ de Bruyn R (ed): *Pediatric Ultrasound: How, Why and When*, 2nd edition (e-book). Philadelphia, Churchill Livingstone/Elsevier, 2010, pp 348–349.

▶ Rumack CM, Levine D (eds): *Diagnostic Ultrasound*, 5th edition. Philadelphia, Elsevier, 2018, pp 1710, 1714–1715.

▶ Siegel MJ (ed): *Pediatric Sonography*, 4th edition. Philadelphia, Lippincott Williams & Wilkins, 2011, p 175.

138. B. Hypoechoic.

The thymus is a mediastinal bilobed gland that can be easily evaluated with ultrasound in the first decade of life. The thymus gland is located anterior to the aortic arch (great vessels) and trachea. The thymus appears hypoechoic and homogeneous (or slightly heterogeneous) with well-defined smooth borders. Upon Doppler interrogation, the thymus appears hypovascular or nearly avascular. This characteristic often helps to differentiate the normal thymus from a mediastinal mass. The left lobe of the thymus is triangular, and the right lobe has an inverted teardrop shape. The thymus gland varies in size depending on the age of the patient and is largest in the first two years of life. In adulthood, the thymus begins to involute and is progressively replaced by fat.

▶ de Bruyn R (ed): *Pediatric Ultrasound: How, Why and When*, 2nd edition (e-book). Philadelphia, Churchill Livingstone/Elsevier, 2010, p 285.

▶ Rumack CM, Levine D (eds): *Diagnostic Ultrasound*, 5th edition. Philadelphia, Elsevier, 2018, p 1723.

▶ Siegel MJ (ed): *Pediatric Sonography*, 4th edition. Philadelphia, Lippincott Williams & Wilkins, 2011, p 165.

139. D. Bochdalek hernia.

A congenital diaphragmatic hernia is a defect in the diaphragm in which there is incomplete closure of the pleuroperitoneal membrane during the embryologic stage. Bochdalek and Morgagni hernias are two different types of congenital diaphragmatic hernias. Bochdalek hernias occur in the posterolateral portion of the diaphragm, while Morgagni hernias are anterior in location. Bochdalek hernias are more often seen in the left side, and there can be herniation of the left lobe of the liver, spleen, stomach, intestines, and left kidney. A Spigelian hernia is a defect of the anterior abdominal wall lateral to the rectus abdominus. A hiatal hernia is a defect in which part of the stomach is herniated through the diaphragm into the chest. Hiatal hernias are not a type of congenital diaphragmatic defect.

▶ de Bruyn R (ed): *Pediatric Ultrasound: How, Why and When*, 2nd edition (e-book). Philadelphia, Churchill Livingstone/Elsevier, 2010, p 344.

▶ Siegel MJ (ed): *Pediatric Sonography*, 4th edition. Philadelphia, Lippincott Williams & Wilkins, 2011, p 188.

140. **A. Anterior.**

The mediastinum is a cavity that separates the lungs. The mediastinum is divided into anterior, middle, posterior, and superior. The anterior mediastinum contains the thymus and lymph nodes. The middle mediastinum contains the heart, the proximal great vessels, lymph nodes, the right and left phrenic nerves, and the trachea. The posterior mediastinum contains the esophagus, the descending aorta, the azygos veins, and lymph nodes. The superior mediastinum contains the superior vena cava (SVC), the right and left brachiocephalic vein, the brachiocephalic artery, the aortic arch, the left common carotid and subclavian arteries, the trachea, and the esophagus.

▶ Marsh P, Jones J: Mediastinum. Available from Radiopaedia at https://radiopaedia.org/articles/mediastinum.

▶ Rumack CM, Levine D (eds): *Diagnostic Ultrasound*, 5th edition. Philadelphia, Elsevier, 2018, p 1723.

▶ Siegel MJ (ed): *Pediatric Sonography*, 4th edition. Philadelphia, Lippincott Williams & Wilkins, 2011, pp 165–166.

141. **C. Transudative pleural effusion.**

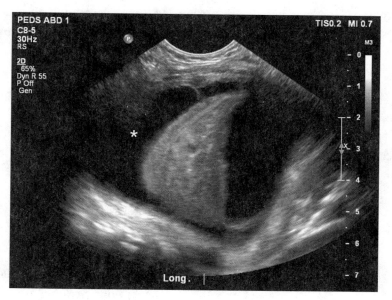

Pleural effusion is the accumulation of fluid within the pleural cavity. Two different types of effusions are transudative, *consisting of clear serous fluid, and* exudative, *consisting of purulent and loculated fluid. In this image, clear anechoic fluid—marked with an asterisk (*)—is seen in the pleural space, representing a transudative pleural effusion.* Empyema *and* hemothorax *are complex types of pleural effusion in which there is accumulation of pus and blood respectively.*

The most common type of pleural effusion in childhood is the parapneumonic effusion, which is most commonly caused by bacterial pneumonias.

▸ de Bruyn R (ed): *Pediatric Ultrasound: How, Why and When*, 2nd edition (e-book). Philadelphia, Churchill Livingstone/Elsevier, 2010, pp 348–351.
▸ Rumack CM, Levine D (eds): *Diagnostic Ultrasound*, 5th edition. Philadelphia, Elsevier, 2018, p 1702.
▸ Siegel MJ (ed): *Pediatric Sonography*, 4th edition. Philadelphia, Lippincott Williams & Wilkins, 2011, pp 171–173.

142. **C. Diaphragm.**

The diaphragm *is a dome-shaped sheet of muscle and tendons that border the inferior portion of the chest, separating it from the abdominal cavity. The diaphragm incorporates the most important muscle used for respiration. Sonographically, the diaphragm appears as a hyperechoic smooth band that can be visualized in longitudinal and axial planes. The right hemidiaphragm is higher than the left and easier to image due to the scanning window that the liver provides. The left hemidiaphragm can be difficult to see due to gas from the stomach and colon. Both hemidiaphragms can be evaluated at the same time in an axial plane for motion during inspiration and expiration. The* thymus *is a mediastinal gland of lymphoid tissue and produces hormones that stimulate the development of T-cells. The* pleura *is a serous membrane that covers the walls of the thoracic cavity and the lungs. The* mediastinum *is the space in the middle of the chest between the two pleural sacs.*

▸ de Bruyn R (ed): *Pediatric Ultrasound: How, Why and When*, 2nd edition (e-book). Philadelphia, Churchill Livingstone/Elsevier, 2010, pp 344–347.
▸ Siegel MJ (ed): *Pediatric Sonography*, 4th edition. Philadelphia, Lippincott Williams & Wilkins, 2011, pp 166, 169–170.

143. **A. Bronchopulmonary sequestration.**

Bronchopulmonary sequestration *is a condition resulting in a nonfunctional mass of pulmonary tissue that has no communication with the tracheobronchial tree. This mass receives its blood supply directly from the aorta (systemic supply) in about 75% of the cases. Ultrasound can be used to demonstrate the blood supply with the use of color Doppler, which helps in the confirmation of the diagnosis.* Congenital pulmonary airway malformation *(CPAM, formerly known as congenital cystic adenomatoid malformation of the lung or CCAML) is a mass of abnormal lung tissue that receives its* blood supply from the pulmonary circulation (normal vascular supply). Teratomas *are complex masses that on Doppler interrogation appear hypovascular or avascular. A* pulmonary arteriovenous malformation *(PAVM) refers to an abnormal communication between a pulmonary artery and vein.*

▸ de Bruyn R (ed): *Pediatric Ultrasound: How, Why and When*, 2nd edition (e-book). Philadelphia, Churchill Livingstone/Elsevier, 2010, pp 28, 343–344.
▸ Rumack CM, Levine D (eds): *Diagnostic Ultrasound*, 5th edition. Philadelphia, Elsevier, 2018, pp 1715–1716.
▸ Siegel MJ (ed): *Pediatric Sonography*, 4th edition. Philadelphia, Lippincott Williams & Wilkins, 2011, pp 178–184.

144. **B. Anterior.**

    A Morgagni hernia *is a type of congenital diaphragmatic hernia that occurs in the anterior portion of the diaphragm. Morgagni hernias are more commonly seen in the right hemidiaphragm and can contain liver, transverse colon, and omentum. Morgagni hernias are associated with trisomy 21 and pentalogy of Cantrell.*

    ▸ de Bruyn R (ed): *Pediatric Ultrasound: How, Why and When*, 2nd edition (e-book). Philadelphia, Churchill Livingstone/Elsevier, 2010, p 344.
    ▸ Siegel MJ (ed): *Pediatric Sonography*, 4th edition. Philadelphia, Lippincott Williams & Wilkins, 2011, pp 188–189.

145. **D. Lymphoma.**

    Lymphomas *are among the most common malignant mediastinal masses encountered in childhood. Lymphomas of the chest are typically located in the anterior mediastinum, which is rarely the site of primary involvement. Hodgkin lymphomas are more common than non-Hodgkin. Mediastinal lymphomas can cause lymphadenopathy and large pleural effusions.* Pleuropulmonary blastomas *are rare neoplasms in children and can arise from the lungs and pleura.* Congenital pulmonary airway malformation *(CPAM, formerly known as congenital cystic adenomatoid malformation of the lung or CCAML) is a pulmonary (not mediastinal) mass.* Thymomas *are rare tumors of the thymus gland, located in the anterior mediastinum; they grow slowly and are usually benign but can be malignant.*

    ▸ de Bruyn R (ed): *Pediatric Ultrasound: How, Why and When*, 2nd edition (e-book). Philadelphia, Churchill Livingstone/Elsevier, 2010, pp 347–348.
    ▸ Rumack CM, Levine D (eds): *Diagnostic Ultrasound*, 5th edition. Philadelphia, Elsevier, 2018, pp 1723–1724.
    ▸ Siegel MJ (ed): *Pediatric Sonography*, 4th edition. Philadelphia, Lippincott Williams & Wilkins, 2011, pp 178, 182–184.

146. D. Gastroesophageal reflux.

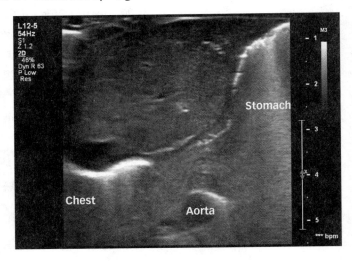

Gastroesophageal reflux *is the retrograde flow of fluid from the stomach into the esophagus. When a patient is referred for ultrasound to rule out pyloric stenosis, one of the differential diagnoses is gastroesophageal reflux. On ultrasound, fluid can be seen moving backward from the stomach into the esophagus at the esophageal junction. Gastroesophageal reflux is usually best demonstrated with real-time (dynamic) imaging. If the transducer is placed in the subxiphoid area, the gastroesophageal junction will be seen anterior to the aorta. Because the evaluation of the esophagus is limited on ultrasound, fluoroscopy and endoscopy are the modalities of choice to make this diagnosis.*

▸ de Bruyn R (ed): *Pediatric Ultrasound: How, Why and When*, 2nd edition (e-book). Philadelphia, Churchill Livingstone/Elsevier, 2010, p 184.
▸ Rumack CM, Levine D (eds): *Diagnostic Ultrasound*, 5th edition. Philadelphia, Elsevier, 2018, p 1834.
▸ Siegel MJ (ed): *Pediatric Sonography*, 4th edition. Philadelphia, Lippincott Williams & Wilkins, 2011, pp 168, 339.

147. C. Pleura.

The pleura *is a serous membrane that covers the walls of the thoracic cavity and the lungs. There are two pleural layers, the visceral pleura and the parietal pleura. The visceral pleura lines the lungs, while the parietal pleura lines the thoracic cavity. Both of these layers mark the border of the pleural cavity. A* synovial membrane *is a membrane formed by connective tissue that covers the joint cavities. The* peritoneum *is the serous membrane that lines the abdominal cavity. The* pericardium *is the serous membrane that surrounds the heart.*

▸ Siegel MJ (ed): *Pediatric Sonography*, 4th edition. Philadelphia, Lippincott Williams & Wilkins, 2011, pp 166–168.

148. B. Diaphragmatic paralysis.

Diaphragmatic paralysis is most commonly associated with phrenic nerve injury. Some of the causes of phrenic nerve injury are thoracic surgery and trauma. Diaphragmatic paralysis refers to an absent or paradoxical (opposite to normal) movement of the diaphragm. In normal breathing, the diaphragm moves downward with inspiration and upward with expiration. Evaluation of the movement of both hemidiaphragms can be performed by placing the transducer transverse in the subxiphoid window and angling upward toward the diaphragm. This method allows visualization of both sides for comparison purposes. Acquiring a cineloop and using M-mode imaging are also helpful tools when evaluation of the diaphragmatic motion is needed.

▶ de Bruyn R (ed): *Pediatric Ultrasound: How, Why and When*, 2nd edition (e-book). Philadelphia, Churchill Livingstone/Elsevier, 2010, pp 345–347.
▶ Rumack CM, Levine D (eds): *Diagnostic Ultrasound*, 5th edition. Philadelphia, Elsevier, 2018, p 1716.
▶ Siegel MJ (ed): *Pediatric Sonography*, 4th edition. Philadelphia, Lippincott Williams & Wilkins, 2011, pp 190–191.

149. A. Thoracentesis.

Thoracentesis is an invasive procedure in which a needle with a syringe is inserted into the chest with the purpose of aspirating a fluid collection. Ultrasound can be used before the procedure to help determine the type of fluid collection to be drained. Ultrasound is also helpful for guidance during the procedure and for site marking. Paracentesis *is a similar procedure, in which the fluid is aspirated from the abdominal cavity.* Amniocentesis *refers to the aspiration of amniotic fluid from a pregnant patient.* Pericardiocentesis *is the aspiration of pericardial fluid. All these procedures can be done for diagnostic or therapeutic purposes and need to be performed in a clean, sterile area using sterile technique.*

▶ Rumack CM, Levine D (eds): *Diagnostic Ultrasound*, 5th edition. Philadelphia, Elsevier, 2018, pp 1724–1725.
▶ Siegel MJ (ed): *Pediatric Sonography*, 4th edition. Philadelphia, Lippincott Williams & Wilkins, 2011, pp 686–687, 692–693.

150. B. Lung consolidation.

Lung consolidation *occurs when the lung is filled with liquid instead of air, causing swelling or hardening of the lung tissue. Consolidation can occur as a result of pneumonia, as blood cells and exudate accumulate within the lung bronchi* and alveoli. Liquid-filled bronchi appear as cystic tubular structures within the lung, and the use of color Doppler helps to differentiate them from blood vessels. The fact that the lungs are filled with liquid, not air, allows transmission of the ultrasound beam, causing "hepatization" of the lung. Atelectasis *occurs when there is partial or complete collapse of the lung (not fluid-filled lung). This condition also allows ultrasound transmission.* Bronchopulmonary sequestration *refers to a mass of nonfunctional lung tissue that receives its blood supply from the systemic circulation (aorta).* Pneumothorax *is a condition in which the pleural space is filled with air, which will not allow ultrasound transmission.*

▸ de Bruyn R (ed): *Pediatric Ultrasound: How, Why and When*, 2nd edition (e-book). Philadelphia, Churchill Livingstone/Elsevier, 2010, p 348.
▸ Siegel MJ (ed): *Pediatric Sonography*, 4th edition. Philadelphia, Lippincott Williams & Wilkins, 2011, pp 175–177, 179.

151. **C. Thymoma.**

Thymomas *are rare and most commonly benign anterior mediastinal masses that affect the thymus. Thymomas are uncommon masses in children and usually affect adults in their fourth and fifth decades of life.* Neuroblastomas, ganglioneuromas, *and* ganglioneuroblastomas *are neurogenic tumors that affect the posterior mediastinum. Posterior mediastinal masses are more common in young infants.*

▸ Rumack CM, Levine D (eds): *Diagnostic Ultrasound*, 5th edition. Philadelphia, Elsevier, 2018, pp 1723–1724.
▸ Siegel MJ (ed): *Pediatric Sonography*, 4th edition. Philadelphia, Lippincott Williams & Wilkins, 2011, p 185.
▸ Stöppler MC: Thymoma. Available at https://www.medicinenet.com/thymoma/article.htm.

152. **D. Congenital pulmonary airway malformation (CPAM).**

Congenital pulmonary airway malformation *(CPAM, formerly known as congenital cystic adenomatoid malformation of the lung or CCAML), is a congenital abnormality where a benign mass of abnormal lung tissue has normal communication with the bronchial tree. This abnormality is usually detected prenatally, and in the postnatal stage ultrasound plays a much smaller role. CPAM can have multiple appearances, ranging from single or multiple large or small cysts (most common) to a solid lesion composed of microscopic cysts; regardless* of cystic structure, CPAM is always avascular in appearance on ultrasound. Lymphomas most commonly involve the mediastinum in older children and adolescents. Thymic cysts are also mediastinal lesions and are typically unilocular. Lymphangiomas are, like CPAM, congenital but arise mostly from the posterior mediastinum.

▸ de Bruyn R (ed): *Pediatric Ultrasound: How, Why and When*, 2nd edition (e-book). Philadelphia, Churchill Livingstone/Elsevier, 2010, pp 27–28, 344.
▸ Rumack CM, Levine D (eds): *Diagnostic Ultrasound*, 5th edition. Philadelphia, Elsevier, 2018, pp 1715–1716.
▸ Siegel MJ (ed): *Pediatric Sonography*, 4th edition. Philadelphia, Lippincott Williams & Wilkins, 2011, pp 178, 184–185.

153. C. Gliding sign.

The sonographic appearance of normal free movement between the visceral pleura/lung and the parietal pleura during respiration is known as the "gliding sign." Evaluation of this movement is important because in cases of pneumothorax, this gliding motion disappears. The characteristic comet-tail artifact is also replaced by homogeneous posterior acoustic shadowing. Normally, pneumothorax can be diagnosed easily with plain chest radiography.

▸ Husain LF, Hagopian L, Wayman D, et al: Sonographic diagnosis of pneumothorax. J Emerg Trauma Shock 5:76–81, 2012.
▸ Siegel MJ (ed): *Pediatric Sonography*, 4th edition. Philadelphia, Lippincott Williams & Wilkins, 2011, pp 166, 175.
▸ Tsai T-H, Yan P-C: Ultrasound diagnosis and management of plural disease. Curr Opin Pulm Med 4:282[en]290, 2003.

154. A. Lungs.

The mediastinum is the space between the lungs, and it contains all the chest viscera except the pleura and the lungs. Some of the main structures located within the mediastinum are the heart, the origin of the great vessels, the esophagus, the trachea, the thymus, and lymph nodes. The superior mediastinum is easy to evaluate on ultrasound, especially in very young children.

▸ de Bruyn R (ed): *Pediatric Ultrasound: How, Why and When*, 2nd edition (e-book). Philadelphia, Churchill Livingstone/Elsevier, 2010, pp 342–343, 347–348.
▸ Siegel MJ (ed): *Pediatric Sonography,* 4th edition. Philadelphia, Lippincott Williams & Wilkins, 2011, p 183.

155. **D. Bacterial pneumonia.**

Bacterial pneumonias *can lead to exudative (complex) and transudative (serous) pleural effusions. The most common causes of pleural effusions in childhood are bacteria such as* Staphylococcus aureus *and* Streptococcus pneumoniae. Congestive heart failure, renal failure, *and* cirrhosis *are conditions that can cause transudative pleural effusions.*

▶ Siegel MJ (ed): *Pediatric Sonography*, 4th edition. Philadelphia, Lippincott Williams & Wilkins, 2011, p 171.

PART 5

Liver

156. B. Glisson's capsule.

Glisson's capsule *is the name of the protective outer capsule of the liver. The connective tissue surrounds the liver, bile ducts, portal vein, and hepatic artery. Francis Glisson, a medical professor in Cambridge, England, first gave the account of his discovery in 1654.* Gerota's fascia *is connective tissue that encapsulates the kidneys.* Peritoneum *is not made of connective tissue but instead is a serous membrane.* Mesentery *is a ligamentous structure that connects the small bowel and portions of the colon to the back of the abdominal wall.*

▸ Launois B, Jamieson GG: The importance of Glisson's capsule and its sheaths in the intrahepatic approach to resection of the liver. Surg Gynecol Obstet 174:7–10, 1992. Available at https://www.ncbi.nlm.nih.gov/pubmed/1729755/.

▸ Siegel MJ (ed): *Pediatric Sonography*, 4th edition. Philadelphia, Lippincott Williams & Wilkins, 2011, pp 323, 435.

157. B. Umbilical vein.

During fetal development, the right and left lobes of the fetal liver are about the same size until the umbilical vein starts supplying the right lobe with nutrient-rich, oxygenated blood from the placenta. In utero, the umbilical vein enters the fetal liver in the left branch of the portal vein in what is called the umbilical recess. *The umbilical vein runs along the lower margin of the falciform ligament, which extends from the fetal umbilicus to the liver. After birth, the umbilical vein will close and become the echogenic* ligamentum teres, *also known as the* round ligament. *The* umbilical arteries *take oxygen-depleted blood from the fetus back to the placenta. The* hepatic artery *and* vein *do not play a full role prenatally, since the liver is not yet fully functional and the majority of blood flows into the liver through the umbilical vein.*

▸ de Bruyn R (ed): *Pediatric Ultrasound: How, Why and When*, 2nd edition (e-book). Philadelphia, Churchill Livingstone/Elsevier, 2010, pp 132, 182.

▸ Rumack CM, Levine D (eds): *Diagnostic Ultrasound*, 5th edition. Philadelphia, Elsevier, 2018, p 1059.

▸ Siegel MJ (ed): *Pediatric Sonography*, 4th edition. Philadelphia, Lippincott Williams & Wilkins, 2011, pp 215, 217.

158. C. Celiac axis.

A The Abdominal Vasculature

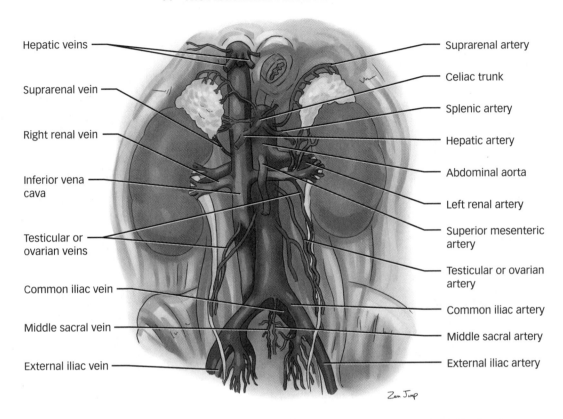

See Color Plate 13 on page xxxviii.

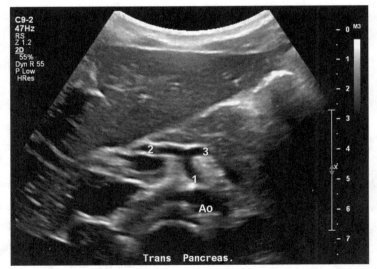

A *Diagram of the abdominal vasculature.* ***B*** *In this transverse image of the epigastric region, the celiac axis (1) is seen arising from the anterior wall of the aorta and branching into the hepatic artery (2) and the splenic artery (3). The superior mesenteric artery (SMA) arises from the anterior wall of the aorta. The SMA runs parallel to the aorta, unlike the celiac*

axis, which runs perpendicular to the aorta. The SMA would be visualized posterior to the body of the pancreas and the splenic vein in the transverse plane.

▸ Rumack CM, Levine D (eds): *Diagnostic Ultrasound*, 5th edition. Philadelphia, Elsevier, 2018, p 211.

▸ Siegel MJ (ed): *Pediatric Sonography*, 4th edition. Philadelphia, Lippincott Williams & Wilkins, 2011, p 219.

159. **D. Riedel lobe.**

Usually, the right lobe of the liver will extend just to, or slightly below, the right kidney. The Riedel lobe *is a common anatomic variant consisting of a tongue-like projection of the right lobe of the liver extending farther below the right kidney than normal. It is important to be aware of its morphology and sonographic appearance, since it can often be confused with an abdominal mass or hepatomegaly.* The quadrate lobe *(Couinaud segment 4B) is located in the mid undersurface of the right liver, inferior to the portal vein.* The caudate lobe *(Couinaud segment 1) is a smaller, midline liver lobe located superior to the portal vein.* A succenturiate lobe *is a variant accessory placental lobe sometimes seen in obstetric sonography.*

▸ de Bruyn R (ed): *Pediatric Ultrasound: How, Why and When*, 2nd edition (e-book). Philadelphia, Churchill Livingstone/Elsevier, 2010, p 134.

▸ Rumack CM, Levine D (eds): *Diagnostic Ultrasound*, 5th edition. Philadelphia, Elsevier, 2018, p 80.

▸ Siegel MJ (ed): *Pediatric Sonography*, 4th edition. Philadelphia, Lippincott Williams & Wilkins, 2011, pp 214–215.

160. **A. Albumin.**

In the event of liver damage or disease, albumin levels are decreased, not increased. Albumin *is a protein made in the liver that helps to keep fluid in the bloodstream from leaking out of the vessels and into surrounding tissues. Albumin can carry medicines, hormones, and enzymes through the body to help it function properly.* Alanine transaminase *(ALT),* aspartate transaminase *(AST), and* alkaline phosphatase *(ALP) are liver enzymes that are elevated in the presence of liver damage or disease. ALT and AST are specific markers for liver function. ALP is an enzyme made in the liver, bones, and intestines and aids in breaking down proteins.*

▸ Keough J: *Nursing Laboratory and Diagnostic Tests Demystified*, 2nd edition. New York, McGraw-Hill, 2017, pp 9–10, 144–147, 152–155.

161. B. Situs inversus.

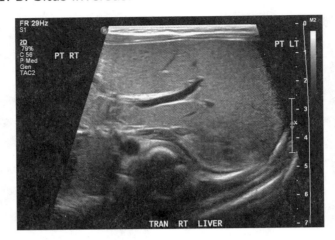

Situs solitus *is the normal positioning of the abdominal and thoracic organs.* Situs inversus, *as seen here, is the "flipped" or mirror image of the anatomy, opposite to the normal positioning of the abdominal and thoracic contents. In situs inversus, the liver and gallbladder are on the left side of the body and the stomach and spleen are on the right. Situs inversus is seen in a very small percentage of the population and can be an isolated incident or can occur with a syndrome.* Riedel lobe *is the term for an anatomic variant of the liver, when the right lobe has a tongue-like projection extending below the right kidney.* Hemihypertrophy *describes the overgrowth of one side of the body and is a genetic disorder.*

▶ de Bruyn R (ed): *Pediatric Ultrasound: How, Why and When*, 2nd edition (e-book). Philadelphia, Churchill Livingstone/Elsevier, 2010, pp 134, 143, 166.

▶ Rumack CM, Levine D (eds): *Diagnostic Ultrasound*, 5th edition. Philadelphia, Elsevier, 2018, p 80.

▶ Siegel MJ (ed): *Pediatric Sonography*, 4th edition. Philadelphia, Lippincott Williams & Wilkins, 2011, p 225.

162. D. Ligamentum teres.

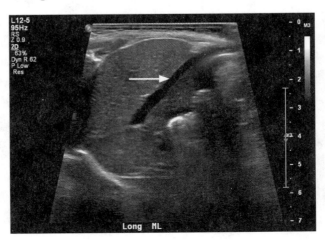

The fetal umbilical vein remnant (arrow) appears as an anechoic patent structure before it turns into the hyperechoic fibrous band known as the ligamentum teres *or round ligament. The ligamentum teres divides the left lobe of the liver into medial and lateral segments. It lies within the free edge of the falciform ligament. In cases of portal hypertension, the fetal umbilical vein remnant may recanalize and become a collateral for portal circulation. The* ligamentum venosum *is a remnant of the fetal ductus venosus. The fetal* urachus *is a canal between the fetal umbilicus and the bladder.*

▶ de Bruyn R (ed): *Pediatric Ultrasound: How, Why and When*, 2nd edition (e-book). Philadelphia, Churchill Livingstone/Elsevier, 2010, p 132.

▶ Siegel MJ (ed): *Pediatric Sonography*, 4th edition. Philadelphia, Lippincott Williams & Wilkins, 2011, pp 215, 450.

163. C. 10 mm.

Portal vein diameter and velocity may fluctuate with respiration and eating. In the pediatric setting, the portal vein diameter should not exceed 10 mm in a normal patient. In cases of portal hypertension, the portal vein will increase in diameter in the early stages, then later show decreased flow and pulsatility.

▶ de Bruyn R (ed): *Pediatric Ultrasound: How, Why and When*, 2nd edition (e-book). Philadelphia, Churchill Livingstone/Elsevier, 2010, p 135.

▶ Rumack CM, Levine D (eds): *Diagnostic Ultrasound*, 5th edition. Philadelphia, Elsevier, 2018, p 1750.

▶ Siegel MJ (ed): *Pediatric Sonography*, 4th edition. Philadelphia, Lippincott Williams & Wilkins, 2011, pp 222, 248–249.

164. D. Arteriovenous malformation (AVM).

In pediatric cases, arteriovenous malformations *(AVMs) within the liver are typically congenital abnormalities, but in the adult they are most often caused by a penetrating wound or biopsy. An AVM is formed when there are multiple blood vessels that have direct arteriovenous communication and shunting. Pediatric AVMs are usually located within one lobe or segment of the liver. The common malformations are portal vein to hepatic vein, portal vein to inferior vena cava, and hepatic artery to portal vein.* Focal nodular hyperplasia *(FNH) is a benign mass of the liver with a central fibrous scar.* Cirrhosis *and* cavernous transformation *are seen in advanced stages of liver disease. FNH, cirrhosis, and cavernous transformation are not congenital conditions.*

▶ Siegel MJ (ed): *Pediatric Sonography*, 4th edition. Philadelphia, Lippincott Williams & Wilkins, 2011, pp 257, 259.

165. B. Gastroesophageal varices.

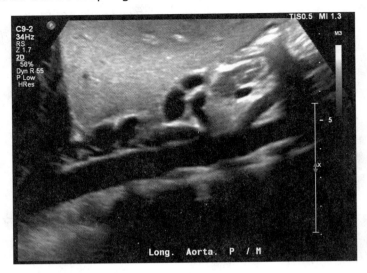

Gastroesophageal varices *are collateral vessels that occur in the gastroesophageal junction near the diaphragm, left lobe of the liver, and proximal aorta. Gastroesophageal varices result from portal hypertension, when the left gastric artery and branches of the splenic vein enlarge. On ultrasound, these varices appear as hypoechoic or anechoic tortuous vessels in the gastroesophageal junction.* Dilated bile ducts and cavernous transformation *would occur in the porta hepatis region.* Budd-Chiari syndrome *affects the hepatic veins.*

▸ de Bruyn R (ed): *Pediatric Ultrasound: How, Why and When*, 2nd edition (e-book). Philadelphia, Churchill Livingstone/Elsevier, 2010, pp 151–152.
▸ Rumack CM, Levine D (eds): *Diagnostic Ultrasound*, 5th edition. Philadelphia, Elsevier, 2018, p 1761.
▸ Siegel MJ (ed): *Pediatric Sonography*, 4th edition. Philadelphia, Lippincott Williams & Wilkins, 2011, pp 250–251, 255–256.

166. C. Fasting.

Fasting is the best exam preparation to help minimize abdominal gas. When a gallbladder is present, fasting assists the gallbladder to be well distended for abdominal sonography. The required time of NPO status (nil per os, or nothing by mouth—i.e., fasting) is dependent on the patient's age and can range from 2 to 8 hours.

▸ de Bruyn R (ed): *Pediatric Ultrasound: How, Why and When*, 2nd edition (e-book). Philadelphia, Churchill Livingstone/Elsevier, 2010, pp 183–184.
▸ Siegel MJ (ed): *Pediatric Sonography*, 4th edition. Philadelphia, Lippincott Williams & Wilkins, 2011, p 214.

167. **B. Right lateral decubitus.**

Patients can be positioned in a supine, left lateral decubitus, or left posterior oblique position when you are scanning the liver. Acoustic windows include subcostal and intercostal approaches. Due to the close proximity of the liver and diaphragm, it may be helpful to have the patient hold his or her breath to avoid motion on the images. The right lateral decubitus position is not optimal because it places the liver farthest from the transducer and also positions the liver beneath the stomach.

▶ de Bruyn R (ed): *Pediatric Ultrasound: How, Why and When*, 2nd edition (e-book). Philadelphia, Churchill Livingstone/Elsevier, 2010, pp 133, 136.
▶ Siegel MJ (ed): *Pediatric Sonography*, 4th edition. Philadelphia, Lippincott Williams & Wilkins, 2011, p 214.

168. **A. Undifferentiated embryonal sarcoma.**

Undifferentiated embryonal sarcoma of the liver is a rare malignant tumor also known as malignant mesenchymoma and hepatic mesenchymal sarcoma. Thought to be the malignant version of mesenchymal hamartoma, these sarcomas occur mainly between ages of 5 and 15. Clinical symptoms include abdominal mass and pain. The patient will usually have a normal AFP level. The sonographic appearance is a large, solitary, solid and complex-appearing mass. The prognosis for undifferentiated embryonal sarcoma is poor, with most patients surviving less than a year. The remaining choices are not rare tumors. Hepatoblastoma and hepatocellular carcinoma are the two most common liver malignancies in children. Hemangioendothelioma is the most common benign liver tumor in children.

▶ de Bruyn R (ed): *Pediatric Ultrasound: How, Why and When*, 2nd edition (e-book). Philadelphia, Churchill Livingstone/Elsevier, 2010, p 159.
▶ Rumack CM, Levine D (eds): *Diagnostic Ultrasound*, 5th edition. Philadelphia, Elsevier, 2018, pp 1746, 1748.
▶ Siegel MJ (ed): *Pediatric Sonography*, 4th edition. Philadelphia, Lippincott Williams & Wilkins, 2011, p 230.

169. D. Portal vein.

See Color Plate 13, "The Abdominal Vasculature," on page xxxviii.

The portal vein *carries blood from the spleen, mesentery, pancreas, and gallbladder to the liver. The portal vein provides the liver with up to 75% of its blood supply. The main portal vein divides into the right and left portal veins. The right portal vein divides into anterior and posterior branches. Portal vein flow should be antegrade (hepatopetal) and monophasic. In a normal sonogram, retrograde flow should be visualized only in the posterior branch of the right portal vein, as the flow is traveling away from the transducer during imaging. When compared to hepatic veins, portal veins have echogenic walls. Hepatic veins transport blood from the liver to the inferior vena cava. The* superior mesenteric vein *(SMV) drains blood from the intestines into the portal venous system at the portal splenic confluence. The* inferior mesenteric vein *carries blood from the large intestine and drains into the splenic vein.*

▸ de Bruyn R (ed): *Pediatric Ultrasound: How, Why and When*, 2nd edition (e-book). Philadelphia, Churchill Livingstone/Elsevier, 2010, pp 151–152.
▸ Rumack CM, Levine D (eds): *Diagnostic Ultrasound*, 5th edition. Philadelphia, Elsevier, 2018, pp 1731–1734.
▸ Siegel MJ (ed): *Pediatric Sonography*, 4th edition. Philadelphia, Lippincott Williams & Wilkins, 2011, pp 215–222.

170. B. Budd-Chiari syndrome.

Budd-Chiari syndrome *is characterized by the signs and symptoms of acute hepatic vein occlusion. In the acute stage, the patient has ascites, abdominal pain, jaundice, and hepatomegaly. Echogenic thrombus can be seen within the hepatic veins or at the level of the inferior vena cava. Budd-Chiari syndrome is a rare finding in children and may cause postsinusoidal hypertension.* Veno-occlusive disease *refers to the obstruction of smaller sublobular veins within the liver and is not generally visualized with ultrasound.* Portal vein thrombosis *and* cavernous transformation *occur within the portal vein, not the hepatic veins.*

▸ de Bruyn R (ed): *Pediatric Ultrasound: How, Why and When*, 2nd edition (e-book). Philadelphia, Churchill Livingstone/Elsevier, 2010, pp 134, 153.
▸ Rumack CM, Levine D (eds): *Diagnostic Ultrasound*, 5th edition. Philadelphia, Elsevier, 2018, pp 1762–1763.
▸ Siegel MJ (ed): *Pediatric Sonography*, 4th edition. Philadelphia, Lippincott Williams & Wilkins, 2011, pp 255–257.

171. A. Ligamentum venosum.

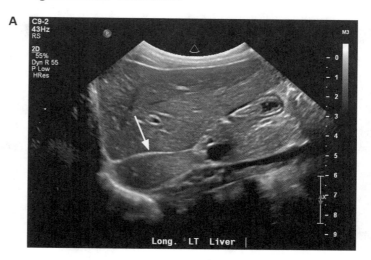

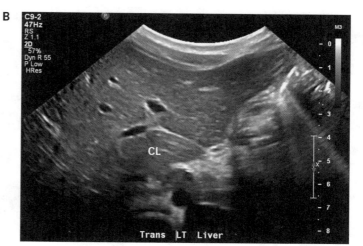

The ligamentum venosum *is a remnant of the ductus venosus. In image **A**, it is demonstrated in the longitudinal plane and appears as a hyperechoic linear structure (arrow). Its path courses along the inferior surface of the liver between the caudate lobe (segment 1) and the lateral segment of the left lobe (segment 2). On the transverse image (image **B**) it is seen anterior to the caudate lobe (CL). The* ligamentum teres, *also known as the* round ligament, *is a remnant of the umbilical vein and extends from the umbilicus to the anterior surface of the liver, running along the falciform ligament. The* falciform ligament, *also known as the* broad ligament, *is a peritoneal fold aiding in the attachment of the anterior surface of the liver to the anterior body wall.*

▶ de Bruyn R (ed): *Pediatric Ultrasound: How, Why and When*, 2nd edition (e-book). Philadelphia, Churchill Livingstone/Elsevier, 2010, pp 132–133.

▶ Rumack CM, Levine D (eds): *Diagnostic Ultrasound*, 5th edition. Philadelphia, Elsevier, 2018, p 1731.

▶ Siegel MJ (ed): *Pediatric Sonography*, 4th edition. Philadelphia, Lippincott Williams & Wilkins, 2011, pp 215–217.

172. **B. Hepatoblastoma.**

Hepatoblastoma is the most common malignant liver tumor in children. Fewer than 10% of hepatoblastomas occur in children over the age of 5; most occur before age 2. Hepatocellular carcinoma *is the second most common liver malignancy in children.* Embryonal sarcoma *is a rare tumor of mesenchymal origin.* Liver metastasis *is a secondary neoplasm most often seen with Wilms tumor, neuroblastoma, rhabdomyosarcoma, and lymphoma.*

▶ de Bruyn R (ed): *Pediatric Ultrasound: How, Why and When*, 2nd edition (e-book). Philadelphia, Churchill Livingstone/Elsevier, 2010, pp 139–141, 157.

▶ Rumack CM, Levine D (eds): *Diagnostic Ultrasound*, 5th edition. Philadelphia, Elsevier, 2018, pp 1746–1747.

▶ Siegel MJ (ed): *Pediatric Sonography*, 4th edition. Philadelphia, Lippincott Williams & Wilkins, 2011, pp 226–230.

173. **A. Bilirubin.**

The liver forms bilirubin *from the breakdown of red blood cells. Indirect/unconjugated bilirubin, which is not soluble in water, is carried to the liver by blood. Once in the liver, it is turned into direct/conjugated bilirubin, which is soluble in water and can then be excreted. Conjugated bilirubin lends its pigment to bile and gives feces its brown color.* Hemoglobin *provides the pigment to red blood cells.* Plasma *is the clear or straw-colored fluid component of blood.* Proteins *are molecular structures within the blood that form the structural components of cells or facilitate chemical reactions and do not affect the color of bile or feces.*

▶ Keough J: *Nursing Laboratory and Diagnostic Tests Demystified*, 2nd edition. New York, McGraw-Hill, 2017, pp 155–158.

174. **B. More echogenic than the right kidney cortex.**

After infancy, the normal liver parenchyma should appear more echogenic than the right kidney cortex. Prior to 6 months of age, it is considered normal for the liver to appear isoechoic to the right kidney cortex. The echogenicity of the renal medulla is not generally characterized as similar to the echogenicity of liver tissue, since it is more echogenic. Primarily, it is the renal cortex, not the renal medulla, that is compared to the liver and spleen, since the cortical tissue is adjacent to those organs. At all ages, the normal liver echotexture should appear smooth and homogeneous.

▸ de Bruyn R (ed): *Pediatric Ultrasound: How, Why and When*, 2nd edition (e-book). Philadelphia, Churchill Livingstone/Elsevier, 2010, p 134.

▸ Siegel MJ (ed): *Pediatric Sonography*, 4th edition. Philadelphia, Lippincott Williams & Wilkins, 2011, p 224.

175. **C. Pancreatic duct.**

See Color Plate 14 on page xxxix.

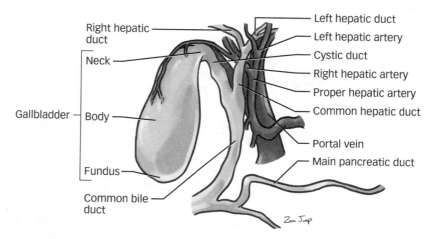

The Biliary Tree

The biliary tree *is made up of those organs and ducts that create and store bile to be released into the small intestine—the* common bile duct, common hepatic duct, *and* intrahepatic ducts. *The intrahepatic ducts are usually too small to be seen with sonography. Bile is drained from the gallbladder through the cystic duct. The* common hepatic duct *(CHD) is formed by the joining of the main right and left hepatic ducts; the CHD is intrahepatic. The cystic duct and the CHD combine to form the* common bile duct *(CBD). The CBD is extrahepatic and lies anterior and to the right of the main portal vein. The CBD and the main pancreatic duct unite at the ampulla of Vater. The intrahepatic ducts form the* portal triad *with the portal veins and hepatic arteries.*

▸ PubMed Health: Biliary tract. Available at https://www.ncbi.nlm.nih.gov/pubmedhealth/PMHT0018956/.

▸ Siegel MJ (ed): *Pediatric Sonography*, 4th edition. Philadelphia, Lippincott Williams & Wilkins, 2011, pp 276, 291.

176. A. Focal nodular hyperplasia (FNH).

Focal nodular hyperplasia (FNH) occurs in a very small percentage of children and is more common in adult females. It is usually asymptomatic, but when it is present in small children they can present with an abdominal mass. FNH is a hyperplastic tumor composed of hepatocytes, Kupffer cells, and bile ducts. On ultrasound, FNH appears as a solitary, well-circumscribed mass. It is usually isoechoic to the liver and has an echogenic fibrous or stellate scar within the center of the mass. Hemangiomas appear echogenic but do not contain a central stellate scar. Hemangioendotheliomas and hamartomas appear complex and can contain cystic spaces. Of these choices, only FNH displays a central stellate scar.

▸ de Bruyn R (ed): *Pediatric Ultrasound: How, Why and When*, 2nd edition (e-book). Philadelphia, Churchill Livingstone/Elsevier, 2010, pp 159–160.

▸ Rumack CM, Levine D (eds): *Diagnostic Ultrasound*, 5th edition. Philadelphia, Elsevier, 2018, p 1746.

▸ Siegel MJ (ed): *Pediatric Sonography*, 4th edition. Philadelphia, Lippincott Williams & Wilkins, 2011, pp 226–228.

177. D. Right hepatic vein.

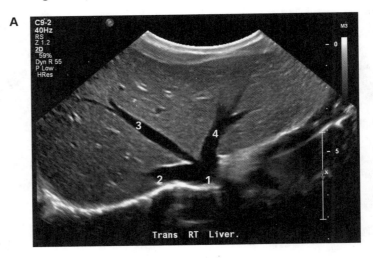

See Color Plate 16 on page xxxix.

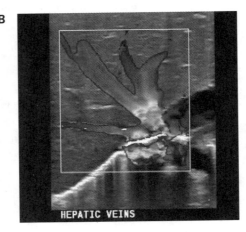

See Color Plate 13, "The Abdominal Vasculature," on page xxxviii.

A B-mode and **B** color Doppler images demonstrating the hepatic veins. The right hepatic vein (2), mid hepatic vein (3), and left hepatic vein (4) deliver blood from the liver into the cardiovascular circulation (visualized by color Doppler in image B) by draining into the inferior vena cava or IVC (1). Hepatic veins are best visualized from a subxiphoid approach. Their waveforms are normally triphasic, display hepatofugal flow, and can be affected by respiration.

▶ de Bruyn R (ed): *Pediatric Ultrasound: How, Why and When*, 2nd edition (e-book). Philadelphia, Churchill Livingstone/Elsevier, 2010, pp 134–135.

▶ Rumack CM, Levine D (eds): *Diagnostic Ultrasound*, 5th edition. Philadelphia, Elsevier, 2018, pp 1733–1734.

▶ Siegel MJ (ed): *Pediatric Sonography*, 4th edition. Philadelphia, Lippincott Williams & Wilkins, 2011, pp 219–223.

178. A. 1.

In the Couinaud system of hepatic segmental anatomy, the liver is divided into eight segments. The right and left lobes each have four segments. The caudate lobe is number 1 and the divisions are made and numbered in a clockwise direction from there. This numbering system was devised to assist surgeons performing liver resections.

▶ Rumack CM, Levine D (eds): *Diagnostic Ultrasound*, 5th edition. Philadelphia, Elsevier, 2018, pp 1731–1733.

▶ Siegel MJ (ed): *Pediatric Sonography*, 4th edition. Philadelphia, Lippincott Williams & Wilkins, 2011, pp 214–215.

179. C. Steatosis.

Steatosis is the replacement of damaged hepatocytes with fat cells, resulting in fatty infiltration of the liver. Causes include enzyme deficiencies, medications, metabolic disorders, and malnutrition. Effects may be reversible. *Fibrosis and cirrhosis occur when there is scarring and destruction of the hepatic parenchyma. Hepatitis is a viral disorder that causes liver inflammation and damage.* On ultrasound, fibrosis, cirrhosis, and hepatitis have a more diffuse effect on the liver parenchyma, whereas fatty infiltration secondary to steatosis can appear focal or diffuse.

▶ de Bruyn R (ed): *Pediatric Ultrasound: How, Why and When*, 2nd edition (e-book). Philadelphia, Churchill Livingstone/Elsevier, 2010, pp 149–150.

▶ Rumack CM, Levine D (eds): *Diagnostic Ultrasound*, 5th edition. Philadelphia, Elsevier, 2018, p 1740.

▶ Siegel MJ (ed): *Pediatric Sonography*, 4th edition. Philadelphia, Lippincott Williams & Wilkins, 2011, pp 240, 244, 247.

180. **D. Decreased flow of the hepatic artery.**

Sonographic signs of portal vein hypertension include decreased portal venous inflow, which causes the portal vein diameter to dilate, portosystemic collaterals to appear, diminished portal vein pulsatility, and bidirectional or reversed portal vein flow. In an effort to continue supplying the liver with adequate blood perfusion, the hepatic artery diameter and velocity will increase, not decrease.

▶ de Bruyn R (ed): *Pediatric Ultrasound: How, Why and When*, 2nd edition (e-book). Philadelphia, Churchill Livingstone/Elsevier, 2010, pp 151–152.
▶ Rumack CM, Levine D (eds): *Diagnostic Ultrasound*, 5th edition. Philadelphia, Elsevier, 2018, pp 1750, 1752–1755.
▶ Siegel MJ (ed): *Pediatric Sonography*, 4th edition. Philadelphia, Lippincott Williams & Wilkins, 2011, pp 248–252.

181. **B. Inferior vena cava (IVC).**

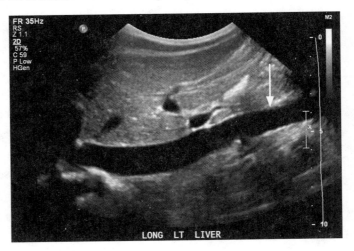

The inferior vena cava (IVC) lies within the retroperitoneum. It courses from the confluence of the common iliac veins and extends across the liver to drain into the right atrium of the heart. The IVC lies anterior to the right renal artery and posterior to the liver, duodenum, and pancreas. The walls of the IVC are less echogenic than the aorta and portal vein. The diameter of the IVC will increase with inspiration and decrease with expiration. With Doppler, the proximal IVC is triphasic near the hepatic veins. As sampling is done more distally, the waveform becomes less pulsatile and can become monophasic. The aorta is a midline structure that also lies within the retroperitoneum but does not traverse the liver. Within the peritoneum, the portal vein lies within the porta hepatis near the posterior surface of the right lobe of the liver.

In congenital absence or obstruction of the IVC, an enlarged azygos vein may be present as a collateral vessel. The azygos vein runs parallel to the IVC, to the right of the thoracic vertebrae.

▸ de Bruyn R (ed): *Pediatric Ultrasound: How, Why and When*, 2nd edition (e-book). Philadelphia, Churchill Livingstone/Elsevier, 2010, p 135.
▸ Rumack CM, Levine D (eds): *Diagnostic Ultrasound*, 5th edition. Philadelphia, Elsevier, 2018, pp 456–457.
▸ Siegel MJ (ed): *Pediatric Sonography*, 4th edition. Philadelphia, Lippincott Williams & Wilkins, 2011, pp 495–497.

182. C. Jaundice.

Jaundice occurs when there is excess bilirubin in the bloodstream. Bilirubin is the yellow pigment released from red blood cells. In the first few weeks of life, infants cannot remove bilirubin from the liver and into the intestinal tract through the bloodstream fast enough, so physiologic jaundice may occur. After early infancy, the liver is matured and jaundice would be an uncommon occurrence, raising the suspicion for hepatobiliary disease. Neonatal hepatitis, cholestasis, and biliary obstruction or atresia may be causes.

▸ de Bruyn R (ed): *Pediatric Ultrasound: How, Why and When*, 2nd edition (e-book). Philadelphia, Churchill Livingstone/Elsevier, 2010, pp 142–144.
▸ Mayo Clinic: Infant jaundice. Available at https://www.mayoclinic.org/diseases conditions/infant jaundice/symptoms causes/syc 20373865.
▸ Rumack CM, Levine D (eds): *Diagnostic Ultrasound*, 5th edition. Philadelphia, Elsevier, 2018, pp 1734–1740.
▸ Siegel MJ (ed): *Pediatric Sonography*, 4th edition. Philadelphia, Lippincott Williams & Wilkins, 2011, pp 240, 291–292.

183. B. Air in the portal vein.

Air in the portal vein or portal venous gas can occur in neonates following necrotizing enterocolitis (NEC). NEC may be seen within the first month of neonatal life and can range from mucosal injury to perforation or even death of bowel segments. Infarcted bowel in older children may also exhibit air in the portal vein on ultrasound. The sonographic appearance of portal venous gas is echogenic foci moving within the walls of the portal vein. Reverberation or shadowing artifacts may also be seen. With perforated bowel, gas may be seen within the walls of the gallbladder as well. NEC is not associated with portal vein thrombosis, hypertension, or obstruction.

▸ de Bruyn R (ed): *Pediatric Ultrasound: How, Why and When*, 2nd edition (e-book). Philadelphia, Churchill Livingstone/Elsevier, 2010, p 198.

▶ Rumack CM, Levine D (eds): *Diagnostic Ultrasound*, 5th edition. Philadelphia, Elsevier, 2018, p 1855.

▶ Siegel MJ (ed): *Pediatric Sonography*, 4th edition. Philadelphia, Lippincott Williams & Wilkins, 2011, p 261.

184. D. Cirrhosis.

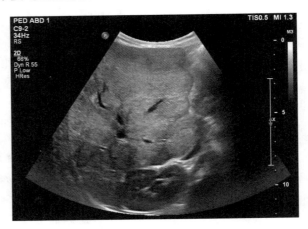

Cirrhosis *is the term used to describe the parenchymal scarring and destruction of the liver caused by chronic disease processes. Fibrosis and nodular changes occur. On ultrasound (as seen here), the liver parenchyma has a coarse, heterogeneous appearance with an increased echogenicity. The echotexture makes it difficult to penetrate with the sound beam. Caudate lobe enlargement is common. Liver borders may appear nodular. The vascular channels within the liver can become obstructed due to the scarring. Ascites and portal hypertension may be present in severe cases. Clinical symptoms include hepatomegaly, abdominal distention, and jaundice. Sonographically,* liver metastases, hydatid disease, and hepatic granulomas *would all demonstrate focal, well-circumscribed lesions within the liver margins and not diffuse parenchymal destruction or nodular liver borders.*

▶ de Bruyn R (ed): *Pediatric Ultrasound: How, Why and When*, 2nd edition (e-book). Philadelphia, Churchill Livingstone/Elsevier, 2010, pp 149–150.

▶ Rumack CM, Levine D (eds): *Diagnostic Ultrasound*, 5th edition. Philadelphia, Elsevier, 2018, pp 1741–1742.

▶ Siegel MJ (ed): *Pediatric Sonography*, 4th edition. Philadelphia, Lippincott Williams & Wilkins, 2011, pp 230, 242, 243, 247–248.

185. A. *Echinococcus granulosus*.

The parasitic adult tapeworm Echinococcus granulosus *is the source of hydatid disease. This parasite lives in the intestines of dogs. The eggs of the parasite are carried through the dog's feces and transmitted to livestock and humans. This disease is more often seen in the Middle East, northern Canada,* and the southern United States. With hydatid disease, the sonographic appearance of the liver includes multiple complex cysts of varying sizes within the liver parenchyma. These lesions are treated medically or surgically. Percutaneous aspiration or drainage may be necessary. Amoebae and Ascaris lumbricoides *(roundworm)* cause hepatic abscesses. Schistosomae *(flatworms)* have a more diffuse effect on the liver, causing a granulomatous response that leads to portal hypertension and portal vein occlusion.

▶ de Bruyn R (ed): *Pediatric Ultrasound: How, Why and When*, 2nd edition (e-book). Philadelphia, Churchill Livingstone/Elsevier, 2010, pp 155–156.

▶ Rumack CM, Levine D (eds): *Diagnostic Ultrasound*, 5th edition. Philadelphia, Elsevier, 2018, pp 1747–1748.

▶ Siegel MJ (ed): *Pediatric Sonography*, 4th edition. Philadelphia, Lippincott Williams & Wilkins, 2011, pp 242–243.

186. **B. Lymphoproliferative disorder.**

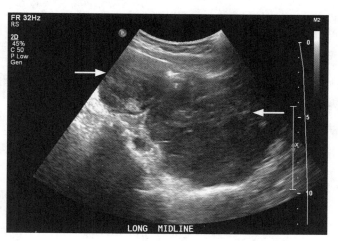

Due to patient immunosuppression, one of the complications following liver or kidney transplants is post-transplant lymphoproliferative disorder *(PTLD)*. The sonographic appearance of PTLD includes heterogeneous, infiltrative, solid focal lesions *(arrows)*. Seromas and bilomas may occur as post-transplant complications that appear simple, anechoic, and well circumscribed. Right adrenal hemorrhage is a complication of liver transplantation that can occur during the anastomoses stage and will appear as a right-sided suprarenal, complex, or echogenic mass.

▶ Borhani A, Hosseinzadeh K, Almusa O, et al: Imaging of posttransplantation lymphoproliferative disorder after solid organ transplantation. *RadioGraphics* 29:981–1000, 2009. Available at https://doi.org/10.1148/rg.294095020.

▶ Heller M: Liver transplant ultrasound. Available at https://iame.com/online/liver_transplant_ultrasound/content.php.

▶ Shum DF, Kim T, Poder L: Sonographic evaluation of abdominal transplants: a practical approach. Applied Radiology, July 2013. Available at http://appliedradiology.com/articles/sonographic-evaluation-of-abdominal-transplants-a-practical-approach.
▶ Siegel MJ (ed): *Pediatric Sonography*, 4th edition. Philadelphia, Lippincott Williams & Wilkins, 2011, pp 268, 447.

187. **C. Falciform ligament.**

The falciform ligament *is often seen in transverse as a hyperechoic linear structure at the junction of the right and left hepatic lobes. The falciform ligament is vertically oriented and connects the anterior surface of the liver to the anterior body wall. On a transverse image, the* ligamentum teres, *also known as the* round ligament, *appears hyperechoic and round just to the right of midline and the head of the pancreas. The* ligamentum venosum *will appear as a more horizontally positioned linear echogenicity anterior to the caudate lobe in the transverse view of the liver.*

▶ de Bruyn R (ed): *Pediatric Ultrasound: How, Why and When*, 2nd edition (e-book). Philadelphia, Churchill Livingstone/Elsevier, 2010, pp 132, 182, 201.
▶ Rumack CM, Levine D (eds): *Diagnostic Ultrasound*, 5th edition. Philadelphia, Elsevier, 2018, pp 1731–1732.
▶ Siegel MJ (ed): *Pediatric Sonography*, 4th edition. Philadelphia, Lippincott Williams & Wilkins, 2011, pp 215–217.

188. **B. Middle hepatic vein.**

Before Couinaud segmental anatomy, the hepatic lobes were divided into right and left lobes by the plane made up of the middle hepatic vein and gallbladder fossa. The left lobe was further divided into medial and lateral segments by the left hepatic vein. The right lobe of the liver was further divided into anterior and posterior segments by the right hepatic vein.

▶ de Bruyn R (ed): *Pediatric Ultrasound: How, Why and When*, 2nd edition (e-book). Philadelphia, Churchill Livingstone/Elsevier, 2010, pp 132–135.
▶ Rumack CM, Levine D (eds): *Diagnostic Ultrasound*, 5th edition. Philadelphia, Elsevier, 2018, pp 1733–1734.
▶ Siegel MJ (ed): *Pediatric Sonography*, 4th edition. Philadelphia, Lippincott Williams & Wilkins, 2011, p 215.

189. **A. Polycystic liver.**

Isolated liver cysts are generally uncommon in children. However, a polycystic liver where multiple cysts are present is associated with inherited autosomal dominant diseases.

Von Hippel–Lindau, tuberous sclerosis, and autosomal dominant polycystic kidney disease (ADPKD) are all disorders associated with polycystic kidneys and liver.

▶ de Bruyn R (ed): *Pediatric Ultrasound: How, Why and When*, 2nd edition (e-book). Philadelphia, Churchill Livingstone/Elsevier, 2010, p 155.

▶ Siegel MJ (ed): *Pediatric Sonography*, 4th edition. Philadelphia, Lippincott Williams & Wilkins, 2011, pp 239, 407, 410.

190. C. Cavernous transformation.

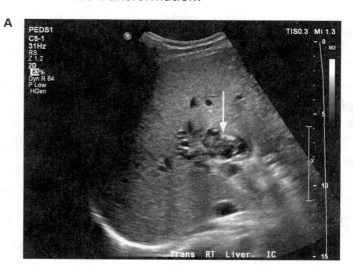

See Color Plate 17 on page xl.

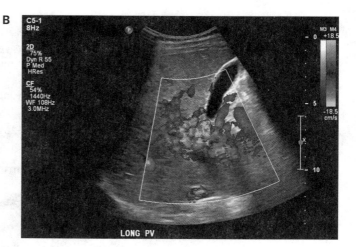

A *Multiple tortuous vessels seen within the porta hepatis that obscure the main portal vein are known as* cavernous transformation *or* portal cavernoma *(arrow). Portal vein thrombosis can be caused by various disease processes, tumors, or simple thrombosis. In acute portal vein thrombosis, the flow within the portal vein is diminished, causing stasis to occur. When the condition is chronic, collaterals will*

form to assist in delivering blood to the liver. Antegrade or bidirectional flow can be seen within the periportal collaterals using color Doppler, as demonstrated in image **B**. Other collaterals or varices may form in the gastroesophageal, intrahepatic, or splanchnic regions. Budd-Chiari syndrome *is obstruction of the hepatic veins.* Arteriovenous malformations (AVMs) of the liver are typically a congenital abnormality associated with portal hypertension.

▶ de Bruyn R (ed): *Pediatric Ultrasound: How, Why and When*, 2nd edition (e-book). Philadelphia, Churchill Livingstone/Elsevier, 2010, p 152.
▶ Rumack CM, Levine D (eds): *Diagnostic Ultrasound*, 5th edition. Philadelphia, Elsevier, 2018, pp 1757, 1761.
▶ Siegel MJ (ed): *Pediatric Sonography*, 4th edition. Philadelphia, Lippincott Williams & Wilkins, 2011, pp 255–257.

191. **B. Cirrhosis.**

Intrahepatic portal hypertension can be caused by cirrhosis. The scarring in cirrhosis will create an increased resistance and prevent portal venous flow into the liver, causing the portal vein to dilate. Portosystemic collaterals form to divert blood flow away from the liver and relieve the pressure. Splenic vein thrombosis is a prehepatic cause of portal hypertension. Posthepatic causes of portal hypertension are hepatic vein obstruction and congestive heart failure.

▶ de Bruyn R (ed): *Pediatric Ultrasound: How, Why and When*, 2nd edition (e-book). Philadelphia, Churchill Livingstone/Elsevier, 2010, p 152.
▶ Rumack CM, Levine D (eds): *Diagnostic Ultrasound*, 5th edition. Philadelphia, Elsevier, 2018, p 1752.
▶ Siegel MJ (ed): *Pediatric Sonography*, 4th edition. Philadelphia, Lippincott Williams & Wilkins, 2011, pp 248–249.

192. **A. Hemoperitoneum.**

See Color Plate 18 on page xl.

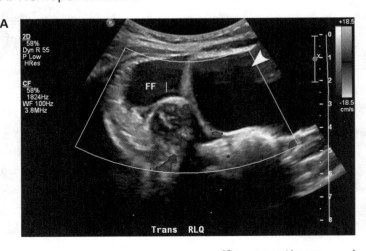

(figure continues . . .)

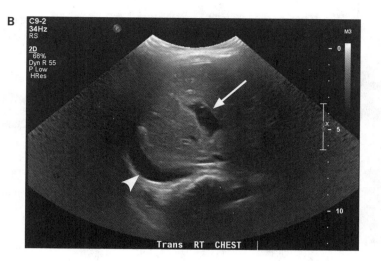

The focused abdominal sonogram for trauma, or FAST sonogram, is commonly used in emergency departments. It is a four-quadrant scanning technique to evaluate for hemoperitoneum in acute injuries and trauma. In children with blunt abdominal trauma, the liver is the most commonly affected organ. Causes of blunt trauma typical for children are sports injuries, falls, and accidents involving cars, bicycles, all-terrain vehicles, and skateboards. The images seen here were obtained from a patient who experienced trauma resulting in a liver contusion. Image **A** demonstrates hemoperitoneum (FF) located in the right lower quadrant adjacent to the bladder (arrowhead). In image **B** the liver contusion (arrow) is seen within the right lobe of the liver. Pleural effusion (arrowhead) is also seen in image **B**.

▶ Rumack CM, Levine D (eds): *Diagnostic Ultrasound*, 5th edition. Philadelphia, Elsevier, 2018, p 508.

▶ Siegel MJ (ed): *Pediatric Sonography*, 4th edition. Philadelphia, Lippincott Williams & Wilkins, 2011, pp 262–263.

193. D. Hepatocellular carcinoma.

Hepatocellular carcinoma *is the second most common childhood liver malignancy following hepatoblastoma. Over half of the patients diagnosed with hepatocellular carcinoma have preexisting liver disease, such as glycogen storage disease, alpha-1 antitrypsin deficiency, or tyrosinemia. Hepatocellular carcinoma typically occurs between the ages of 5 and 15, most often in the right lobe of the liver. Clinical symptoms include right upper quadrant mass, abdominal distention, and an elevated serum alpha-fetoprotein (AFP) level. On ultrasound, the tumor will appear as an echogenic heterogeneous, focal mass with a hypoechoic rim caused by its fibrous capsule.*

Liver vasculature can be disrupted by tumor invasion and metastases may be present. Hepatoblastoma, undifferentiated embryonal sarcoma, *and* angiosarcoma *are not associated with preexisting liver disease and are primary neoplasms.*

▶ de Bruyn R (ed): *Pediatric Ultrasound: How, Why and When*, 2nd edition (e-book). Philadelphia, Churchill Livingstone/Elsevier, 2010, pp 149–150, 157–159.

▶ Rumack CM, Levine D (eds): *Diagnostic Ultrasound*, 5th edition. Philadelphia, Elsevier, 2018, p 1746.

▶ Siegel MJ (ed): *Pediatric Sonography*, 4th edition. Philadelphia, Lippincott Williams & Wilkins, 2011, pp 226–230.

194. A. Hepatic fibrosis.

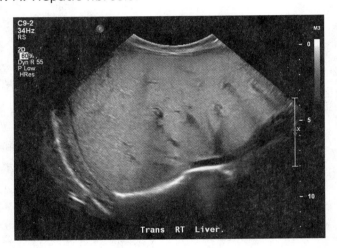

Hepatic fibrosis *is the buildup of scar tissue or fibrous bands. These bands can cause ductal dilatation and portal hypertension by compressing and restricting the flow of bile, blood, and lymph. The chronic presentation of hepatic fibrosis usually precedes cirrhosis. Hepatic fibrosis can be an isolated finding or associated with congenital conditions such as Meckel-Gruber and Caroli disease. Sonographically, the liver will be enlarged and echogenic, containing dilated bile ducts.* Focal nodular hyperplasia *(FNH) appears as a solitary tumor. With* metastatic disease of the liver, *focal lesions may be present throughout the parenchyma and the liver may be enlarged, but it is an unlikely cause of cirrhosis.* Veno-occlusive disease *is the obstruction of small sublobular hepatic veins and is not directly visualized on ultrasound. Portal hypertension is not demonstrated in this image but may be caused by cirrhosis.*

▶ de Bruyn R (ed): *Pediatric Ultrasound: How, Why and When*, 2nd edition (e-book). Philadelphia, Churchill Livingstone/Elsevier, 2010, pp 74–75, 76, 145.

▶ Siegel MJ (ed): *Pediatric Sonography*, 4th edition. Philadelphia, Lippincott Williams & Wilkins, 2011, p 246.

195. B. Subcapsular hematoma.

A subcapsular liver hematoma is a lenticular (lens-shaped) fluid collection. The mass effect of the hematoma flattens or indents the underlying liver. Subcapsular hematomas are most commonly seen on the anterior surface of the right liver. Parenchymal hematomas occur within the liver margins. The sonographic appearance of hematomas will vary with the age of the injury. Hepatic lacerations *and hepatic fractures will appear as linear parenchymal defects.*

▶ Siegel MJ (ed): *Pediatric Sonography*, 4th edition. Philadelphia, Lippincott Williams & Wilkins, 2011, p 262.

196. B. Hepatitis B.

Healthcare workers have an increased risk for hepatitis B. In the healthcare profession, there is a higher risk of exposure to blood, and for that reason the hepatitis B vaccine is offered to the employees of many hospitals and clinics. Hepatitis is an infection of the liver, usually viral in origin, but can also be due to infections resulting from bacteria, parasites, drug abuse, metabolic conditions, or systemic causes. Hepatitis A is the most common form of hepatitis in the United States. Hepatitis A and E are transmitted through the fecal-oral route and do not become chronic. Hepatitis B, C, and D are bloodborne infections that can progress to chronic liver disease. On ultrasound, the liver will appear normal in mild cases of hepatitis. In more severe acute forms, hepatomegaly, decreased parenchymal echogenicity, and the "starry sky" appearance of the echogenic portal venule walls will be present. Chronic hepatitis causes the liver to have an increased parenchymal echogenicity and a coarse, heterogeneous texture.

▶ de Bruyn R (ed): *Pediatric Ultrasound: How, Why and When*, 2nd edition (e-book). Philadelphia, Churchill Livingstone/Elsevier, 2010, p 153.

▶ Siegel MJ (ed): *Pediatric Sonography*, 4th edition. Philadelphia, Lippincott Williams & Wilkins, 2011, pp 240–241.

197. D. Percutaneous biopsy.

Percutaneous biopsy *of the liver is performed on liver parenchyma to diagnose hepatic disease. Usually, a sample of the right lobe is taken under sterile conditions with a 16- to 18-gauge needle. Focal lesions are also biopsied to determine tumor etiology.* Elastography *is a sonographic procedure that measures tissue stiffness.* Abscess drainage *is performed on a focal liver lesion.* Contrast ultrasound *is used primarily to improve liver mass detection or to differentiate focal liver lesions.*

▶ de Bruyn R (ed): *Pediatric Ultrasound: How, Why and When*, 2nd edition (e-book). Philadelphia, Churchill Livingstone/Elsevier, 2010, pp 155, 364.
▶ Rumack CM, Levine D (eds): *Diagnostic Ultrasound*, 5th edition. Philadelphia, Elsevier, 2018, p 1962.
▶ Siegel MJ (ed): *Pediatric Sonography*, 4th edition. Philadelphia, Lippincott Williams & Wilkins, 2011, p 684.

198. C. Hepatic artery.

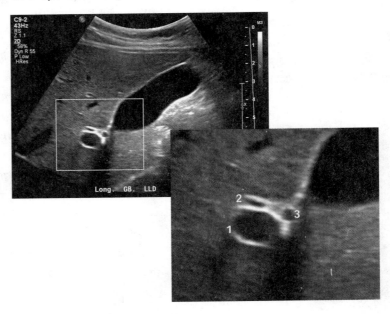

See Color Plate 14, "The Biliary Tree," on page xxxix.

The boxed portion of the image on the left is enlarged on the right. The portal triad *is made up of the portal vein (1), common bile duct (2), and proper hepatic artery (3). This arrangement is commonly referred to as the "Mickey Mouse" sign. The hepatic artery (left "ear") is anterior and medial to the portal vein, and the common bile duct (right ear) lies anterior and lateral to the portal vein (head). The hepatic artery and portal vein will show flow on color Doppler, while the bile duct will not. With spectral Doppler, the hepatic artery has antegrade low-resistance flow. After the patient eats there can be an increase in the resistive index. The proper hepatic artery divides into the right and left hepatic arteries. The common bile duct is formed by the joining of the common hepatic duct and the cystic duct.*

▶ Rumack CM, Levine D (eds): *Diagnostic Ultrasound*, 5th edition. Philadelphia, Elsevier, 2018, pp 1733–1734, 1753.
▶ Siegel MJ (ed): *Pediatric Sonography*, 4th edition. Philadelphia, Lippincott Williams & Wilkins, 2011, pp 220, 224.

199. **A. Granulomas.**

Resulting from widespread inflammation or disease, abnormal clumps of cells can form granulomas *within the liver. The cause of granulomas may be systemic (cholangitis, sarcoidosis), a drug reaction, a bacterial infection (TB), a viral infection (hepatitis C, cytomegalovirus), or a parasitic infection (schistosomiasis). Granulomas are usually asymptomatic and rarely disrupt liver function. On ultrasound, granulomas appear as focal lesions with clear borders and the echogenicity of the liver parenchyma is not affected. Their echogenicity can vary. Diagnosis is made by biopsy. Infectious or drug-related granulomas resolve after treatment.* Hemangiomas *are vascular masses made up of mesenchymal tissue.* Lipomas *are composed of adipose tissue.* Sarcomas *are malignant lesions.*

▶ de Bruyn R (ed): *Pediatric Ultrasound: How, Why and When*, 2nd edition (e-book). Philadelphia, Churchill Livingstone/Elsevier, 2010, p 156.

▶ Herrine SK: Hepatic granulomas. Available at https://www.merckmanuals.com/professional/hepatic-and-biliary-disorders/liver-masses-and-granulomas/hepatic-granulomas.

▶ Rumack CM, Levine D (eds): *Diagnostic Ultrasound*, 5th edition. Philadelphia, Elsevier, 2018, p 1748.

200. **C. Mesenchymal hamartoma.**

Mesenchymal hamartomas *are considered a rare congenital abnormality arising from the periportal connective tissue or mesenchyme. Other names include* lymphangioma, bile cell fibroadenoma, *and* cystic hamartoma. *Most commonly occurring between the ages of 1 and 3, mesenchymal hamartomas are slightly less common in girls. The clinical sign is often a palpable mass or right abdominal enlargement. The sonographic appearance is a large encapsulated and multilocular mass. If internal cystic spaces are present and rupture occurs, ascites may be seen.* Hemangiomas *are composed of mesenchymal tissue but are vascular and are not rare.* Hemangioendotheliomas *are the most common benign liver tumor of children.* Hepatic adenomas *associated with metabolic liver disease are not uncommon.*

▶ de Bruyn R (ed): *Pediatric Ultrasound: How, Why and When*, 2nd edition (e-book). Philadelphia, Churchill Livingstone/Elsevier, 2010, p 157.

▶ Rumack CM, Levine D (eds): *Diagnostic Ultrasound*, 5th edition. Philadelphia, Elsevier, 2018, p 1744.

▶ Siegel MJ (ed): *Pediatric Sonography*, 4th edition. Philadelphia, Lippincott Williams & Wilkins, 2011, pp 232–234.

201. D. Hepatopetal low-resistance flow.

Arteries traveling toward the liver in a preprandial state, such as the proper hepatic artery, should display continuous hepatopetal flow with a low resistance. After a meal (postprandially), vasoconstriction can occur, leading to high-resistance flow. The decrease of diastolic blood flow will cause an increase in the resistive index of the hepatic artery. Note should be made of the patient's NPO status so as to not mistake the elevated RI with liver disease. Hepatopetal flow would be coursing toward the liver. Hepatofugal flow indicates blood flow away from the liver.

▶ Rumack CM, Levine D (eds): *Diagnostic Ultrasound*, 5th edition. Philadelphia, Elsevier, 2018, pp 1752–1754.

▶ Siegel MJ (ed): *Pediatric Sonography*, 4th edition. Philadelphia, Lippincott Williams & Wilkins, 2011, p 224.

202. B. Hepatoblastoma.

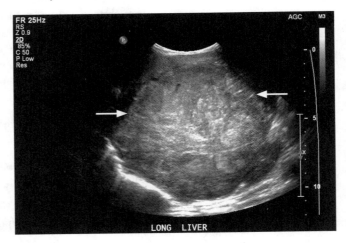

Hepatoblastoma *is the most common malignant liver tumor of childhood. Less than 10% of cases are seen over the age of 5, and most occur in the first 2 years of life. Clinically hepatoblastomas are often asymptomatic, but symptoms can include abdominal mass, pain, anorexia, weight loss, and jaundice. Levels of alpha-fetoprotein (AFP) are elevated in 90% of patients. Signs of precocious puberty may be present with the release of chorionic gonadotropins. Hepatoblastoma is associated with Beckwith-Wiedemann syndrome. On ultrasound, a hepatoblastoma will appear as a large, well-defined focal mass in the right lobe of the liver (arrows). The tumor can be echogenic or heterogeneous and contain calcium or necrotic areas. Vascular invasion is most often seen into the portal system. Treatment is chemotherapy and partial hepatectomy. Focal nodular hyperplasia (FNH,*

usually seen in adult females) and undifferentiated embryonal sarcoma *(in children over the age of 5) are rare occurrences in young children.* Cirrhosis *can occur in children with existing hepatobiliary disease; however, it is a diffuse parenchymal disease of the liver and not a focal neoplasm.*

▶ de Bruyn R (ed): *Pediatric Ultrasound: How, Why and When,* 2nd edition (e-book). Philadelphia, Churchill Livingstone/Elsevier, 2010, pp 139, 140–141, 157–158.

▶ Rumack CM, Levine D (eds): *Diagnostic Ultrasound,* 5th edition. Philadelphia, Elsevier, 2018, pp 1746–1747.

▶ Siegel MJ (ed): *Pediatric Sonography,* 4th edition. Philadelphia, Lippincott Williams & Wilkins, 2011, pp 226–229, 230, 237, 247.

203. **A. Elastography.**

Elastography *is a noninvasive test performed with ultrasound to measure liver stiffness. On newer software systems, the vibrations of elastic shear waves can be measured and averaged. The velocity of the shear waves relates to the stiffness of the liver. An increase in shear wave velocity is equal to an increase in liver stiffness or fibrosis. An* abdominal vascular study *is an ultrasound Doppler test that evaluates the flow direction, velocity, and resistive index of abdominal vessels to evaluate for liver function, portal hypertension, and obstruction.* Liver function tests *consist of a panel of enzymes obtained from bloodwork; in the presence of liver disease these enzymes will be elevated.* Contrast-enhanced ultrasound (CEUS) *is used primarily to improve liver mass detection or to differentiate focal liver lesions.*

▶ Rumack CM, Levine D (eds): *Diagnostic Ultrasound,* 5th edition. Philadelphia, Elsevier, 2018, pp 1764–1765.

▶ Siegel MJ (ed): *Pediatric Sonography,* 4th edition. Philadelphia, Lippincott Williams & Wilkins, 2011, pp 427–428, 684.

204. **D. Portal vein.**

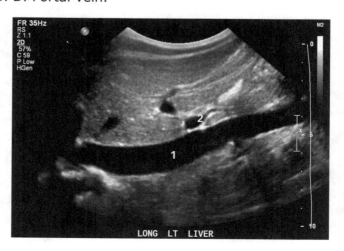

The portal triad consists of the common bile duct, hepatic artery, and portal vein and is located within the porta hepatis, which is a deep fissure or hilum of the liver. In a longitudinal scan plane (as seen in this image), the portal vein (2) is seen anterior to the inferior vena cava (1). The portal vein is then demonstrated in the transverse plane.

▶ de Bruyn R (ed): *Pediatric Ultrasound: How, Why and When*, 2nd edition (e-book). Philadelphia, Churchill Livingstone/Elsevier, 2010, pp 132–136.

▶ Siegel MJ (ed): *Pediatric Sonography*, 4th edition. Philadelphia, Lippincott Williams & Wilkins, 2011, p 220.

▶ Tirumani SH, Shanbhogue AKP, Vikram R, et al: Imaging of the porta hepatis: spectrum of disease. Available at https://pubs.rsna.org/doi/pdf/10.1148/rg.341125190.

205. B. Hemangioma.

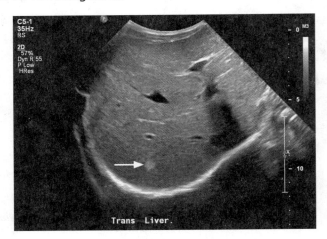

Hemangiomas *account for almost 40% of liver masses. This mass is typically solitary and hypovascular with slow blood flow. On ultrasound, hemangiomas (arrow) are moderately echogenic or hyperechoic and homogeneous, with well-defined borders. Smaller hemangiomas tend to be more echogenic and larger hemangiomas can appear more complex. Larger hemangiomas that demonstrate blood-filled vascular spaces are referred to as* cavernous hemangiomas. *Hemangiomas are an uncommon cause of abdominal masses in neonates and infants and more likely to be seen in children and adolescents. The older age of the patient in this example rules out hemangioendothelioma, hepatoblastoma (not benign), and mesenchymal hamartoma—which all occur under the age of 5.*

▶ Regier TS, Ramji FG: Pediatric Hepatic hemangioma. Available at https://pubs.rsna.org/doi/full/10.1148/rg.246035188.

▶ Rumack CM, Levine D (eds): *Diagnostic Ultrasound*, 5th edition. Philadelphia, Elsevier, 2018, pp 233–235.

▶ Siegel MJ (ed): *Pediatric Sonography*, 4th edition. Philadelphia, Lippincott Williams & Wilkins, 2011, pp 1742–1744.

206. **D. 30-degree vessel-beam angle.**

To accurately calculate velocity and flow within a vessel, there should be as small a vessel-beam angle as possible, ideally 60 degrees or less. At a perpendicular angle of 90 degrees, no flow can be detected toward or away from the transducer, so there will not be a detectable Doppler shift. Pediatric vessels generally have lower flow within them than do adult vessels. Setting the pulse repetition frequency (PRF) and the wall filter as low as possible (less than 5 MHz) will best demonstrate presence or absence of flow. Having the Doppler gain down too low will also hinder signal identification.

▶ Rumack CM, Levine D (eds): *Diagnostic Ultrasound*, 5th edition. Philadelphia, Elsevier, 2018, p 1754.

▶ Siegel MJ (ed): *Pediatric Sonography*, 4th edition. Philadelphia, Lippincott Williams & Wilkins, 2011, pp 15–17.

207. **A. Adenoma.**

Pediatric hepatic adenomas are rare unless they accompany metabolic liver disease. Hepatic adenomas in children are associated with glycogen storage disease type 1, oral contraceptive use, and anabolic steroid therapy for Fanconi's anemia. Hepatic adenomas have such a varying appearance and are so nonspecific that imaging modalities such as ultrasound, computed tomography (CT), and magnetic resonance imaging (MRI) have a difficult time discriminating between adenomas and other hepatic malignancies. Hamartomas, hemangiomas, and lymphomas do not have any association with preexisting metabolic liver disease.

▶ de Bruyn R (ed): *Pediatric Ultrasound: How, Why and When*, 2nd edition (e-book). Philadelphia, Churchill Livingstone/Elsevier, 2010, pp 149, 159.

▶ Rumack CM, Levine D (eds): *Diagnostic Ultrasound*, 5th edition. Philadelphia, Elsevier, 2018, p 1746.

▶ Siegel MJ (ed): *Pediatric Sonography*, 4th edition. Philadelphia, Lippincott Williams & Wilkins, 2011, p 238.

208. **C. Right portal vein.**

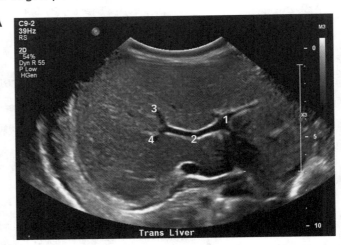

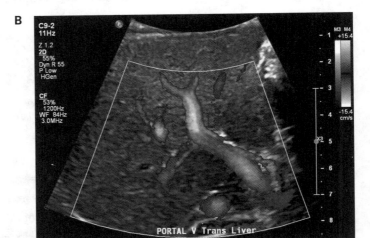

See Color Plate 19 on page xl.

A *The main portal vein enters the liver and divides into the left portal vein (1) and the right portal vein (2). This division takes place within the porta hepatis. The left portal vein then branches into an anterior and a more cephalad branch. The right portal vein branches into an anterior (3) and a posterior (4) branch. Portal venous blood flow is continuous, monophasic, and hepatopetal (toward the liver/transducer).*
B *Color Doppler imaging demonstrates the hepatopetal flow of the main portal vein. In a normal liver, the only vessel not showing antegrade flow on color Doppler should be the posterior branch of the right portal vein because it travels away from the transducer. The walls of the portal vein are thicker and more echogenic than those of the inferior vena cava.*

▶ de Bruyn R (ed): *Pediatric Ultrasound: How, Why and When*, 2nd edition (e-book). Philadelphia, Churchill Livingstone/Elsevier, 2010, pp 132–136.
▶ Rumack CM, Levine D (eds): *Diagnostic Ultrasound*, 5th edition. Philadelphia, Elsevier, 2018, pp 1731–1734.
▶ Siegel MJ (ed): *Pediatric Sonography*, 4th edition. Philadelphia, Lippincott Williams & Wilkins, 2011, pp 215–218, 222.

209. **D. Pyogenic abscess.**

Pyogenic abscesses usually occur in immunocompromised children or cases of septic spread from other organs. On ultrasound, pyogenic abscesses appear round with thickened, irregular walls and can contain small air bubbles that cause artifacts such as reverberation (ring-down) artifacts. Their complex internal appearance can vary and include debris, fluid levels, and septations. Most are located in the posterior right lobe of the liver. The most common cause in neonates is the bacterium Escherichia coli *(E. coli). In infants and children,* Staphylococcus aureus *(S. aureus) is the main cause. Hemangioma, lymphoma, and hepatic cysts do not have thick walls or contain air.*

▶ de Bruyn R (ed): *Pediatric Ultrasound: How, Why and When*, 2nd edition (e-book). Philadelphia, Churchill Livingstone/Elsevier, 2010, pp 155, 168.
▶ Rumack CM, Levine D (eds): *Diagnostic Ultrasound*, 5th edition. Philadelphia, Elsevier, 2018, pp 1746–1747, 1751.
▶ Siegel MJ (ed): *Pediatric Sonography*, 4th edition. Philadelphia, Lippincott Williams & Wilkins, 2011, pp 233, 238–239, 241.

210. **B. Portal vein thrombosis.**

Portal vein thrombosis is the restriction of blood flow into the liver. The slow flow into the liver causes blood stasis or accumulation and blocks the flow. Collaterals may form in the hepatic, splenic, or renal hilum to help get blood into the liver. This backup in blood flow can cause splenomegaly, not hepatomegaly. Hepatomegaly is the enlargement of the liver. Inflammation, infection, storage diseases, tumors, congestion of blood in the liver (Budd-Chiari), and biliary obstruction are all possible causes.

▶ de Bruyn R (ed): *Pediatric Ultrasound: How, Why and When*, 2nd edition (e-book). Philadelphia, Churchill Livingstone/Elsevier, 2010, pp 132–133, 152, 163.
▶ Rumack CM, Levine D (eds): *Diagnostic Ultrasound*, 5th edition. Philadelphia, Elsevier, 2018, pp 1756–1759.
▶ Siegel MJ (ed): *Pediatric Sonography*, 4th edition. Philadelphia, Lippincott Williams & Wilkins, 2011, pp 226–230, 233, 237–238, 240, 244, 247–253.
▶ University of Chicago: Hepatomegaly. Available at https://pedclerk.bsd.uchicago.edu/page/hepatomegaly.

211. **D. Veno-occlusive disease.**

Veno-occlusive disease is the term used for the obstruction of small sublobular hepatic veins and is not usually diagnosed by ultrasound. This obstruction is associated with chemotherapy, radiation, toxins, and bone marrow transplant. Ultrasound signs preceding veno-occlusive disease include slow or reversed portal venous and hepatic artery blood flow, monophasic waveforms of the hepatic veins, and/or an elevated resistive index of the hepatic artery. Filling defects or thrombus may be present in the hepatic veins. The caudate lobe can become enlarged. Ascites, gallbladder wall thickening, and hepatomegaly may also be present. Portal hypertension, arteriovenous malformation (AVM), and Budd-Chiari syndrome can all be demonstrated by ultrasound.

▶ de Bruyn R (ed): *Pediatric Ultrasound: How, Why and When*, 2nd edition (e-book). Philadelphia, Churchill Livingstone/Elsevier, 2010, pp 152, 153–154.

▶ Ghersin E, Brook OR, Gaitini D, et al: Color Doppler demonstration of segmental portal flow reversal: an early sign of hepatic veno-occlusive disease in an infant. J Ultrasound Med 22:1103–1106, 2003.

▶ Siegel MJ (ed): *Pediatric Sonography*, 4th edition. Philadelphia, Lippincott Williams & Wilkins, 2011, pp 257–258.

212. A. Hemangioendotheliomas.

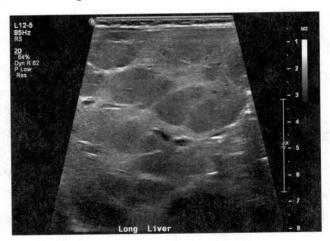

Hemangioendothelioma *is the most common childhood benign liver tumor. Only 15% of cases occur after 6 months of age, making it predominantly an infantile condition. This mass is typically found on a screening ultrasound for asymptomatic hepatomegaly. Hemangioendotheliomas can be single or multiple. Single masses tend to be larger and complex with well-defined, round or lobular borders. When multiple smaller masses are present—as seen in this image—they are round, homogeneous, and hypoechoic. Hemangioendotheliomas will typically regress and involute, therefore requiring only medical management.*

▶ de Bruyn R (ed): *Pediatric Ultrasound: How, Why and When*, 2nd edition (e-book). Philadelphia, Churchill Livingstone/Elsevier, 2010, pp 137–141.

▶ Rumack CM, Levine D (eds): *Diagnostic Ultrasound*, 5th edition. Philadelphia, Elsevier, 2018, pp 1743–1745.

▶ Siegel MJ (ed): *Pediatric Sonography*, 4th edition. Philadelphia, Lippincott Williams & Wilkins, 2011, pp 232–233.

PART 6

Gallbladder and Biliary Ducts

213. **B. Alkaline phosphatase (ALP).**

   Alkaline phosphatase *(ALP) is an enzyme found within the liver, bile ducts, and bone. An increase in ALP may indicate liver or gallbladder inflammation or disease.* Amylase *is an enzyme that assists in turning starch into sugar and is associated with the pancreas.* Albumin *is a protein made in the liver that is decreased in the presence of liver disease.* Aldosterone *is a hormone produced by the adrenal gland that helps conserve sodium and stabilize blood pressure.*

   ▶ Keough J: *Nursing Laboratory and Diagnostic Tests Demystified*, 2nd edition. New York, McGraw-Hill, 2017, pp 9–10, 54–55, 147–150.

214. **C. Interlobar fissure.**

   The interlobar fissure *is located anterior to the right portal vein and courses medially toward the neck of the gallbladder. It appears linear and hyperechoic. This fissure is a landmark for locating the gallbladder. The* ligamentum teres *and* ligamentum venosum *are associated with the left branch of the portal vein. The* cystic duct *drains the gallbladder and joins the common hepatic duct to form the common bile duct. The cystic duct would not appear hyperechoic.*

   ▶ Rumack CM, Levine D (eds): *Diagnostic Ultrasound*, 5th edition. Philadelphia, Elsevier, 2018, p 1801.

   ▶ Siegel MJ (ed): *Pediatric Sonography*, 4th edition. Philadelphia, Lippincott Williams & Wilkins, 2011, pp 215, 275–276.

215. **D. Phrygian cap.**

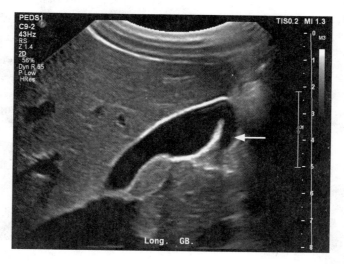

The folding of the gallbladder fundus is a normal anatomic variant known as the Phrygian cap. Junctional folds are present at the junction of the body and neck of the gallbladder. Gallbladder folds can produce a shadowing artifact that may cause concern for a gallstone. To rule out a stone, it is important to scan the patient in multiple positions and from different angles. A septate gallbladder is a congenital anomaly that causes a honeycomb appearance within the gallbladder. Gallbladder fissure is not an anatomic term.

▶ Siegel MJ (ed): *Pediatric Sonography*, 4th edition. Philadelphia, Lippincott Williams & Wilkins, 2011, pp 277–278.

216. A. Jaundice.

Jaundice is the most common indication for pediatric gallbladder and biliary tree imaging. Most common causes of pediatric cholestasis and jaundice include biliary atresia, neonatal hepatitis syndrome, and choledochal cyst. These can commonly be identified on ultrasound. Abdominal pain, nausea and vomiting, and a family history of gallstones are other reasons for performing gallbladder ultrasound.

▶ de Bruyn R (ed): *Pediatric Ultrasound: How, Why and When*, 2nd edition (e-book). Philadelphia, Churchill Livingstone/Elsevier, 2010, p 142.
▶ Rumack CM, Levine D (eds): *Diagnostic Ultrasound*, 5th edition. Philadelphia, Elsevier, 2018, p 1737.
▶ Siegel MJ (ed): *Pediatric Sonography*, 4th edition. Philadelphia, Lippincott Williams & Wilkins, 2011, p 291.

217. B. Middle hepatic vein.

The middle hepatic vein and the gallbladder fossa course along the same plane. Locating the middle hepatic vein can help identify the gallbladder fossa. The middle hepatic vein also lies within the interlobar fissure and on ultrasound visually divides the liver into right and left lobes. The right hepatic vein lies within the right hepatic fissure. The left hepatic vein is always located anterior to the left portal vein, which courses away from the gallbladder fossa.

▶ Rumack CM, Levine D (eds): *Diagnostic Ultrasound*, 5th edition. Philadelphia, Elsevier, 2018, p 1801.
▶ Siegel MJ (ed): *Pediatric Sonography*, 4th edition. Philadelphia, Lippincott Williams & Wilkins, 2011, p 275.

218. C. Choledochal cyst.

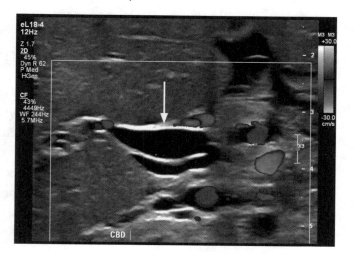

See Color Plate 2 on page xxxiii.

The congenital abnormality consisting of a dilated common bile duct associated with biliary obstruction is known as a choledochal cyst (arrow). One theory of causation is that cyst formation occurs when cholangitis weakens the bile duct wall. There are multiple classifications of choledochal cysts based on their location and severity. The most common clinical sign is jaundice, but abdominal mass and pain can occur. More than half of the diagnoses of choledochal cysts will occur before age 10. If the cyst becomes large enough, duodenal obstruction can occur. Other complications include ascending cholangitis, stone formation, pancreatitis, biliary cirrhosis, and abscess. On ultrasound a well-defined cystic structure can be seen in the porta hepatis separate from the gallbladder but continuous with the extrahepatic bile ducts. Intrahepatic biliary duct dilatation visualized in this image can be seen in half of the cases. Choledocholithiasis is a stone within a biliary duct. A hydropic gallbladder would not be continuous with the common bile duct. A fluid-filled duodenum would be located inferior and medial to the gallbladder.

▶ Mieli-Vergani G, Hadzic N: Biliary atresia and neonatal disorders of the bile ducts. In Wyllie R, Hyams JS, Kay M (eds): *Pediatric Gastrointestinal and Liver Disease*, 5th edition. Philadelphia, Elsevier, 2016, pp 838–851.

▶ Rumack CM, Levine D (eds): *Diagnostic Ultrasound*, 5th edition. Philadelphia, Elsevier, 2018, pp 168–170, 1735–1736.

▶ Siegel MJ (ed): *Pediatric Sonography*, 4th edition. Philadelphia, Lippincott Williams & Wilkins, 2011, pp 294–296.

219. A. Cholestasis.

Cholestasis *is the primary cause of acalculous cholecystitis. Over a prolonged period of time, the bile thickens and leads to obstruction of the cystic duct. Bacteria within the gallbladder can cause inflammation of the mucosa and wall. Clinical symptoms are fever, right upper quadrant (RUQ) pain, and vomiting. The sonographic appearance is the same as that of acute cholecystitis, but* without *gallstones (acalculous). Acalculous cholecystitis is an uncommon condition associated with burn victims, recent surgery, sepsis, and debilitating conditions. Trauma of the gallbladder usually results in contusion, laceration, or perforation.* Cholangitis *is an infection of the bile ducts.*

▸ Rumack CM, Levine D (eds): *Diagnostic Ultrasound*, 5th edition. Philadelphia, Elsevier, 2018, pp 176, 200.

▸ Siegel MJ (ed): *Pediatric Sonography*, 4th edition. Philadelphia, Lippincott Williams & Wilkins, 2011, pp 287, 290, 299.

220. B. Supine and left lateral decubitus.

The most common scanning positions for gallbladder imaging are supine and left lateral decubitus. Rolling a patient onto the left side will demonstrate the mobility of gallstones or sludge. The left posterior oblique position may also be used. It is important to image in two positions in case there are gallstones located too inferior to be seen in the supine position. Longitudinal and transverse views of all gallbladder segments should be obtained. Patients should be held NPO to better visualize the distended gallbladder and its contents. For larger patients a low-frequency transducer may be necessary to allow for greater beam penetration to the region of interest.

▸ de Bruyn R (ed): *Pediatric Ultrasound: How, Why and When*, 2nd edition (e-book). Philadelphia, Churchill Livingstone/Elsevier, 2010, p 133.

▸ Siegel MJ (ed): *Pediatric Sonography*, 4th edition. Philadelphia, Lippincott Williams & Wilkins, 2011, p 275.

221. D. Bilirubin.

Bilirubin *is the end product of the metabolic breakdown of hemoglobin. It is the substance produced by the breakdown of old red blood cells within the liver. Bilirubin is excreted in stool and gives feces color. Increased levels of bilirubin cause jaundice.* Unconjugated *or* indirect bilirubin *is carried to the* liver via blood and is not soluble in water. Conjugated or direct bilirubin has been converted by the liver to a water-soluble form:

Total bilirubin − direct bilirubin = indirect bilirubin

Biliverdin *is a green bile pigment from hemoglobin catabolism. It accounts for the green color seen in bruises.* Hematocrit *is a lab value that shows the percentage of red blood cells within the blood volume.*

▸ Keough J: *Nursing Laboratory and Diagnostic Tests Demystified*, 2nd edition. New York, McGraw-Hill, 2017, pp 147, 155.

222. **B. Main right and left hepatic ducts.**

The *common hepatic duct (CHD) is formed by the union of the main right and left hepatic ducts. The CHD is the intrahepatic portion of the hepatic duct system and joins with the cystic duct. The CHD is most commonly found anterior and to the right of the main portal vein and hepatic artery. The* common bile duct *(CBD) is the extrahepatic portion located at the junction of the cystic duct with the CHD, extending to the ampulla of Vater, where it connects with the main pancreatic duct.* Intrahepatic bile ducts *join to form the main right and left hepatic ducts. Intrahepatic bile ducts are normally not visualized on ultrasound due to their small size.*

▸ Rumack CM, Levine D (eds): *Diagnostic Ultrasound*, 5th edition. Philadelphia, Elsevier, 2018, p 166.

▸ Siegel MJ (ed): *Pediatric Sonography*, 4th edition. Philadelphia, Lippincott Williams & Wilkins, 2011, p 291.

223. **A. Reverberation and ring-down artifact.**

Air within the gallbladder will cause a bright ring-down artifact *and* reverberation, *also known as "dirty shadowing." These artifacts will interfere with the visualization of the posterior gallbladder wall and lumen and may be mistaken for the presence of gallstones.* Clean shadowing *would be found behind a gallstone.* Posterior enhancement *is an artifact that can appear during imaging of a normal distended gallbladder and is not related to the presence or absence of air in the gallbladder.*

▸ Rumack CM, Levine D (eds): *Diagnostic Ultrasound*, 5th edition. Philadelphia, Elsevier, 2018, p 198.

▸ Siegel MJ (ed): *Pediatric Sonography*, 4th edition. Philadelphia, Lippincott Williams & Wilkins, 2011, p 283.

224. C. 3 mm.

The upper limit of normal for gallbladder wall thickness in a fasting patient is 3 mm. If the patient is not fasting, the wall can appear thicker. Note should be made if the patient is postprandial. The gallbladder may also be contracted if the patient has eaten prior to the study. Fasting times vary based on pediatric age.

▸ Rumack CM, Levine D (eds): *Diagnostic Ultrasound*, 5th edition. Philadelphia, Elsevier, 2018, p 4235.

▸ Siegel MJ (ed): *Pediatric Sonography*, 4th edition. Philadelphia, Lippincott Williams & Wilkins, 2011, p 279.

▸ Wolson AH: Ultrasound measurements of the gallbladder. In Goldberg BB, Kurtz AB (eds): *Atlas of Ultrasound Measurements*. Chicago: Year Book Publishers, 1990, pp 108–112.

225. D. Hydropic gallbladder.

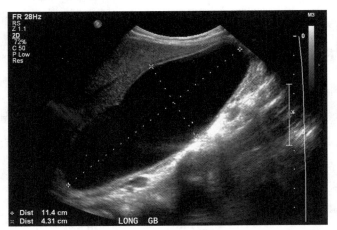

Gallbladder hydrops *is the extreme distention of the gallbladder without inflammation, as seen in this image, in which the gallbladder measures greater than 7 cm in length. No wall thickening or dilated ducts are seen with a hydropic gallbladder. Neonatal causes are hyperalimentation, sepsis, shock, and cystic fibrosis. Dehydration can lead to bile stasis, and the thickened bile can prevent the cystic duct from emptying the gallbladder. Hydropic gallbladders can be seen in older children with Kawasaki disease. A* contracted gallbladder *is usually demonstrated in cases of* chronic cholecystitis. *With* biliary atresia, *the gallbladder is either small or absent.* Micro gallbladders *are defined as less than 2 cm in diameter and are associated with cystic fibrosis.*

▸ de Bruyn R (ed): *Pediatric Ultrasound: How, Why and When*, 2nd edition (e-book). Philadelphia, Churchill Livingstone/Elsevier, 2010, pp 161–162.

▸ Siegel MJ (ed): *Pediatric Sonography*, 4th edition. Philadelphia, Lippincott Williams & Wilkins, 2011, pp 287–288, 292.

226. **B. Cholangitis.**

Cholangitis is the infection of the bile ducts. Cholangitis caused by bacterial organisms is associated with AIDS, choledochal malformations, Kasai procedures, and several syndromes. Sclerosing cholangitis can cause fibrotic changes in the bile ducts, eventually leading to cirrhosis. It is associated with Langerhans cell histiocytosis, chronic irritable bowel syndrome, and AIDS. Clinical symptoms of cholangitis are jaundice, RUQ pain, and abnormal labs. On ultrasound, the intrahepatic ducts will be dilated and have thickened walls. Areas of focal narrowing or strictures within the ducts will be present. The gallbladder wall may be thickened and pericholecystic fluid may be present. *Cholecystitis* is the inflammation of the gallbladder. With *cholestasis* the bile does not flow out of the gallbladder and liver. *Choledocholithiasis* is a stone within a bile duct.

▶ de Bruyn R (ed): *Pediatric Ultrasound: How, Why and When*, 2nd edition (e-book). Philadelphia, Churchill Livingstone/Elsevier, 2010, pp 143, 147.

▶ Rumack CM, Levine D (eds): *Diagnostic Ultrasound*, 5th edition. Philadelphia, Elsevier, 2018, pp 172–174, 176, 195–198.

▶ Siegel MJ (ed): *Pediatric Sonography*, 4th edition. Philadelphia, Lippincott Williams & Wilkins, 2011, pp 286, 299, 300.

227. **C. Porta hepatis.**

Biliary rhabdomyosarcomas are typically seen within the age ranges of 2–6 and 14–18. Almost all patients will present with obstructive jaundice. Biliary rhabdomyosarcomas are most commonly found within the porta hepatis as an echogenic mass with intrahepatic and extrahepatic ductal dilatation.

▶ de Bruyn R (ed): *Pediatric Ultrasound: How, Why and When*, 2nd edition (e-book). Philadelphia, Churchill Livingstone/Elsevier, 2010, p 162.

▶ Rumack CM, Levine D (eds): *Diagnostic Ultrasound*, 5th edition. Philadelphia, Elsevier, 2018, p 1746.

▶ Siegel MJ (ed): *Pediatric Sonography*, 4th edition. Philadelphia, Lippincott Williams & Wilkins, 2011, p 302.

228. **D. Hepatitis**

In children between ages 10 and 19, the most common cause of jaundice is hepatocellular disease such as hepatitis and cirrhosis. Air in the gallbladder does not commonly result in jaundice. Neonatal jaundice is most often the result of biliary atresia and choledochal cyst. Systemic causes such as shock and sepsis can also cause jaundice.

▶ de Bruyn R (ed): *Pediatric Ultrasound: How, Why and When*, 2nd edition (e-book). Philadelphia, Churchill Livingstone/Elsevier, 2010, pp 148, 153.

▶ Rumack CM, Levine D (eds): *Diagnostic Ultrasound*, 5th edition. Philadelphia, Elsevier, 2018, p 1737.

▶ Siegel MJ (ed): *Pediatric Sonography*, 4th edition. Philadelphia, Lippincott Williams & Wilkins, 2011, pp 172–174, 292.

229. **D. Ultrasound.**

Sonography is the imaging modality of choice to determine the presence of gallbladder or biliary tree pathology. Exam preparation requires fasting for best results. The exam time is short and there is no radiation involved.

▶ de Bruyn R (ed): *Pediatric Ultrasound: How, Why and When*, 2nd edition (e-book). Philadelphia, Churchill Livingstone/Elsevier, 2010, p 133.

▶ Rumack CM, Levine D (eds): *Diagnostic Ultrasound*, 5th edition. Philadelphia, Elsevier, 2018, p 165.

▶ Siegel MJ (ed): *Pediatric Sonography*, 4th edition. Philadelphia, Lippincott Williams & Wilkins, 2011, p 275.

230. **A. Retroperitoneal.**

An ectopic gallbladder is a congenital anomaly. The most common locations are retrohepatic (posterior to the right or left lobes), suprahepatic (between the liver and the diaphragm), and intrahepatic. Rarely, an ectopic gallbladder may be located within the retroperitoneum or lower abdomen, but these are not common locations.

▶ Rumack CM, Levine D (eds): *Diagnostic Ultrasound*, 5th edition. Philadelphia, Elsevier, 2018, pp 190, 194.

▶ Siegel MJ (ed): *Pediatric Sonography*, 4th edition. Philadelphia, Lippincott Williams & Wilkins, 2011, pp 277–278.

231. **D. Change the position of the patient.**

Low-level echoes can often be found within the gallbladder from side-lobe artifacts that mimic the appearance of sludge. Repositioning the patient and changing the angle of the sound beam can help to eliminate artifactual echoes. True sludge will layer with a change of position and will have a flat surface.

▶ Rumack CM, Levine D (eds): *Diagnostic Ultrasound*, 5th edition. Philadelphia, Elsevier, 2018, pp 194–195.

▶ Siegel MJ (ed): *Pediatric Sonography*, 4th edition. Philadelphia, Lippincott Williams & Wilkins, 2011, pp 283–285.

232. A. Pericholecystic fluid.

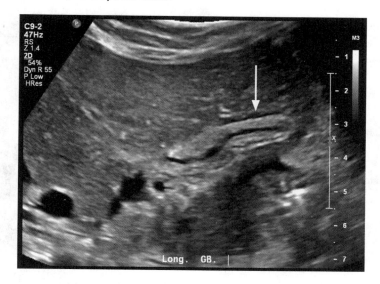

On occasion, a rim of pericholecystic fluid *can be seen with a thickened gallbladder wall, suggesting cholecystitis. It appears as a hypoechoic linear rim around the gallbladder wall.* Intrahepatic ducts *are usually too small to visualize with ultrasound. The* ligamentum venosum *and* interlobar fissure *would appear as a hyperechoic linear structure.*

▶ de Bruyn R (ed): *Pediatric Ultrasound: How, Why and When*, 2nd edition (e-book). Philadelphia, Churchill Livingstone/Elsevier, 2010, p 160.
▶ Rumack CM, Levine D (eds): *Diagnostic Ultrasound*, 5th edition. Philadelphia, Elsevier, 2018, pp 200, 1741.
▶ Siegel MJ (ed): *Pediatric Sonography*, 4th edition. Philadelphia, Lippincott Williams & Wilkins, 2011, p 279.

233. C. Jejunum.

The Kasai procedure *is also known as* hepatoportoenterostomy. *In this procedure, the abnormal bile ducts are removed from the liver and the porta hepatis is exposed to attach a Roux-en-Y loop of jejunum to the porta hepatis (hepaticojejunostomy). The jejunum then becomes the path for bile drainage. The earlier biliary atresia is diagnosed and surgery performed, the better the prognosis. The Kasai procedure is sometimes a temporary repair in children, with liver transplant ultimately the end treatment.*

▶ Rumack CM, Levine D (eds): *Diagnostic Ultrasound*, 5th edition. Philadelphia, Elsevier, 2018, pp 1737–1738.
▶ Siegel MJ (ed): *Pediatric Sonography*, 4th edition. Philadelphia, Lippincott Williams & Wilkins, 2011, p 292.

234. A. Cystic duct.

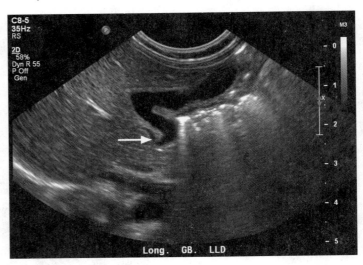

See Color Plate 14, "The Biliary Tree," on page xxxix.

The cystic duct *(arrow) is the adjoining duct that drains the gallbladder. Because of its small size, it is usually not seen with ultrasound in children. If the cystic duct is dilated, the distal part may be visualized near its insertion into the common bile duct. The cystic duct is best appreciated in the longitudinal plane when a patient is supine or in a left posterior oblique position. The* common bile duct, common hepatic duct, *and* intrahepatic ducts *do not have direct contact with the gallbladder.*

▶ de Bruyn R (ed): *Pediatric Ultrasound: How, Why and When*, 2nd edition (e-book). Philadelphia, Churchill Livingstone/Elsevier, 2010, p 132.
▶ Rumack CM, Levine D (eds): *Diagnostic Ultrasound*, 5th edition. Philadelphia, Elsevier, 2018, p 168.
▶ Siegel MJ (ed): *Pediatric Sonography*, 4th edition. Philadelphia, Lippincott Williams & Wilkins, 2011, pp 275, 291.

235. D. Alagille syndrome.

Alagille syndrome *is a hereditary disorder, usually autosomal dominant, in which there is an insufficient number of interlobular bile ducts. The lack of ducts leads to cholestasis and newborn jaundice. Alagille syndrome also includes heart, skeletal, and facial defects. The additional syndrome findings, especially the characteristic facies, help distinguish the cause of jaundice from biliary atresia. Patients will have elevated transaminase and bilirubin levels. Ultrasound findings are inconclusive since there is usually normal echogenicity of the liver parenchyma, no intrahepatic ductal dilatation is seen, and the gallbladder can range in size.* Caroli disease is a congenital anomaly consisting of cystic dilatation of the intrahepatic ducts. Cystic fibrosis (CF) is an autosomal recessive hereditary disorder causing a defect of fluid movement through transmembranes that results in thick secretions. CF patients may demonstrate a micro gallbladder and obstruction of the pancreatic ducts.

▶ de Bruyn R (ed): *Pediatric Ultrasound: How, Why and When*, 2nd edition (e-book). Philadelphia, Churchill Livingstone/Elsevier, 2010, p 143.
▶ Rumack CM, Levine D (eds): *Diagnostic Ultrasound*, 5th edition. Philadelphia, Elsevier, 2018, pp 171, 1736–1738, 1864.
▶ Siegel MJ (ed): *Pediatric Sonography*, 4th edition. Philadelphia, Lippincott Williams & Wilkins, 2011, p 294.

236. B. Contracted.

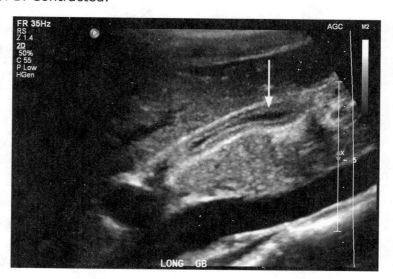

The largest amount of gallbladder emptying occurs postprandially, 45–60 minutes following a meal. The volume of the gallbladder decreases and the gallbladder will appear slit-like with a well-defined thickened wall (arrow) with no increase in blood flow. An acutely inflamed gallbladder would appear distended with a thickened wall. A complication of gangrenous cholecystitis, a perforated gallbladder would also include a thick wall. Septate gallbladders have a honeycomb appearance within a thin wall.

▶ de Bruyn R (ed): *Pediatric Ultrasound: How, Why and When*, 2nd edition (e-book). Philadelphia, Churchill Livingstone/Elsevier, 2010, p 136.
▶ Siegel MJ (ed): *Pediatric Sonography*, 4th edition. Philadelphia, Lippincott Williams & Wilkins, 2011, pp 275, 278, 285, 286.

237. **C. Choledocholithiasis.**

The disorder of stones within the biliary ducts is termed choledocholithiasis. *These stones usually start within the gallbladder and travel distally into the ducts. The majority of obstruction occurs near the level of the pancreatic head. The most common symptom is abdominal pain. Sonographically, a dilated bile duct will be seen proximal to the stone. If large enough, the stone will display shadowing and possibly the color Doppler "twinkle" sign.* Cholestasis *occurs when bile flow is slowed or stopped.* Cholecystitis *is the inflammation of the gallbladder.* Cholangitis *is infection of the bile ducts.*

▸ de Bruyn R (ed): *Pediatric Ultrasound: How, Why and When*, 2nd edition (e-book). Philadelphia, Churchill Livingstone/Elsevier, 2010, p 142.

▸ Rumack CM, Levine D (eds): *Diagnostic Ultrasound*, 5th edition. Philadelphia, Elsevier, 2018, pp 168–170, 172–174, 176, 1735–1736.

▸ Siegel MJ (ed): *Pediatric Sonography*, 4th edition. Philadelphia, Lippincott Williams & Wilkins, 2011, pp 285, 299, 300.

238. **D. Choledochal cyst.**

A choledochal cyst *is a congenital anomaly resulting in dilatation of the common bile duct associated with biliary obstruction. One theory of causation is that cyst formation occurs when cholangitis weakens the bile duct wall. There are multiple classifications of choledochal cysts based on their location and severity. Clinical signs are most commonly jaundice, but abdominal mass and pain can occur. More than half of the diagnosis of choledochal cysts will occur before age 10. If the cyst becomes large enough, duodenal obstruction can occur. Other complications include ascending cholangitis, stone formation, pancreatitis, biliary cirrhosis, and abscess. On ultrasound a well-defined cystic structure can be seen in the porta hepatis separate from the gallbladder but continuous with the extrahepatic bile ducts. Intrahepatic biliary duct dilatation can be seen in half of the cases.* Alagille syndrome *is a genetic disorder of bile duct formation resulting in a paucity of intrahepatic ducts and jaundice.* Cholecystitis *and* chloledocholithiasis *are not congenital anomalies.*

▸ Mieli-Vergani G, Hadzic N: Biliary atresia and neonatal disorders of the bile ducts. In Wyllie R, Hyams JS, Kay M (eds): *Pediatric Gastrointestinal and Liver Disease*, 5th edition. Philadelphia, Elsevier, 2016, pp 838–851.

▸ Rumack CM, Levine D (eds): *Diagnostic Ultrasound*, 5th edition. Philadelphia, Elsevier, 2018, pp 168–170, 1735–1736.

▸ Siegel MJ (ed): *Pediatric Sonography*, 4th edition. Philadelphia, Lippincott Williams & Wilkins, 2011, pp 286, 294–295, 300.

239. A. Head.

The head is <u>not</u> a segment of the gallbladder; it is a segment of the pancreas. The gallbladder fundus is the bulbous, most distal portion of the gallbladder. The body is the middle portion of the gallbladder. The neck is the most proximal portion, and it is the segment that is continuous with the cystic duct.

▶ Siegel MJ (ed): *Pediatric Sonography*, 4th edition. Philadelphia, Lippincott Williams & Wilkins, 2011, p 275.

240. C. Acute cholecystitis.

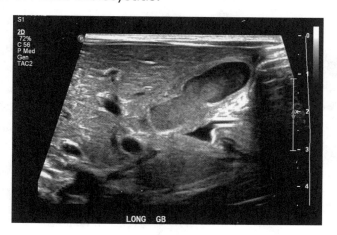

Cholecystitis is inflammation of the gallbladder. One of the symptoms of acute cholecystitis is a positive Murphy's sign, which is performed by an examiner deeply palpating the right subcostal region. The patient is instructed to take in a deep breath, which prompts the gallbladder to descend against the examiner's hand, causing pain to the patient. Other symptoms include epigastric or right upper quadrant tenderness or pain, jaundice, fever, and abnormal labs such as elevated white blood cells (WBC), alkaline phosphatase (ALP), and bilirubin. On ultrasound, gallstones, sludge, gallbladder enlargement, pericholecystic fluid, and hyperemia within a thickened wall may be seen. In chronic cholecystitis, the gallbladder is contracted rather than enlarged, there is no hyperemia within the wall, and the patient will not have a positive Murphy's sign. This image demonstrates a sludge-filled gallbladder with a thickened wall, typical of acute cholecystitis. Acalculous cholecystitis occurs without the presence of stones. Choledocholithiasis is the term for stones within the bile ducts.

▶ de Bruyn R (ed): *Pediatric Ultrasound: How, Why and When*, 2nd edition (e-book). Philadelphia, Churchill Livingstone/Elsevier, 2010, p 160.

▸ Rumack CM, Levine D (eds): *Diagnostic Ultrasound*, 5th edition. Philadelphia, Elsevier, 2018, pp 195–198, 200–202.

▸ Siegel MJ (ed): *Pediatric Sonography*, 4th edition. Philadelphia, Lippincott Williams & Wilkins, 2011, pp 286–288, 300–301.

▸ Urbano FL, Carroll M: Murphy's sign of cholecystitis. Hospital Physician 36:51–52, 2000. Available at http://www.turner-white.com/pdf/hp_nov00_murphy.pdf.

241. **A. Gallbladder agenesis.**

Gallbladder agenesis *is associated with biliary atresia. Although extremely rare, agenesis of the gallbladder is a congenital anomaly that can occur with or without biliary atresia. Gallbladder duplication, ectopic gallbladder, and septate gallbladder are also congenital anomalies. In* gallbladder duplication *a septum divides the gallbladder into two separate compartments. Each compartment will have its own cystic duct.* Ectopic gallbladders *are most often found in other areas around the liver.* Septate gallbladders *contain septations, causing a honeycomb appearance.*

▸ de Bruyn R (ed): *Pediatric Ultrasound: How, Why and When*, 2nd edition (e-book). Philadelphia, Churchill Livingstone/Elsevier, 2010, p 143.

▸ Rumack CM, Levine D (eds): *Diagnostic Ultrasound*, 5th edition. Philadelphia, Elsevier, 2018, pp 190, 194.

▸ Siegel MJ (ed): *Pediatric Sonography*, 4th edition. Philadelphia, Lippincott Williams & Wilkins, 2011, pp 277–278.

242. **B. Underlying disease.**

A high percentage (85%) of gallstones in children occur secondary to underlying disease. Gallstones in the pediatric population are not common, but most occur in adolescents. The more common underlying factors are cystic fibrosis, sickle cell disease, hemolytic anemia, Crohn disease, and liver disease. Gallstones appear as an intraluminal, echogenic focus with a "clean" distal shadow. If they measure less than 3 mm, a shadow may not be seen. Gallstones tend to be gravity dependent and move when patient position is changed. Some gallstones may float or can be immobile if they are adhered to the gallbladder wall. Gallstones are not associated with biliary atresia, low cholesterol levels, or gallbladder hydrops.

▸ de Bruyn R (ed): *Pediatric Ultrasound: How, Why and When*, 2nd edition (e-book). Philadelphia, Churchill Livingstone/Elsevier, 2010, pp 148, 155, 160–161.

▸ Rumack CM, Levine D (eds): *Diagnostic Ultrasound*, 5th edition. Philadelphia, Elsevier, 2018, pp 194, 1741, 1743.

▸ Siegel MJ (ed): *Pediatric Sonography*, 4th edition. Philadelphia, Lippincott Williams & Wilkins, 2011, pp 279–281, 292–293.

See Color Plate 14, "The Biliary Tree," on page xxxix.

243. D. Main pancreatic duct.

The common bile duct is extrahepatic in location. It is the portion of the biliary tree located between the junction of the cystic and common hepatic ducts and the main pancreatic duct at the level of the ampulla of Vater. The main right and left hepatic ducts *merge to form the common hepatic duct. Intrahepatic ducts are located within the liver, and all merge to become the main right and left hepatic ducts.*

▸ de Bruyn R (ed): *Pediatric Ultrasound: How, Why and When*, 2nd edition (e-book). Philadelphia, Churchill Livingstone/Elsevier, 2010, p 172.
▸ Rumack CM, Levine D (eds): *Diagnostic Ultrasound*, 5th edition. Philadelphia, Elsevier, 2018, p 166.
▸ Siegel MJ (ed): *Pediatric Sonography*, 4th edition. Philadelphia, Lippincott Williams & Wilkins, 2011, pp 276, 291.

244. B. Caroli disease.

Caroli disease is a congenital condition consisting of the cystic dilatation of the intrahepatic biliary tree. There are two forms of Caroli disease. Both forms are associated with renal cystic disease and both forms increase the risk for cholangiocarcinoma. One form includes saccular-appearing dilated ducts, cholangitis, and stones. There is no cirrhosis or portal hypertension. Symptoms include pain, fever, and jaundice. The second form is associated with congenital hepatic fibrosis and portal hypertension but does not usually include cholangitis or stones. On ultrasound, multiple dilated ducts are present. The ducts may have linear bands, echogenic protrusions, or a "central dot sign" within the ductal walls. Enlarged, cystic kidneys with echogenic pyramids may also be found. Alagille syndrome and cystic fibrosis are inherited disorders that do not display intrahepatic dilated ducts. Biliary atresia *is congenital, but intrahepatic ducts are not typically seen at all.*

▸ de Bruyn R (ed): *Pediatric Ultrasound: How, Why and When*, 2nd edition (e-book). Philadelphia, Churchill Livingstone/Elsevier, 2010, pp 145–146.
▸ Rumack CM, Levine D (eds): *Diagnostic Ultrasound*, 5th edition. Philadelphia, Elsevier, 2018, pp 171, 1736–1738, 1864.
▸ Siegel MJ (ed): *Pediatric Sonography*, 4th edition. Philadelphia, Lippincott Williams & Wilkins, 2011, pp 292–296.

245. **C. Endoscopic retrograde cholangiopancreatography (ERCP).**

Endoscopic retrograde cholangiopancreatography *(ERCP) is an endoscopic procedure that a gastroenterologist performs. It can be used to diagnose diseases of the biliary system, remove stones from bile ducts, or place a stent within a duct for drainage. For biliary atresia, the* Kasai procedure *is the surgical replacement of the biliary ducts with a portion of the jejunum.* Cholescintography *is a nuclear medicine scan performed to detect gallbladder function or abnormalities.* Magnetic resonance cholangiopancreatography *(MRCP) is an imaging technique to visualize the biliary and pancreatic ducts and is not a therpeutic procedure.*

▶ Orfanidis NT: Imaging tests of the liver and gallbladder. Available at https://www.merckmanuals.com/professional/hepatic-and-biliary-disorders/testing-for-hepatic-and-biliary-disorders/imaging-tests-of-the-liver-and-gallbladder.

▶ Siegel MJ (ed): *Pediatric Sonography*, 4th edition. Philadelphia, Lippincott Williams & Wilkins, 2011, pp 296, 290.

246. **D. Junctional fold.**

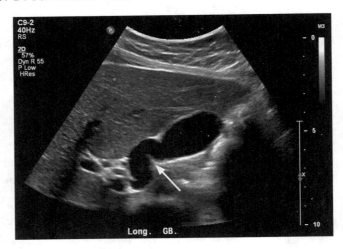

Gallbladder folds *are anatomic variants secondary to kinking or folding of the organ; junctional folds and Phrygian caps are the most common.* Junctional folds *are located between the neck and body segments of the gallbladder.* Phrygian caps *occur when the gallbladder fundus folds over. A* septate gallbladder *would be represented sonographically by a honeycomb appearance within the gallbladder lumen.* Sludge *would also be seen within the gallbladder lumen and would not appear as a linear echogenic fold.*

▶ Siegel MJ (ed): *Pediatric Sonography*, 4th edition. Philadelphia, Lippincott Williams & Wilkins, 2011, pp 277–278, 283–284.

247. **A. Bile stasis.**

Neonates undergoing total parenteral nutrition (TPN) or intravenous (IV) feeds are at a higher risk of gallstone development secondary to bile stasis. Bowel rest and bile stasis induced by IV feeds can lead to the production of sludge and gallstones. Cholangitis is inflammation of the bile duct system and is commonly related to bacterial infections. Cholangitis is not associated with TPN and/or gallstone formation. TPN is not associated with anemia or malnutrition, as it is a special balanced food supplement delivered directly to the bloodstream.

▶ de Bruyn R (ed): *Pediatric Ultrasound: How, Why and When*, 2nd edition (e-book). Philadelphia, Churchill Livingstone/Elsevier, 2010, pp 143, 144, 161–162.

▶ Rumack CM, Levine D (eds): *Diagnostic Ultrasound*, 5th edition. Philadelphia, Elsevier, 2018, pp 1741, 1743.

▶ Siegel MJ (ed): *Pediatric Sonography*, 4th edition. Philadelphia, Lippincott Williams & Wilkins, 2011, p 280.

248. **D. Polyp.**

Gallbladder polyps are typically small nonshadowing, nonmobile, echogenic structures adhered to the gallbladder wall. They protrude from the gallbladder wall into the lumen. Gallstones and sludge are more commonly gravity dependent. Air in the gallbladder wall causes a reverberation shadowing artifact.

▶ Rumack CM, Levine D (eds): *Diagnostic Ultrasound*, 5th edition. Philadelphia, Elsevier, 2018, p 2035.

▶ Siegel MJ (ed): *Pediatric Sonography*, 4th edition. Philadelphia, Lippincott Williams & Wilkins, 2011, pp 283, 289.

249. **C. Thin gallbladder wall.**

Perforation of the gallbladder can occur secondary to trauma or as a complication of extensive cholecystitis or gangrene. The most common site of perforation is the gallbladder fundus. Sonographic signs include a small gallbladder, interruption in the gallbladder wall, pericholecystic fluid, abscess formation, and cholelithiasis.

▶ Siegel MJ (ed): *Pediatric Sonography*, 4th edition. Philadelphia, Lippincott Williams & Wilkins, 2011, pp 200, 286.

250. **B. Murphy's sign and wall hyperemia.**

The two sonographic signs that help differentiate acute from chronic cholecystitis are the sonographic Murphy's sign and wall hyperemia. In acute cholecystitis, Murphy's sign and a thickened hyperemic gallbladder wall are present. In chronic cholecystitis, Murphy's sign and hyperemia are absent. The wall appears thickened in the presence of both acute and chronic cholecystitis, but the increased vascularity helps differentiate acute from chronic. Lab values are elevated in both instances.

▶ de Bruyn R (ed): *Pediatric Ultrasound: How, Why and When*, 2nd edition (e-book). Philadelphia, Churchill Livingstone/Elsevier, 2010, p 160.

▶ Rumack CM, Levine D (eds): *Diagnostic Ultrasound*, 5th edition. Philadelphia, Elsevier, 2018, pp 195–198, 200–202.

▶ Siegel MJ (ed): *Pediatric Sonography*, 4th edition. Philadelphia, Lippincott Williams & Wilkins, 2011, pp 286–287.

251. **C. Hypoalbuminemia.**

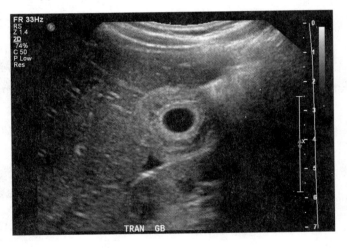

Causes of gallbladder wall thickening include cholecystitis, hepatic dysfunction, pancreatitis, hypoalbuminemia, congestive heart failure, sepsis, bone marrow transplant, cholangiopathy, and eating. Wall thickening can be focal or diffuse, but diffuse is most common. A normal gallbladder should not have a thickened wall when the patient is in a fasting state. Splenomegaly and anemia are not causes of thickening of the gallbladder wall.

▶ Rumack CM, Levine D (eds): *Diagnostic Ultrasound*, 5th edition. Philadelphia, Elsevier, 2018, pp 200, 1741.

▶ Siegel MJ (ed): *Pediatric Sonography*, 4th edition. Philadelphia, Lippincott Williams & Wilkins, 2011, p 279.

252. D. Sludge.

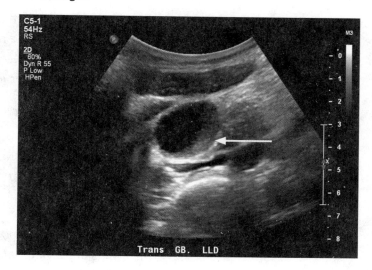

Sludge *(arrow)* is particulate matter of bile within the gallbladder and has a typical sonographic appearance. Lower to medium echoes are seen within the lumen without shadowing. Sludge is gravity dependent and will change position as the patient moves because it is viscous. Acoustic enhancement can still be demonstrated. Although also typically gravity dependent, gallstones and air within the gallbladder will most often display shadowing. Gallbladder polyps are adhered to the wall and do not change position when the patient does.

▶ de Bruyn R (ed): *Pediatric Ultrasound: How, Why and When*, 2nd edition (e-book). Philadelphia, Churchill Livingstone/Elsevier, 2010, p 161.

▶ Rumack CM, Levine D (eds): *Diagnostic Ultrasound*, 5th edition. Philadelphia, Elsevier, 2018, pp 194–196.

▶ Siegel MJ (ed): *Pediatric Sonography*, 4th edition. Philadelphia, Lippincott Williams & Wilkins, 2011, pp 283–284.

253. B. Wall thickening.

Polypoid masses such as adenomas, papillomas, hamartomas, and adenocarcinomas within the gallbladder are uncommon in the pediatric population. Sludge, hydrops, and ductal dilatation may show evidence of obstruction but are not associated with an increased risk for malignancy. The sonographic finding of a thickened gallbladder wall adjacent to the mass increases the likelihood of malignancy.

▶ Rumack CM, Levine D (eds): *Diagnostic Ultrasound*, 5th edition. Philadelphia, Elsevier, 2018, p 203.

▶ Siegel MJ (ed): *Pediatric Sonography*, 4th edition. Philadelphia, Lippincott Williams & Wilkins, 2011, p 289.

254. C. Pancreatitis.

Although it affects only a small percentage (10%) of cases, pancreatitis is the most common complication of pediatric gallstone disease. Cholangitis, perforation, and choledocholithiasis occur less often than pancreatitis.

▸ Fishman DS, Gilger MA: Diseases of the gallbladder. In Wyllie R, Hyams JS, Kay M (eds): *Pediatric Gastrointestinal and Liver Disease*, 5th edition. Philadelphia, Elsevier, 2016, pp 977–989.

▸ Siegel MJ (ed): *Pediatric Sonography*, 4th edition. Philadelphia, Lippincott Williams & Wilkins, 2011, p 280.

255. D. Tumefactive.

Tumefactive sludge, *also known as a* sludge ball, *occurs when the sludge material doesn't form a fluid level but instead combines to form a mass-like structure. Sludge balls are echogenic, nonshadowing, and mobile on decubitus. The mobility is what helps differentiate them from polypoid tumors.*

▸ Rumack CM, Levine D (eds): *Diagnostic Ultrasound*, 5th edition. Philadelphia, Elsevier, 2018, pp 195–196.

▸ Siegel MJ (ed): *Pediatric Sonography*, 4th edition. Philadelphia, Lippincott Williams & Wilkins, 2011, p 284.

256. B. Pancreas.

The primary components of the biliary tree consist of the liver, gallbladder, and bile ducts. The biliary tree makes, stores, and transports bile. The liver is responsible for detoxification, metabolism, storage, and the production of bile. The role of the gallbladder is to store concentrated bile until it is needed for digestion. The pancreas is an exocrine gland that makes insulin and enzymes to aid in digestion.

▸ PubMed Health: Biliary tract. Available at https://www.ncbi.nlm.nih.gov/pubmedhealth/PMHT0018956/.

▸ Siegel MJ (ed): *Pediatric Sonography*, 4th edition. Philadelphia, Lippincott Williams & Wilkins, 2011, p 291.

257. A. Biliary atresia.

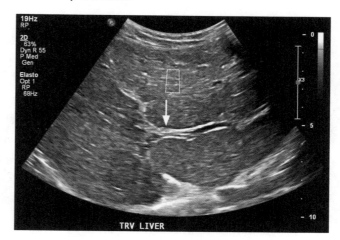

The "triangular cord sign" is an avascular, echogenic, cone- or triangle-shaped thickness located above or anterior to the portal vein bifurcation. This reliable finding, along with an absent or small gallbladder, has a specificity as high as 100% for biliary atresia. In biliary atresia, the liver can appear normal or increased in parenchymal echogenicity. There is typically an enlarged hepatic artery and subcapsular arterial flow extending to the hepatic surface. Intrahepatic ducts are not visualized. Biliary atresia is associated with polysplenia, absent inferior vena cava, and situs inversus. In Caroli disease, the intrahepatic ducts are dilated and cystic. With a choledochal cyst or portal vein thrombosis, the gallbladder is usually unaffected.

▶ de Bruyn R (ed): *Pediatric Ultrasound: How, Why and When*, 2nd edition (e-book). Philadelphia, Churchill Livingstone/Elsevier, 2010, pp 142–143.
▶ Rumack CM, Levine D (eds): *Diagnostic Ultrasound*, 5th edition. Philadelphia, Elsevier, 2018, pp 1737–1738.
▶ Siegel MJ (ed): *Pediatric Sonography*, 4th edition. Philadelphia, Lippincott Williams & Wilkins, 2011, pp 292–293.

258. D. 6 mm.

In children (ages 1–10) and adolescents, the common bile duct (CBD) should measure less than 6 mm. In neonates, the upper limit of normal is much smaller at 1 mm. For infants up to 1 year old, the CBD should measure less than 2 mm. Measurements are taken in a sagittal plane. Post cholecystectomy, it is normal for the CBD to increase in diameter.

▶ Rumack CM, Levine D (eds): *Diagnostic Ultrasound*, 5th edition. Philadelphia, Elsevier, 2018, p 168.
▶ Siegel MJ (ed): *Pediatric Sonography*, 4th edition. Philadelphia, Lippincott Williams & Wilkins, 2011, p 291.

PART 7

Pancreas

259. **A. Uncinate process.**

The pancreas comprises the segmental portions termed the head, neck, body, tail, and uncinate process. The uncinate process is an extension of the head segment and lies more caudal and medial to the head. The uncinate process curls underneath the splenic vein at the level of the portosplenic confluence. The head, body, and tail all lie anterior to the splenic vein.

▶ de Bruyn R (ed): *Pediatric Ultrasound: How, Why and When*, 2nd edition (e-book). Philadelphia, Churchill Livingstone/Elsevier, 2010, p 173.
▶ Rumack CM, Levine D (eds): *Diagnostic Ultrasound*, 5th edition. Philadelphia, Elsevier, 2018, pp 211–212.
▶ Siegel MJ (ed): *Pediatric Sonography*, 4th edition. Philadelphia, Lippincott Williams & Wilkins, 2011, p 478.

260. **D. Insulinoma.**

An *insulinoma is the most common endocrine tumor of the pancreas. Endocrine tumors are known as* islet cell tumors. *These tumors actively produce and secrete hormones. Clinical signs are elevated insulin levels and symptoms of hypoglycemia. An insulinoma will appear as a small (usually 2 cm) homogeneous, hypoechoic mass. Insulinomas may have an echogenic capsule and are hypervascular.* Lymphangiomas *are caused by the obstruction of fetal lymphatics and do not produce or secrete hormones.* Adenocarcinoma *and* pancreatoblastomas *are large and malignant exocrine tumors of the pancreas.*

▶ Rumack CM, Levine D (eds): *Diagnostic Ultrasound*, 5th edition. Philadelphia, Elsevier, 2018, pp 238, 248, 1865.
▶ Siegel MJ (ed): *Pediatric Sonography*, 4th edition. Philadelphia, Lippincott Williams & Wilkins, 2011, pp 483, 486.

261. **A. Hormones.**

The pancreas acts as both an endocrine gland and an exocrine gland. The endocrine function of the pancreas is to secrete the hormones insulin and glucagon directly into the bloodstream to control blood sugar levels. Islet cells (islets of Langerhans) produce insulin, which can raise blood sugar, and glucagon, which can lower blood sugar. The exocrine function of the pancreas produces enzymes that help to break down ingested proteins and fats.

- Columbia University Department of Surgery: The pancreas and its functions. Available at http://columbiasurgery.org/pancreas/pancreas-and-its-functions.
- Hormones of the pancreas. Available at http://www.biology-pages.info/P/Pancreas.html.
- Sargis RM: An overview of the pancreas. Available at https://www.endocrineweb.com/endocrinology/overview-pancreas.

262. **B. Computed tomography (CT).**

Computed tomography (CT) is the method of choice for the evaluation of pancreatic abnormalities such as pancreatitis, trauma, or tumors. Whether the patient is fasting or not, the presence of abdominal gas on ultrasound can hinder the visualization of the pancreas and adjacent structures. Magnetic resonance imaging (MRI) may also be helpful, but it usually takes longer to complete than the faster CT scan. Endoscopic ultrasound (EUS) is used to assess digestive structures and the adjacent pancreas, often following an abnormal CT.

- de Bruyn R (ed): *Pediatric Ultrasound: How, Why and When*, 2nd edition (e-book). Philadelphia, Churchill Livingstone/Elsevier, 2010, pp 174, 176, 179.
- DiMaio CJ: Pancreas endoscopic ultrasound (EUS). Available at https://pancreasfoundation.org/endoscopic-ultrasound-eus/.
- Siegel MJ (ed): *Pediatric Sonography*, 4th edition. Philadelphia, Lippincott Williams & Wilkins, 2011, p 488.

263. **B. Curved 9.5 MHz.**

The highest-frequency transducer with the proper penetration is always the best selection when imaging. In children, the most adequate transducer would be the curved 9.5 MHz. A curved 8 MHz may work well with infants, since the transducer footprint is smaller than that of the curved 9.5 MHz. The linear 12 MHz transducer may work on a neonate, but it will not supply enough penetration on a child. The curved 5 MHz, with a lower frequency that allows greater penetration, would be the proper selection for larger adolescents and teens.

- Rumack CM, Levine D (eds): *Diagnostic Ultrasound*, 5th edition. Philadelphia, Elsevier, 2018, p 211.
- Siegel MJ (ed): *Pediatric Sonography*, 4th edition. Philadelphia, Lippincott Williams & Wilkins, 2011, p 478.

264. **D. Anterior perirenal space.**

Inflammatory spread occurs with the pancreas more than other organs because the pancreas is not surrounded by a fibrous capsule like the liver or kidneys. Fluid collections accompany pancreatitis in about half of patients with this disorder. Inflammatory fluid collections most commonly occur within the anterior perirenal space, where the pancreas is located. The lesser omental sac, located between the pancreas and the stomach, is the second most common location. Other areas that may demonstrate fluid collections are the subphrenic spaces, greater and lesser omentum, transverse colon, perihepatic spaces, and pelvis.

▶ Rumack CM, Levine D (eds): *Diagnostic Ultrasound*, 5th edition. Philadelphia, Elsevier, 2018, pp 219–225, 230–233, 1862–1864.

▶ Siegel MJ (ed): *Pediatric Sonography*, 4th edition. Philadelphia, Lippincott Williams & Wilkins, 2011, pp 488–489.

265. **C. Congenital hyperinsulinism/nesidioblastosis.**

Nesidioblastosis, *now known as* congenital hyperinsulinism *or* hyperinsulinemic hypoglycemia, *is a rare disorder occurring when there is diffuse proliferation of islet cells that results in hyperinsulinism and endocrine hypoglycemia. Symptoms of hypoglycemia are present shortly after birth. Because this condition is typically resistant to medical treatment, a subtotal pancreatectomy is usually performed. Ultrasound does not typically play a role in this diagnosis.* Insulinomas *are the most common type of islet cell tumor made up of beta cells. Patients with insulinomas present with elevated serum insulin levels (hypoglycemia).* Hyperglycemia *is a condition caused by an elevated blood sugar or glucose level.* Schwachman-Diamond syndrome *is an inherited genetic disorder causing pancreatic (exocrine) insufficiency. The pancreas undergoes lipomatosis, the replacement of pancreatic tissue by fat.*

▶ de Bruyn R (ed): *Pediatric Ultrasound: How, Why and When*, 2nd edition (e-book). Philadelphia, Churchill Livingstone/Elsevier, 2010, p 175.

▶ Rumack CM, Levine D (eds): *Diagnostic Ultrasound*, 5th edition. Philadelphia, Elsevier, 2018, pp 248, 1865.

▶ Siegel MJ (ed): *Pediatric Sonography*, 4th edition. Philadelphia, Lippincott Williams & Wilkins, 2011, pp 482–483, 485.

266. A. Superior mesenteric artery (SMA).

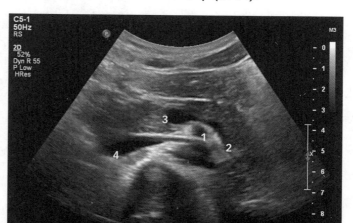

The pancreas lies obliquely within the body between the second portion of the duodenum and the splenic hilum. The pancreatic head lies to the right of the superior mesenteric artery or SMA (1), anterior to the inferior vena cava or IVC (4), and medial to the duodenum. The neck and body lie anterior to the SMA. The tail lies anterior and to the left of the SMA and the portosplenic confluence, which comprises the portal vein (3) and splenic vein (2).

▶ de Bruyn R (ed): *Pediatric Ultrasound: How, Why and When*, 2nd edition (e-book). Philadelphia, Churchill Livingstone/Elsevier, 2010, p 191.

▶ Rumack CM, Levine D (eds): *Diagnostic Ultrasound*, 5th edition. Philadelphia, Elsevier, 2018, pp 211–213.

▶ Siegel MJ (ed): *Pediatric Sonography*, 4th edition. Philadelphia, Lippincott Williams & Wilkins, 2011, p 478.

267. C. 3 mm.

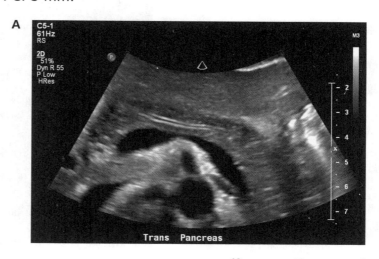

(figure continues . . .)

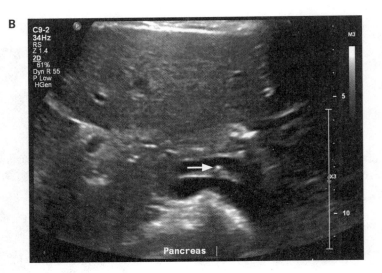

The pancreatic duct is normally visualized in the majority of pediatric cases. The most common area of visualization is within the central body of the pancreas in the transverse plane. The AP diameter of the pancreatic duct should not exceed 3 mm in normal cases. Dilatation of the pancreatic duct is associated with pancreatitis. These images demonstrate **A** a normal pancreatic duct and **B** a dilated pancreatic duct with a stone present within the lumen (arrow).

▸ Rumack CM, Levine D (eds): *Diagnostic Ultrasound*, 5th edition. Philadelphia, Elsevier, 2018, p 218.

▸ Siegel MJ (ed): *Pediatric Sonography*, 4th edition. Philadelphia, Lippincott Williams & Wilkins, 2011, p 479.

268. C. Pseudocyst.

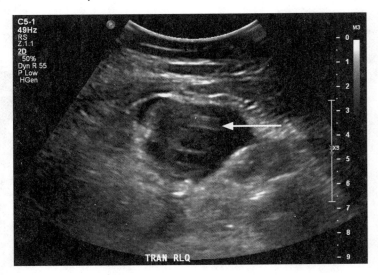

Pseudocyst *is the most common complication of acute pancreatitis. A pseudocyst is termed "pseudo" because it does not have the normal thin epithelial lining that a true cyst has. Instead, its lining is thicker and made up of glandular*

and fibrous tissue. Most often, pseudocysts occur near the pancreas or within the lesser sac, but they can be found in other areas, such as the distal end of a ventriculoperitoneal (VP) shunt. On ultrasound, they appear well circumscribed and may contain septations or debris. They can be anechoic or hypoechoic and demonstrate posterior enhancement. This image shows a pseudocyst with the VP shunt tip (arrow) present within. Pseudocysts usually do not resolve and require percutaneous catheter drainage or surgery. Organ failure, GI bleeding, and decreased calcium levels are complications that occur with chronic pancreatitis.

▶ de Bruyn R (ed): *Pediatric Ultrasound: How, Why and When*, 2nd edition (e-book). Philadelphia, Churchill Livingstone/Elsevier, 2010, pp 147, 167, 176–178, 200.

▶ Rumack CM, Levine D (eds): *Diagnostic Ultrasound*, 5th edition. Philadelphia, Elsevier, 2018, pp 228–229, 1865.

▶ Siegel MJ (ed): *Pediatric Sonography*, 4th edition. Philadelphia, Lippincott Williams & Wilkins, 2011, pp 489–490.

269. **D. Body.**

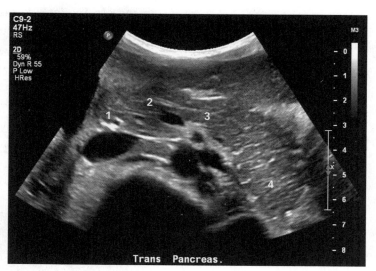

The body of the pancreas is labeled 3. This is the segment of the pancreas where the pancreatic duct is most commonly visualized. The head (1) and neck (2) are located to the right of the body. The tail (4) is located to the left of the body and is closest to the splenic hilum.

▶ Rumack CM, Levine D (eds): *Diagnostic Ultrasound*, 5th edition. Philadelphia, Elsevier, 2018, pp 211–213.

▶ Siegel MJ (ed): *Pediatric Sonography*, 4th edition. Philadelphia, Lippincott Williams & Wilkins, 2011, p 478.

270. **A. Digestion.**

   The exocrine glands within the pancreas produce many enzymes that aid in digestion. Trypsin and chymotrypsin digest proteins. Amylase aids in breaking down carbohydrates and turning them into sugar. Lipase breaks down fats. Along with bile, the pancreatic juices that contain these enzymes are released into the duodenum to aid in the digestion process. Controlling blood sugar is the endocrine function of the pancreas. The production of white blood cells occurs in bone marrow and the spleen. The liver is the organ that detoxifies the blood.

   ▶ Columbia University Department of Surgery: The pancreas and its functions. Available at http://columbiasurgery.org/pancreas/pancreas-and-its-functions.

271. **D. Congenital.**

   Congenital cysts of the pancreas are associated with von Hippel–Lindau disease and autosomal dominant polycystic kidney disease (ADPKD). Both are autosomal dominant disorders and include cysts in various organs. Congenital cysts are simple, thin-walled, and unilocular. Clinical signs include abdominal mass or distention, vomiting, and jaundice from the compression of adjacent structures.

   ▶ Rumack CM, Levine D (eds): *Diagnostic Ultrasound*, 5th edition. Philadelphia, Elsevier, 2018, p 1865.
   ▶ Siegel MJ (ed): *Pediatric Sonography*, 4th edition. Philadelphia, Lippincott Williams & Wilkins, 2011, p 482.

272. **C. Cystic fibrosis.**

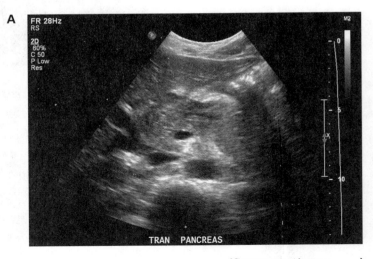

(figure continues . . .)

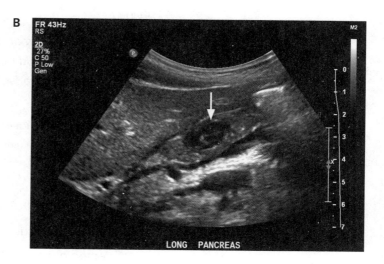

Cystic fibrosis *(see image **A**)* is associated with an echogenic pancreas; other conditions also characterized by an echogenic pancreas are chronic pancreatitis, lipomatosis, and steroid therapy. With acute pancreatitis, inflammation is usually mild and reversible, and the pancreas may appear normal or may enlarge and decrease in echogenicity. As the inflammation progresses to chronic pancreatitis, the pancreas increases in echogenicity due to fatty deposits and/or fibrosis. Calcifications may also be present with chronic pancreatitis. Necrotizing pancreatitis *is the most severe form of acute pancreatitis, where destruction and liquefaction of tissue can occur. Necrosis of the pancreas can be parenchymal or peripancreatic. Image **B** shows parenchymal necrotizing pancreatitis (arrow) within the head of the pancreas. An* annular pancreas *is a congenital anomaly affecting the position of the pancreas, not the echogenicity.*

▶ de Bruyn R (ed): *Pediatric Ultrasound: How, Why and When*, 2nd edition (e-book). Philadelphia, Churchill Livingstone/Elsevier, 2010, pp 174–175.
▶ Rumack CM, Levine D (eds): *Diagnostic Ultrasound*, 5th edition. Philadelphia, Elsevier, 2018, pp 219–225, 230–233, 1862–1864.
▶ Siegel MJ (ed): *Pediatric Sonography*, 4th edition. Philadelphia, Lippincott Williams & Wilkins, 2011, pp 481, 488–491.

273. **B. Anteroposterior.**

The anteroposterior (AP) diameter is the standard dimension for measuring the pancreas because in the transverse plane, the margins of the pancreas are most consistently delineated. The best approach for visualizing the pancreas in its entirety is the subxiphoid approach. Measurements of the different segments are not routinely performed on children when the pancreas is normal. Sagittal, transverse, and volume measurements would not be performed in the different segments due to the lack of definitive borders.

▶ de Bruyn R (ed): *Pediatric Ultrasound: How, Why and When*, 2nd edition (e-book). Philadelphia, Churchill Livingstone/Elsevier, 2010, p 173.
▶ Rumack CM, Levine D (eds): *Diagnostic Ultrasound*, 5th edition. Philadelphia, Elsevier, 2018, pp 211–213.
▶ Siegel MJ (ed): *Pediatric Sonography*, 4th edition. Philadelphia, Lippincott Williams & Wilkins, 2011, pp 479–480.

274. **A. Duct of Wirsung.**

In the embryo, the merging of the dorsal and ventral ducts forms the main pancreatic duct or duct of Wirsung. The main pancreatic duct merges into the common bile duct near the ampulla of Vater before emptying into the duodenum. The duct of Santorini is an accessory pancreatic duct seen in only a portion of the population.

▶ Rumack CM, Levine D (eds): *Diagnostic Ultrasound*, 5th edition. Philadelphia, Elsevier, 2018, p 218.
▶ Siegel MJ (ed): *Pediatric Sonography*, 4th edition. Philadelphia, Lippincott Williams & Wilkins, 2011, p 480.

275. **C. Portal vein.**

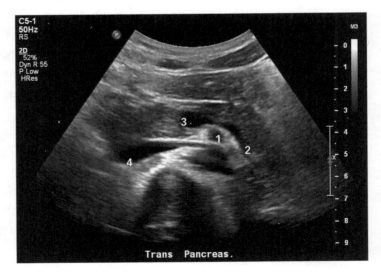

The pancreas lies obliquely within the body between the second portion of the duodenum and the splenic hilum. The pancreatic head lies to the right of the superior mesenteric artery or SMA (1), anterior to the inferior vena cava or IVC (4), and medial to the duodenum. The neck and body lie

anterior to the SMA. The tail lies anterior and to the left of the SMA and portosplenic confluence, which comprises the portal vein (3) and splenic vein (2).

▶ de Bruyn R (ed): *Pediatric Ultrasound: How, Why and When*, 2nd edition (e-book). Philadelphia, Churchill Livingstone/Elsevier, 2010, pp 132, 135.
▶ Rumack CM, Levine D (eds): *Diagnostic Ultrasound*, 5th edition. Philadelphia, Elsevier, 2018, pp 211–213.
▶ Siegel MJ (ed): *Pediatric Sonography*, 4th edition. Philadelphia, Lippincott Williams & Wilkins, 2011, p 478.

276. D. Lymphangioma.

A lymphangioma is a congenital pancreatic mass caused by the blockage of fetal lymphatics. Sonographically, a lymphangioma appears hypoechoic and contains septated areas filled with chylous fluid. If hemorrhagic, it may contain areas of echoes and debris. Teratomas, insulinomas, and lymphomas are not congenital masses.

▶ Chung EM, Travis MD, Conran RM: Pancreatic tumors in children: radiologic-pathologic correlation. Radiographics 26:1211–1238, 2006. Available at https://pubs.rsna.org/doi/full/10.1148/rg.264065012.
▶ Rumack CM, Levine D (eds): *Diagnostic Ultrasound*, 5th edition. Philadelphia, Elsevier, 2018, p 1865.
▶ Siegel MJ (ed): *Pediatric Sonography*, 4th edition. Philadelphia, Lippincott Williams & Wilkins, 2011, p 486.

277. B. GI tract.

Pancreatic tissue separate from the anatomic or vascular channels of the pancreas is termed an "ectopic" pancreas. Ectopic pancreatic tissue is a congenital anomaly and typically asymptomatic. Most of the time, ectopic pancreatic tissue is located in the stomach, duodenum, or jejunum. Other locations include the ileum, liver, splenic hilum, and umbilicus.

▶ de Bruyn R (ed): *Pediatric Ultrasound: How, Why and When*, 2nd edition (e-book). Philadelphia, Churchill Livingstone/Elsevier, 2010, pp 172, 173, 187–188.
▶ Rumack CM, Levine D (eds): *Diagnostic Ultrasound*, 5th edition. Philadelphia, Elsevier, 2018, p 218.
▶ Siegel MJ (ed): *Pediatric Sonography*, 4th edition. Philadelphia, Lippincott Williams & Wilkins, 2011, p 481.

278. C. Caudate.

When you are scanning in the sagittal plane, the head of the pancreas can be visualized inferior to the caudate lobe of the liver. The head of the pancreas is also anterior to the inferior vena cava and right of the superior mesenteric artery (SMA) and vein (SMV). The gastroduodenal artery lies close to the anterior surface of the pancreatic head and neck. The head of the pancreas is inferior to the left lobe of the liver, but not directly. The majority of the right lobe is lateral to the pancreas. The quadrate lobe lies cephalad to the caudate lobe, so it would also not be directly superior to the head of the pancreas.

▶ Rumack CM, Levine D (eds): *Diagnostic Ultrasound*, 5th edition. Philadelphia, Elsevier, 2018, pp 211–213.
▶ Siegel MJ (ed): *Pediatric Sonography*, 4th edition. Philadelphia, Lippincott Williams & Wilkins, 2011, p 478.

279. **A. Annular pancreas.**

Annular pancreas is a congenital anomaly of the pancreas. It is second in occurrence to pancreas divisum. This anomaly occurs when a bifid ventral bud forms during embryonic development. The bifid pancreatic tissue encases the duodenum and can lead to duodenal obstruction. Clinical symptoms can be vomiting, abdominal distention, and a "double bubble" sign on x-ray. On ultrasound, pancreatic tissue is seen surrounding a dilated and fluid-filled descending duodenum. Pancreas divisum is the most common congenital anomaly of the pancreas, occurring when the ventral and dorsal ducts do not fuse into one main pancreatic duct. Ectopic pancreatic tissue, when it occurs, can be found throughout the body but most often is located in the GI tract. Dorsal pancreatic agenesis results in a short pancreas because only the head develops. Dorsal pancreatic agenesis is associated with polysplenia.

▶ de Bruyn R (ed): *Pediatric Ultrasound: How, Why and When*, 2nd edition (e-book). Philadelphia, Churchill Livingstone/Elsevier, 2010, p 172.
▶ Rumack CM, Levine D (eds): *Diagnostic Ultrasound*, 5th edition. Philadelphia, Elsevier, 2018, p 218.
▶ Siegel MJ (ed): *Pediatric Sonography*, 4th edition. Philadelphia, Lippincott Williams & Wilkins, 2011, pp 480–481.

280. **D. Cystic fibrosis.**

Cystic fibrosis is an autosomal recessive inherited disorder caused by a gene on chromosome 7. This gene causes a defect of fluid movement through transmembranes that results in thickened secretions. The thickness of the secretions causes obstruction of the alveoli and pancreatic ducts. Obstruction of the pancreatic ducts leads to the fatty replacement, fibrotic changes, and atrophy of the pancreas. Clinical signs include pain, steatorrhea, and failure to thrive. On ultrasound, fatty infiltration causes an increase in echogenicity and a pancreas that appears smaller if it has atrophied. Microscopic or small cysts and calcifications may be present. Schwachman-Diamond syndrome *is an inherited genetic disorder causing pancreatic (exocrine) insufficiency. With Schwachman-Diamond syndrome, the pancreas undergoes lipomatosis, where the pancreatic tissue is replaced by fat.* Von Hippel–Lindau disease *is associated with pancreatic cysts. Tuberous sclerosis is a multisystem disorder where tumors can be found in multiple organs, although the pancreas would be an uncommon location. Most tumors secondary to tuberous sclerosis occur in the brain, eyes, heart, kidneys, and skin.*

▶ de Bruyn R (ed): *Pediatric Ultrasound: How, Why and When*, 2nd edition (e-book). Philadelphia, Churchill Livingstone/Elsevier, 2010, pp 154–155, 174–175, 192–193.

▶ Rumack CM, Levine D (eds): *Diagnostic Ultrasound*, 5th edition. Philadelphia, Elsevier, 2018, pp 1864–1865.

▶ Siegel MJ (ed): *Pediatric Sonography*, 4th edition. Philadelphia, Lippincott Williams & Wilkins, 2011, pp 481–482.

281. B. Presence of metastasis.

One of the most obvious sonographic differences between a pancreatoblastoma and an adenocarcinoma is the presence of metastasis at the time of discovery. With adenocarcinoma *it is very common that metastasis and tumor extension will already be present. Surgery is required for adenocarcinoma, but usually the entire tumor cannot be resected due to its extension or invasion into other vessels; therefore patients have a poor prognosis.* Pancreatoblastomas *have a lower grade of malignancy with a more favorable outcome. Adenocarcinomas most commonly arise from ductal or, less commonly, acinar cells. Both pancreatoblastomas and adenocarcinomas appear on ultrasound as large masses averaging 10 cm in size and range from hypoechoic to more complex in appearance. Both may be accompanied by ascites and/or obstruction of the common bile or pancreatic duct. Another difference between pancreatoblastoma and adenocarcinoma is that pancreatoblastoma has a well-defined border and adenocarcinoma has an irregular border.*

▶ Rumack CM, Levine D (eds): *Diagnostic Ultrasound*, 5th edition. Philadelphia, Elsevier, 2018, pp 238, 1865.

▶ Siegel MJ (ed): *Pediatric Sonography*, 4th edition. Philadelphia, Lippincott Williams & Wilkins, 2011, p 483.

282. B. Splenic vein.

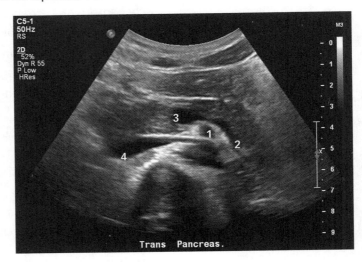

The pancreas lies obliquely within the body between the second portion of the duodenum and the splenic hilum. The pancreatic head lies to the right of the superior mesenteric artery or SMA (1), anterior to the inferior vena cava or IVC (4) and medial to the duodenum. The neck and body lie anterior to the SMA (1). The tail lies anterior and to the left of the SMA (1) and portosplenic confluence, which comprises the portal vein (3) and splenic vein (2).

▶ de Bruyn R (ed): *Pediatric Ultrasound: How, Why and When*, 2nd edition (e-book). Philadelphia, Churchill Livingstone/Elsevier, 2010, pp 171–174.
▶ Rumack CM, Levine D (eds): *Diagnostic Ultrasound*, 5th edition. Philadelphia, Elsevier, 2018, pp 211–213.
▶ Siegel MJ (ed): *Pediatric Sonography*, 4th edition. Philadelphia, Lippincott Williams & Wilkins, 2011, p 478.

283. A. Left lobe of the liver.

The best acoustic window for visualizing the pancreas is the left lobe of the liver. Using the midline subxiphoid approach in the transverse plane, you can visualize the majority of the pancreas in one image. The right subcostal approach using the right lobe of the liver can help you visualize the uncinate process. The tail can be seen coronally using the spleen as a window. The stomach would not be an appropriate acoustic window due to abdominal gas.

▶ Rumack CM, Levine D (eds): *Diagnostic Ultrasound*, 5th edition. Philadelphia, Elsevier, 2018, pp 211–213.
▶ Siegel MJ (ed): *Pediatric Sonography*, 4th edition. Philadelphia, Lippincott Williams & Wilkins, 2011, p 478.

284. C. Pancreas divisum.

Pancreas divisum *is the most common congenital anomaly of the pancreas, with annular pancreas following. With pancreas divisum, the dorsal and ventral ducts don't fuse during embryonic development. Because the duct of Santorini is too small to allow the flow of pancreatic secretions, buildup can occur, leading to pancreatitis. On ultrasound, pancreas size may be normal or the pancreatic head may be enlarged. Pancreas divisum is best seen with magnetic resonance imaging (MRI).* Annular pancreas *occurs when two segments of pancreatic tissue encase the duodenum, which can lead to duodenal obstruction.* Congenital cysts *are associated with other cystic disorders, such as von Hippel–Lindau disease and autosomal dominant polycystic kidney disease (ADPKD).* Ectopic pancreatic tissue *is most commonly found within the upper GI tract.*

▶ de Bruyn R (ed): *Pediatric Ultrasound: How, Why and When*, 2nd edition (e-book). Philadelphia, Churchill Livingstone/Elsevier, 2010, p 172.
▶ Rumack CM, Levine D (eds): *Diagnostic Ultrasound*, 5th edition. Philadelphia, Elsevier, 2018, p 218.
▶ Siegel MJ (ed): *Pediatric Sonography*, 4th edition. Philadelphia, Lippincott Williams & Wilkins, 2011, pp 480–481.

285. A. Pancreatoblastoma.

Pancreatoblastoma *is an infantile pancreatic exocrine malignancy. Exocrine tumors arise from or occur within the ducts or exocrine cells of the pancreas. The mean age of diagnosis is approximately 4 years, but it can occur in neonates or infants. Neonatal and infantile pancreatoblastomas have been associated with Beckwith-Wiedemann syndrome. Clinical signs are a large abdominal mass, pain, nausea, vomiting, and jaundice in the presence of common bile duct obstruction from the tumor. Pancreatoblastomas are large, solitary tumors that average 10 cm but can reach 20 cm in size. Sonographically, they are well defined and can range from hypoechoic to hyperechoic in appearance. These are low-grade malignancies with a favorable outcome; it is rare for metastasis, vessel invasion, or spread to lymph nodes to occur.* An insulinoma *is the most common endocrine tumor of the pancreas. Endocrine tumors are known as islet cell tumors.* Lymphomas *of the pancreas are rare in children and are not exocrine tumors.* An adenocarcinoma *is a malignant exocrine tumor of the pancreas* but is not histologically infantile in nature. Adenocarcinomas are also large masses, but they have irregular borders and are more aggressive tumors, with metastasis and vascular invasion commonly seen at the time of diagnosis.

▶ Rumack CM, Levine D (eds): *Diagnostic Ultrasound*, 5th edition. Philadelphia, Elsevier, 2018, pp 248, 1865.

▶ Siegel MJ (ed): *Pediatric Sonography*, 4th edition. Philadelphia, Lippincott Williams & Wilkins, 2011, pp 483, 485, 486–487.

286. **B. Insulinoma.**

An insulinoma *is the most common endocrine tumor of the pancreas. Insulinomas do not occur as a result of trauma.* Hematomas, lacerations, *and* fractures *of the pancreas can be seen following any blunt abdominal trauma such as that caused by a motor vehicle accident, bicycle accident, or child abuse.* Pancreatitis *can also be caused by a traumatic pancreas injury, resulting in an inflamed, enlarged pancreas with intapancreatic or extrapancreatic fluid collections. Leaking pancreatic enzymes can lead to peritonitis and erosion. Computed tomography (CT) is the preferred imaging modality for abdominal trauma.*

▶ de Bruyn R (ed): *Pediatric Ultrasound: How, Why and When*, 2nd edition (e-book). Philadelphia, Churchill Livingstone/Elsevier, 2010, p 178.

▶ Siegel MJ (ed): *Pediatric Sonography*, 4th edition. Philadelphia, Lippincott Williams & Wilkins, 2011, p 491.

287. **A. Bilirubin.**

Bilirubin *is a biomarker that, when elevated, indicates liver and biliary disease.* Amylase *is an enzyme within saliva and pancreatic fluid that converts starch into simple sugars.* Lipase *is an enzyme that breaks down fats into fatty acids and glycerol. Amylase and lipase are involved in the exocrine function of the pancreas and will be elevated with pancreatitis.* Glucose *is significant to the endocrine function of the pancreas. Insulin is released by the pancreas to regulate glucose levels within the blood. Glucose levels can be increased or decreased, leading to hyperglycemia when elevated and hypoglycemia when low.*

288. **C. Isoechoic to the liver.**

In a normal patient, the pancreas should be isoechoic to the liver. The pancreas will be well marginated and homogeneous. In the presence of pancreatic disease, the pancreas will appear more hyperechoic than the liver.

▸ Rumack CM, Levine D (eds): *Diagnostic Ultrasound*, 5th edition. Philadelphia, Elsevier, 2018, p 1862.

▸ Siegel MJ (ed): *Pediatric Sonography*, 4th edition. Philadelphia, Lippincott Williams & Wilkins, 2011, p 478.

289. **D. Tail.**

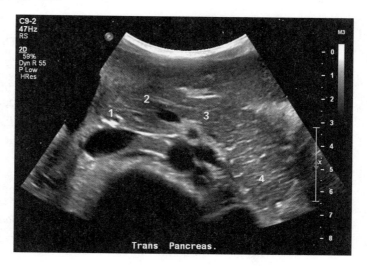

The tail *of the pancreas is labeled 4. The tail is located anterior and to the left of the superior mesenteric artery (SMA) and vein (SMV) and the portosplenic confluence. It is anterior to the left kidney and superior and posterior to the splenic hilum. The* head *(1) and* neck *(2) are located to the right of the body. The* body *(3) lies anterior to the SMA and SMV.*

▸ Rumack CM, Levine D (eds): *Diagnostic Ultrasound*, 5th edition. Philadelphia, Elsevier, 2018, pp 211–213.

▸ Siegel MJ (ed): *Pediatric Sonography*, 4th edition. Philadelphia, Lippincott Williams & Wilkins, 2011, p 478.

PART 8

Spleen

290. **B. Smooth muscle.**

The spleen *is the largest organ of lymphoid tissue within the body. Surrounded by a fibrous capsule, the spleen consists of red blood cells, reticuloendothelial cells, and lymphoid tissue. The tissue pulp of the spleen is divided into red pulp and white pulp. The* white pulp *is made up of lymphoid tissue that includes arteries, lymphatic follicles, and the reticuloendothelial cells. The white pulp aids in initiating the immune response. The* red pulp *consists of blood-filled sinusoids and mononuclear phagocytic cells that filter out abnormal red blood cells and foreign material. The spleen produces all types of blood cells in the fetal stage but performs no hematopoiesis after birth. Smooth muscle is found within the digestive tract.*

▶ Cesta MF: Normal structure, function, and histology of the spleen. Toxicol Pathol 34:455–465, 2006. Available at http://journals.sagepub.com/doi/full/10.1080/01926230600867743.

▶ Siegel MJ (ed): *Pediatric Sonography*, 4th edition. Philadelphia, Lippincott Williams & Wilkins, 2011, p 305.

291. **A. Abscess.**

Cat scratch fever is a bacterial disease caused by the gram-negative bacillus Bartonella henselae. *It can be transmitted to humans through a scratch by an infected cat. The spread of infection results in painful lymphadenopathy at the scratch site, and a small percentage of patients will develop multiple pyogenic abscesses in the spleen. On ultrasound, the abscesses will appear hypoechoic and small. If the patient has been treated, calcifications may be present within the focal lesions. Cysts, hemangiomas, and lymphangiomas are not associated with lymphadenopathy.*

▶ Paterson A, Frush DP, Donnelly LF, et al: A pattern-oriented approach to splenic imaging in infants and children. RadioGraphics 19:1465–1485, 1999. Available at https://pubs.rsna.org/doi/full/10.1148/radiographics.19.6.g99no231465.

▶ Rumack CM, Levine D (eds): *Diagnostic Ultrasound*, 5th edition. Philadelphia, Elsevier, 2018, p 1769.

▶ Siegel MJ (ed): *Pediatric Sonography*, 4th edition. Philadelphia, Lippincott Williams & Wilkins, 2011, pp 311–314, 318.

292. B. Hemangioma.

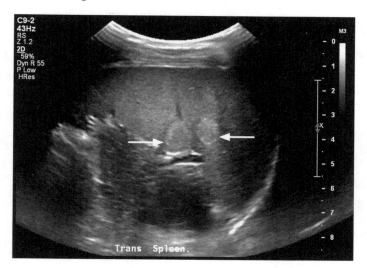

Hemangiomas *are the most common primary splenic neoplasm in children. Consisting of vascular channels filled with red blood cells, hemangiomas are benign and encased within a single endothelial layer. Hemangiomas are at risk for rupture. Two syndromes are associated with splenic hemangiomas: Beckwith-Wiedemann and Klippel-Trenaunay syndromes.* Beckwith-Wiedemann syndrome *consists of hemihypertrophy, macroglossia, and anterior abdominal wall defects.* Klippel-Trenaunay syndrome *consists of port wine stains, venous varicosities, and extremity overgrowth of soft tissue and occasionally bone. Sonographically, hemangiomas appear well defined, homogeneous, and increased in echogenicity in comparison to the spleen. They can demonstrate arterial flow, and when pressure is applied with the transducer, the arterial flow will diminish with compression, then return when the pressure is released. If large, hemangiomas may appear complex with cystic and solid components.* Lymphangiomas *and* hamartomas *are also benign neoplasms, but both are typically hypoechoic, and lymphangiomas are also multilocular.* Lymphomas *are malignant neoplasms that also appear hypoechoic or anechoic.*

▶ de Bruyn R (ed): *Pediatric Ultrasound: How, Why and When*, 2nd edition (e-book). Philadelphia, Churchill Livingstone/Elsevier, 2010, pp 137–140.

▶ Siegel MJ (ed): *Pediatric Sonography*, 4th edition. Philadelphia, Lippincott Williams & Wilkins, 2011, pp 313–317.

293. **A. Posterior to the pancreatic tail.**

The spleen is an intraperitoneal organ with a fibrous capsule. It is located posterior and lateral to the stomach. The pancreatic tail is medial to the splenic hilum. The splenic vein and artery course transversely posterior to the pancreatic tail and anterior to the left kidney. These vessels are located posterior to the stomach and superior to the transverse colon.

▶ de Bruyn R (ed): *Pediatric Ultrasound: How, Why and When*, 2nd edition (e-book). Philadelphia, Churchill Livingstone/Elsevier, 2010, p 173.
▶ Siegel MJ (ed): *Pediatric Sonography*, 4th edition. Philadelphia, Lippincott Williams & Wilkins, 2011, p 305.

294. **C. Wandering spleen.**

A wandering spleen *occurs when the gastrosplenic and splenorenal ligaments holding the spleen are longer than normal or absent. This results in greater mobility of the spleen and can cause rotation, torsion, or the appearance of an abdominal mass. Treatment is splenopexy. On ultrasound, the spleen is not seen within the splenic fossa but may appear as a "mass" resembling a spleen and located somewhere else in the body. Signs of torsion include an increased size, heterogeneous parenchyma, twisted pedicle, whorled appearance of the tail of the pancreas, and ascites. Torsion can lead to an infarction. With infarction, there will be no arterial flow at the hilum or within the parenchyma. Over time, anechoic areas of necrosis and liquefaction will appear and splenic size will decrease.* Sequestration *occurs when blood pools within the sinusoids.* Splenosis *occurs after splenic rupture when splenic tissue is found in different areas of the body. An* accessory spleen *is a common anatomic variant consisting of a single, small additional portion of splenic tissue found near the hilum.*

▶ de Bruyn R (ed): *Pediatric Ultrasound: How, Why and When*, 2nd edition (e-book). Philadelphia, Churchill Livingstone/Elsevier, 2010, p 166.
▶ Paterson A, Frush DP, Donnelly LF, et al: A pattern-oriented approach to splenic imaging in infants and children. RadioGraphics 19:1465–1485, 1999. Available at https://pubs.rsna.org/doi/full/10.1148/radiographics.19.6.g99no231465.
▶ Siegel MJ (ed): *Pediatric Sonography*, 4th edition. Philadelphia, Lippincott Williams & Wilkins, 2011, pp 307–308, 311.

295. D. Mononucleosis.

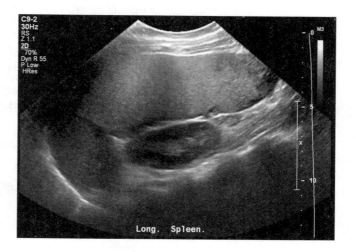

Splenomegaly *is enlargement of the spleen. The spleen is considered enlarged when it extends below the inferior margin of the left kidney. Most facilities use the length of the spleen based on pediatric age more than the volume. Many factors can cause splenomegaly. Causes such as infection (viral, such as mononucleosis, or bacterial, such as cat scratch fever and parasitic malaria) and hematologic malignancies (leukemia and lymphoma) can result in hypoechoic lesions along with splenomegaly. Sickle cell disease and inherited blood disorders are hemoglobinopathies that can cause splenomegaly. Storage disorders (Gaucher and Niemann-Pick diseases), portal vein thrombosis, and portal hypertension also can cause splenomegaly. Gaucher disease is the most common lysomal storage disorder affecting lipid metabolism. Gaucher disease type 1 is most common and is known to cause hepatosplenomegaly. One of the most common noninfectious causes of splenomegaly in children is portal hypertension.* Tuberous sclerosis *is a multisystem genetic disease that causes benign tumors of the kidneys, heart, eyes, liver, skin, and lungs and does not affect the spleen. Heterotaxy is associated with asplenia or polysplenia, not splenomegaly. When acute, a splenic infarct appears as a hypoechoic, wedge-shaped lesion in the periphery of the organ. As an infarct becomes chronic, the spleen will become echogenic and smaller in size as it atrophies.*

▶ de Bruyn R (ed): *Pediatric Ultrasound: How, Why and When*, 2nd edition (e-book). Philadelphia, Churchill Livingstone/Elsevier, 2010, pp 166–167.

▶ Paterson A, Frush DP, Donnelly LF, et al: A pattern-oriented approach to splenic imaging in infants and children. RadioGraphics 19:1465–1485, 1999. Available at https://pubs.rsna.org/doi/full/10.1148/radiographics.19.6.g99no231465.

▶ Rumack CM, Levine D (eds): *Diagnostic Ultrasound*, 5th edition. Philadelphia, Elsevier, 2018, pp 1769–1770.

▶ Siegel MJ (ed): *Pediatric Sonography*, 4th edition. Philadelphia, Lippincott Williams & Wilkins, 2011, pp 310–311.

296. D. Acute sequestration.

Patients with sickle cell anemia are at risk for sequestration *and typically present with a low hematocrit, lethargy, and abdominal pain. The pain is the result of the rapid enlargement of the spleen. The sickle-shaped cells can block the flow of blood, causing it to pool within the sinusoids and enlarge the spleen. Sequestration can become life-threatening and requires immediate treatment.* Sarcoidosis *is a multisystem disease resulting in splenomegaly with multiple granulomatous nodules, abdominal lymphadenopathy, and hepatomegaly.* Peliosis *is rare and associated with human immunodeficiency virus (HIV). On ultrasound, peliosis appears as multiple small hypoechoic lesions composed of blood-filled spaces without epithelial linings.* Infection *would cause splenomegaly and pain, but it would be accompanied by a fever and the presence of an abscess would be expected.*

▶ Rumack CM, Levine D (eds): *Diagnostic Ultrasound*, 5th edition. Philadelphia, Elsevier, 2018, pp 1769–1770.

▶ Siegel MJ (ed): *Pediatric Sonography*, 4th edition. Philadelphia, Lippincott Williams & Wilkins, 2011, pp 311, 313–314, 318, 322.

297. C. Lymphoma.

Lymphoma *is the most common malignancy of the spleen in children with non-Hodgkin or Hodgkin disease. On ultrasound, lymphoma appears as solitary or multiple hypoechoic or anechoic, avascular masses. Lymphadenopathy can be present in the hilar region, mesentery, or retroperitoneum. The spleen may be normal in size or have a varying range of splenomegaly. With* leukemia, *the spleen usually enlarges prior to treatment, but focal masses are rare.* Metastatic disease *within the spleen is an uncommon finding.* Hamartomas *are benign lesions appearing isoechoic or hyperechoic to the parenchyma of the spleen.*

▶ de Bruyn R (ed): *Pediatric Ultrasound: How, Why and When*, 2nd edition (e-book). Philadelphia, Churchill Livingstone/Elsevier, 2010, p 168.

▶ Siegel MJ (ed): *Pediatric Sonography*, 4th edition. Philadelphia, Lippincott Williams & Wilkins, 2011, pp 315–318.

298. B. Infarction.

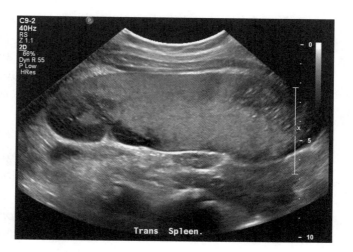

When there is occlusion of the splenic artery or branches, splenic infarction *and ischemia occur. Causes include leukemia, lymphoma, Gaucher disease, emboli, and portal hypertension. More common causes are sickle cell anemia and sickle thalassemia. Larger infarcts cause pain and fever, but smaller infarcts tend to be asymptomatic. Acute infarcts on ultrasound are classically wedge-shaped, hypoechoic areas appearing in the periphery of the spleen, as seen in this image. They can also be round or irregular in shape. Gas within the tiny vessels can look like linear echogenic striations. There will be an absence of hilar flow. A* hematoma *appears as a well-defined hypoechoic, heterogeneous mass and is not associated with leukemia.* Infection *may cause splenomegaly or abscess.* Sequestration *causes rapid enlargement and a heterogeneous echotexture of the spleen.*

▶ de Bruyn R (ed): *Pediatric Ultrasound: How, Why and When*, 2nd edition (e-book). Philadelphia, Churchill Livingstone/Elsevier, 2010, pp 169–170.
▶ Siegel MJ (ed): *Pediatric Sonography*, 4th edition. Philadelphia, Lippincott Williams & Wilkins, 2011, pp 311, 318–320, 322.

299. A. Potassium.

Lab tests performed when the spleen is in question can include a complete blood count (CBC) that includes values for hemoglobin, hematocrit, red blood cells, white blood cells, and platelets. Clotting factors, liver function tests, viral-antibody titers, and cultures may also be obtained. Potassium is included in an electrolyte panel. Abnormal potassium levels are associated with kidney disease, heart disease, and high blood pressure but not with splenic disorders.

300. **D. Epithelial lining.**

Splenic cysts are usually congenital, infectious, or post-traumatic. Congenital cysts *are solitary unilocular "true" cysts with an epithelial lining and a fibrous capsule.* Post-traumatic cysts *do not have an epithelial lining, making them "false" (pseudo) cysts. Both congenital and post-traumatic cysts are typically well circumscribed, round, and either hypoechoic or anechoic. They both have smooth walls and posterior enhancement on ultrasound. Splenic tissue will be seen surrounding the cysts.* Infectious cysts *of the spleen are more common in countries where sanitation and drinking water infrastructures are compromised. With echinococcal infections, daughter cysts within larger cysts can be visualized. Post-traumatic and echinococcal infectious cysts can have calcifications within the rim of the cyst.*

▸ Dachman AH, Ros PF, Murari PJ, et al: Nonparasitic splenic cysts: a report of 52 cases with radiologic-pathologic correlation. Am J Roentgenol 147:537–542, 1986.

▸ de Bruyn R (ed): *Pediatric Ultrasound: How, Why and When*, 2nd edition (e-book). Philadelphia, Churchill Livingstone/Elsevier, 2010, p 167.

▸ Siegel MJ (ed): *Pediatric Sonography*, 4th edition. Philadelphia, Lippincott Williams & Wilkins, 2011, p 311.

301. **C. More echogenic than the renal cortex.**

A normal spleen should appear more echogenic than the renal cortex. When compared to the liver, it will be isoechoic or slightly more echogenic. Although normal adrenal glands are not commonly visible on ultrasound after about 1 month of age, when the adrenal gland can *be seen the pancreas should be more echogenic than the adrenal gland. When normal, the pancreas should appear more echogenic than the spleen.*

▸ de Bruyn R (ed): *Pediatric Ultrasound: How, Why and When*, 2nd edition (e-book). Philadelphia, Churchill Livingstone/Elsevier, 2010, pp 115–117, 164.

▸ Siegel MJ (ed): *Pediatric Sonography*, 4th edition. Philadelphia, Lippincott Williams & Wilkins, 2011, p 305.

302. **B. Splenosis.**

Splenosis *is the term used for splenic tissue found throughout the body following splenic rupture. This usually occurs secondary to trauma or surgery. If splenosis occurs, the most common locations are within the peritoneum and/or retroperitoneum.* Sequestration *can be seen in sickle cell disease and occurs when blood pools within the sinusoids,* enlarging the spleen. Polysplenia *is associated with thoracic and abdominal anomalies. Polysplenia can be identified as multiple echogenic splenic nodules and is commonly found in the right upper quadrant, but it is not a result of trauma or rupture. Polysplenia and asplenia are included in the heterotaxy and cardiosplenic syndromes. A wandering spleen occurs when the ligaments holding the spleen are abnormally long or absent, resulting in the spleen's shifting to an ectopic location.*

▸ Paterson A, Frush DP, Donnelly LF, et al: A pattern-oriented approach to splenic imaging in infants and children. RadioGraphics 19:1465–1485, 1999. Available at https://pubs.rsna.org/doi/full/10.1148/radiographics.19.6.g99no231465.

▸ Rumack CM, Levine D (eds): *Diagnostic Ultrasound*, 5th edition. Philadelphia, Elsevier, 2018, p 1770.

▸ Siegel MJ (ed): *Pediatric Sonography*, 4th edition. Philadelphia, Lippincott Williams & Wilkins, 2011, pp 307–309, 311.

303. D. Accessory spleen.

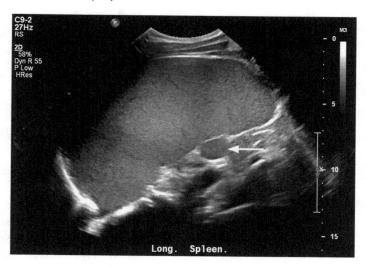

An accessory spleen, *also known as a* splenule *or* splenunculus, *is the most common anatomic variant of the spleen, occurring when embryonic buds of mesenchyme fail to fuse in the dorsal mesogastrium. The majority of accessory spleens are located near the splenic hilum. Usually seen as single, small, and round, they are most often an incidental finding. There can be more than one accessory spleen, but multiple accessory spleens are not as common as solitary ones. The typical size is 2–3 cm. If not removed in splenectomy patients, they may enlarge. If torsion occurs, they may appear as a thick-walled hypoechoic mass with a twisted vascular pedicle.* Lymphangiomas *appear as multilocular complex cysts within*

the spleen. Polysplenia *would appear similar to an accessory spleen on ultrasound but would be found within the right upper quadrant. A* splenic lobule *is a variant that extends medially from the inferior aspect of the spleen and is found anterior to the upper pole of the left kidney.*

▸ de Bruyn R (ed): *Pediatric Ultrasound: How, Why and When*, 2nd edition (e-book). Philadelphia, Churchill Livingstone/Elsevier, 2010, pp 165–166.

▸ Siegel MJ (ed): *Pediatric Sonography*, 4th edition. Philadelphia, Lippincott Williams & Wilkins, 2011, pp 307–309, 314.

304. **B. Peritoneal inclusion cyst.**

A peritoneal inclusion cyst *is not associated with splenic trauma.* Peritoneal inclusion cysts occur in females when pelvic adhesions wall off fluid released by the ovaries, forming a cystic mass. Blunt abdominal trauma involving the spleen is best imaged with computed tomography (CT) when patients are stable. Sonography is applicable for locating hematomas, lacerations, and hemoperitoneum. Hematomas can be intraparenchymal or subcapsular. *Acute intraparenchymal hematomas appear echogenic initially, then become more hypoechoic as the clot liquefies.* Subscapular hematomas appear crescent-shaped and will push down and flatten the surface of the spleen; a high-frequency transducer may be helpful in demonstrating subcapsular hematomas. Fractures course through the entire parenchyma, whereas lacerations usually occur on the lateral border of the spleen. Other signs of trauma include splenomegaly, perisplenic fluid, and left pleural effusion.

▸ Rumack CM, Levine D (eds): *Diagnostic Ultrasound*, 5th edition. Philadelphia, Elsevier, 2018, pp 1770–1772.

▸ Siegel MJ (ed): *Pediatric Sonography*, 4th edition. Philadelphia, Lippincott Williams & Wilkins, 2011, pp 322–323, 327.

305. **C. Asplenia.**

See also the answer to question 302.

Asplenia *is the absence of splenic tissue and occurs more commonly in males.* While nuclear medicine imaging is the diagnostic tool of choice, on ultrasound the left lobe of the liver can be seen crossing the midline and extending into the splenic fossa—concerning for splenic agenesis. Both asplenia and polysplenia are associated with multiple thoracic and abdominal anomalies such as situs inversus, heterotaxy, malrotation, renal anomalies, transverse liver, and heart *and lung defects. Patients with asplenia require prophylactic antibiotics due to their increased risk of sepsis. Spleen lobules, wandering spleen, and accessory spleen are not associated with other anomalies.*

▸ de Bruyn R (ed): *Pediatric Ultrasound: How, Why and When*, 2nd edition (e-book). Philadelphia, Churchill Livingstone/Elsevier, 2010, p 166.

▸ Paterson A, Frush DP, Donnelly LF, et al: A pattern-oriented approach to splenic imaging in infants and children. RadioGraphics 19:1465–1485, 1999. Available at https://pubs.rsna.org/doi/full/10.1148/radiographics.19.6.g99no231465.

▸ Siegel MJ (ed): *Pediatric Sonography*, 4th edition. Philadelphia, Lippincott Williams & Wilkins, 2011, pp 307–309.

306. **A. Lymphangioma.**

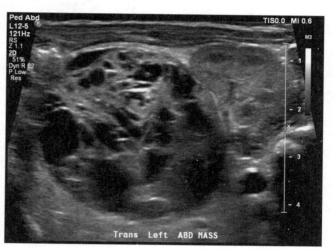

A lymphangioma *is a benign congenital malformation involving the lymphatic system. The masses can be single or multiple and contain lymph separated by fibrous bands and lined with endothelium. Sonographically, lymphangiomas appear as hypoechoic or anechoic multilocular cysts with echogenic septations. The walls or septations may contain calcifications. Lymphangiomas are mostly avascular, but vessels may be seen within the septations. A complex cyst can have characteristics similar to those of a lymphangioma, but it is not a congenital malformation. Hemangiomas are not multiloculated; they are homogeneous. Lymphoma is the most common malignant neoplasm involving the pediatric spleen, appearing hypoechoic or anechoic on ultrasound.*

▸ de Bruyn R (ed): *Pediatric Ultrasound: How, Why and When*, 2nd edition (e-book). Philadelphia, Churchill Livingstone/Elsevier, 2010, p 168.

▸ Siegel MJ (ed): *Pediatric Sonography*, 4th edition. Philadelphia, Lippincott Williams & Wilkins, 2011, pp 311, 313–314, 317.

307. B. Pyogenic abscess.

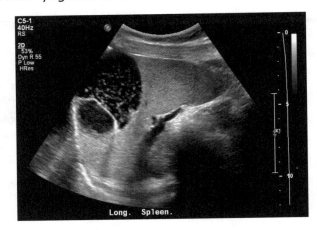

Pyogenic abscesses *result from infection or sepsis. Organisms that may cause these infections are* Staphylococcus aureus, Streptococcus, *and* Salmonella. *Amebic dysentery, otitis media, peritonsillar abscess, and mastoiditis are also causes. Symptoms can include fever, left shoulder pain, abdominal pain, and splenomegaly. On ultrasound, a pyogenic abscess appears hypoechoic and complex. It can contain fluid-fluid levels, septations, and gas. Margins can be smooth or irregular. Fungal abscesses of the spleen have a different appearance, typically multiple, hypoechoic, and small, with a "bull's-eye" or "wheel-within-a-wheel" appearance. A splenic cyst can be simple or complex but would not be expected to present with a fever. Clinical signs of lymphangioma of the spleen do not include fever.*

▶ de Bruyn R (ed): *Pediatric Ultrasound: How, Why and When*, 2nd edition (e-book). Philadelphia, Churchill Livingstone/Elsevier, 2010, pp 167–168.

▶ Paterson A, Frush DP, Donnelly LF, et al: A pattern-oriented approach to splenic imaging in infants and children. RadioGraphics 19:1465–1485, 1999. Available at https://pubs.rsna.org/doi/full/10.1148/radiographics.19.6.g99no231465.

▶ Siegel MJ (ed): *Pediatric Sonography*, 4th edition. Philadelphia, Lippincott Williams & Wilkins, 2011, pp 311, 314, 318–319.

308. D. Pancreatitis.

In children, splenic vein thrombosis most commonly results from pancreatitis. *Pancreatitis can cause vascular complications such as pseudoaneurysms and thrombosis elsewhere in the body. On ultrasound, splenomegaly and echogenic thrombus within the splenic vein are usually visualized. In certain cases, the splenic vein may not be visualized at all. Varices may develop secondary to splenic vein thrombosis.*

▶ Siegel MJ (ed): *Pediatric Sonography*, 4th edition. Philadelphia, Lippincott Williams & Wilkins, 2011, p 320.

309. **C. Initiates the immune response.**

The spleen has many functions. It filters and recycles red blood cells, and it stores blood. The white pulp assists with fighting infections by initiating the immune response. Regulation of blood pressure is performed by the kidneys.

▸ Children's Hospital of Pittsburgh of UPMC: What does the spleen do? Available at http://www.chp.edu/our-services/transplant/liver/education/organs/spleen-information.

▸ Siegel MJ (ed): *Pediatric Sonography*, 4th edition. Philadelphia, Lippincott Williams & Wilkins, 2011, p 305.

PART 9

Urinary Tract

310. **D. Psoas major.**

The psoas major *muscle lies medial to and deeper than the kidneys. It extends from the lumbar vertebrae into the lesser pelvis. The* quadratus lumborum *muscle is seen posterior to the kidneys and is the deepest of the abdominal muscles; it is associated with lower back or flank pain. The* latissimus dorsi *is one of the largest muscles in the upper back. The* oblique muscles *lie anterior to the kidneys and are located outside the abdominal cavity. All these muscles are paired, bilateral muscles.*

▶ de Bruyn R (ed): *Pediatric Ultrasound: How, Why and When*, 2nd edition (e-book). Philadelphia, Churchill Livingstone/Elsevier, 2010, p 44.
▶ Lazo DL: *Fundamentals of Sectional Anatomy: An Imaging Approach*, 2nd edition. Stamford, CT, Cengage Learning, 2015, pp 222–223.
▶ Rumack CM, Levine D (eds): *Diagnostic Ultrasound*, 5th edition. Philadelphia, Elsevier, 2018.
▶ Siegel MJ (ed): *Pediatric Sonography*, 4th edition. Philadelphia, Lippincott Williams & Wilkins, 2011, pp 498–499.

311. **A. Duplex kidney.**

A duplex kidney *(also known as* duplication of the renal pelvis*) contains two collecting systems and is an anomaly of different variations. The duplication occurs during the embryonic stage when two ureteral buds arise from the wolffian ducts of the mesoderm during organogenesis. On ultrasound, a duplex kidney will be visualized as having two renal pelves separated by normal renal parenchyma, typically one in the upper pole and one in the lower pole. One variation consists of two complete ureters that course from the kidney to the bladder. Another variation involves two ureters connecting at some point along the course to the bladder, creating a Y-shaped ureter. This Y-shaped ureter is known as a* bifid ureter. Crossed-fused ectopia *refers to the condition where two kidneys are fused together and located on the same side of the body. Within the intravesical segments of the ureter, a cystic dilatation may occur, known as a* ureterocele. Ureteroceles *are associated with single or duplex ureters.*

An ectopic ureter *does not empty into the normal location of the bladder at the trigone but inserts more distally within the bladder, bladder neck, urethra, vagina, or perineum.*

▶ de Bruyn R (ed): *Pediatric Ultrasound: How, Why and When*, 2nd edition (e-book). Philadelphia, Churchill Livingstone/Elsevier, 2010, pp 31, 44–46.
▶ Rumack CM, Levine D (eds): *Diagnostic Ultrasound*, 5th edition. Philadelphia, Elsevier, 2018, pp 1360, 1783–1785, 1904–1905.
▶ Siegel MJ (ed): *Pediatric Sonography*, 4th edition. Philadelphia, Lippincott Williams & Wilkins, 2011, pp 391, 393, 399–401.

312. B. Medulla.

The medulla *is the central innermost portion of the kidney and is divided into sections known as the* pyramids. *The pyramids appear more prominent and hypoechoic in infant kidneys than in adult kidneys. The* renal sinus *is the more centrally located echogenic cavity within the kidney. The renal sinus is occupied by the renal pelvis and collecting system, renal calyces, major renal vessels, nerves, and fat. The* renal cortex *is the outermost, peripheral renal tissue that contains the glomeruli. The* renal columns *are the portions of the cortical tissue that extend between the renal pyramids.*

▶ de Bruyn R (ed): *Pediatric Ultrasound: How, Why and When*, 2nd edition (e-book). Philadelphia, Churchill Livingstone/Elsevier, 2010, pp 49–50, 52.
▶ Rumack CM, Levine D (eds): *Diagnostic Ultrasound*, 5th edition. Philadelphia, Elsevier, 2018, p 1783.
▶ Siegel MJ (ed): *Pediatric Sonography*, 4th edition. Philadelphia, Lippincott Williams & Wilkins, 2011, p 386.

313. C. Hypertrophied column of Bertin.

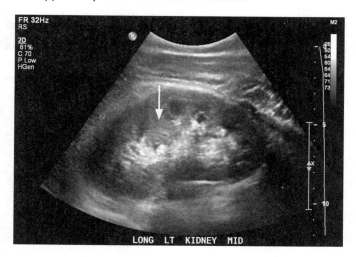

A hypertrophied column of Bertin *is a normal renal variant demonstrating a thick, hypertrophic layer of cortex extending between two renal pyramids toward the renal sinus.*

Sonographically, a hypertrophied column of Bertin can appear isoechoic or slightly more echogenic than the other areas of renal cortex. A column of Bertin can mimic a mass because it may appear round or oval. A fetal lobulation, also known as a renunculus, appears as an indented or scalloped margin bordering the kidney that eventually smooths out postnatally. Junctional parenchymal defects are echogenic fusion lines usually found within the upper two-thirds of the kidney. Fusion lines can be mistaken for renal scarring. A dromedary hump is also made up of renal tissue but will appear as an area of cortex bulging outward from the center of the lateral aspect of the left kidney, usually just beyond the splenic tip.

▸ Rumack CM, Levine D (eds): *Diagnostic Ultrasound*, 5th edition. Philadelphia, Elsevier, 2018, p 1781.

▸ Siegel MJ (ed): *Pediatric Sonography*, 4th edition. Philadelphia, Lippincott Williams & Wilkins, 2011, pp 389–390.

314. B. 0.7.

See Color Plate 20 on page xli.

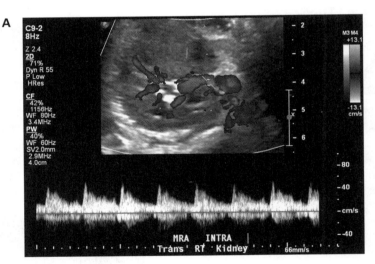

See Color Plate 21 on page xli.

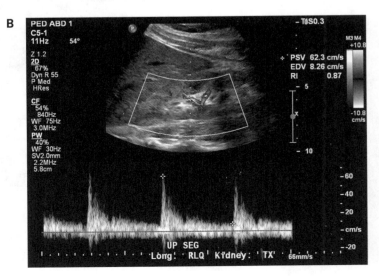

The resistive index (RI) is a calculation used to estimate arterial resistance. The formula for the RI is peak systolic frequency shift (or peak systolic velocity, PSV) minus minimum diastolic frequency shift (or end-diastolic velocity, EDV) divided by the PSV.

$$RI = \frac{PSV - EDV}{PSV}$$

A A normal, low-resistance renal artery waveform has a sharp systolic upstroke to peak. There should be continuous flow with a gradual drop-off in diastole toward the baseline. The early systolic peak is a notch seen in systole in the normal intrarenal arterial waveform. **B** An abnormal, higher-resistance waveform demonstrates a narrowed systolic upstroke, typically with a higher velocity, and a more sudden descent toward the baseline.

Flow should always remain above the baseline. Renal Doppler examinations are routinely performed to evaluate renal disease, renal vein thrombosis, renal arterial stenosis, and renal vascular hypertension. The upper limit of normal for the RI in children over the age of 1 year is 0.7. Preterm infants and neonates up to 4 months of age can have an RI as high as 0.9 normally.

▶ Goldberg B, McGahan J: *Atlas of Ultrasound Measurements*, 2nd edition. Philadelphia, Elsevier Mosby, 2006, pp 394–398.
▶ Rumack CM, Levine D (eds): *Diagnostic Ultrasound*, 5th edition. Philadelphia, Elsevier, 2018, p 1876.
▶ Siegel MJ (ed): *Pediatric Sonography*, 4th edition. Philadelphia, Lippincott Williams & Wilkins, 2011, pp 385, 387–388.

315. **A. Posterior urethral valves (PUV).**

Posterior urethral valves *(PUV)* are the result of a congenital anomaly—an extra flap of mucosal membrane obstructing the urethra and thus keeping it from emptying. This leads to prenatal oligohydramnios, bladder distention, and bilateral hydronephrosis. The flap acts like a windsock, ballooning or distending the urethra and preventing urine outflow. The dilated urethra and bladder will create the "keyhole" appearance. PUV is a common cause of urinary obstruction in male neonates. Another congenital anomaly, ureteropelvic junction *(UPJ)* obstruction, occurs when the junction of the renal pelvis and the proximal ureter is blocked, causing urine to build up within the kidney. Vesicoureteral reflux *(VUR)* is an anatomic or functional disorder where there is reversed flow of urine from the bladder back into the ureters.

Multicystic dysplastic kidney *(MCDK)* predominantly displays a unilateral nonfunctioning, dysplastic kidney. Bilateral MCDK is uncommon and lethal. PUV, UPJ, and VUR are treatable conditions.

▸ de Bruyn R (ed): *Pediatric Ultrasound: How, Why and When*, 2nd edition (e-book). Philadelphia, Churchill Livingstone/Elsevier, 2010, pp 32, 48–50, 62–64.
▸ Rumack CM, Levine D (eds): *Diagnostic Ultrasound*, 5th edition. Philadelphia, Elsevier, 2018, pp 1340, 1788, 1905–1906.
▸ Siegel MJ (ed): *Pediatric Sonography*, 4th edition. Philadelphia, Lippincott Williams & Wilkins, 2011, pp 390, 394–395, 397–398, 400–403, 429.

316. C. Superior.

The kidneys are located within the retroperitoneal space between the T12 and L3 vertebrae. The upper poles are positioned more medial and posterior than the lower poles. The left kidney is typically more superior than the right kidney due to the larger size of the liver than the spleen. Because the left kidney lies more superior in location, it is helpful to place the patient in a right lateral decubitus (RLD) position for better visualization while scanning.

▸ Lazo DL: *Fundamentals of Sectional Anatomy: An Imaging Approach*, 2nd edition. Stamford, CT, Cengage Learning, 2015, p 224.
▸ Siegel MJ (ed): *Pediatric Sonography*, 4th edition. Philadelphia, Lippincott Williams & Wilkins, 2011, pp 384–385, 461.

317. B. Gerota's fascia.

Gerota's fascia is the renal fascia or layer of thin, fibrous connective tissue that encapsulates the kidneys, adrenal glands, and perinephric fat. Scarpa's fascia *is a superficial, anterior abdominal wall fascia. The* extraperitoneal fascia *lies on top of or outside of Gerota's fascia.* Psoas fascia *covers the psoas muscle and also lies outside of Gerota's fascia.*

▸ Rumack CM, Levine D (eds): *Diagnostic Ultrasound*, 5th edition. Philadelphia, Elsevier, 2018, p 314.
▸ Siegel MJ (ed): *Pediatric Sonography*, 4th edition. Philadelphia, Lippincott Williams & Wilkins, 2011, p 435.

318. D. Calyces.

Renal calyces are cup-shaped cavities located within the renal sinus. Two or three minor calyces drain into one major calyx. Urine drains from the calyces into the renal pelvis. A nephron is the functioning unit of the kidney. Nephrons regulate water and salt concentration in the body, excreting what is not needed as urine. Glomeruli are located within the cortex and filter the blood. The renal pyramids contain the tubules that transport urine from the outer cortex, where urine is produced, to the calyces within the renal sinus.

▸ Rumack CM, Levine D (eds): *Diagnostic Ultrasound*, 5th edition. Philadelphia, Elsevier, 2018, p 1354.

▸ Siegel MJ (ed): *Pediatric Sonography*, 4th edition. Philadelphia, Lippincott Williams & Wilkins, 2011, p 386.

319. C. Angiomyolipomas.

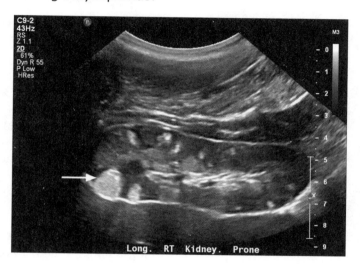

Angiomyolipomas *are benign tumors often seen in adolescents and adults with the genetic disease tuberous sclerosis. Of children with tuberous sclerosis, 80% will have angiomyolipomas, and they are usually multiple in number. Angiomyolipomas are composed of fat cells, smooth muscle cells, and blood vessels. They appear within the renal cortices of both kidneys as small, round, and echogenic.* Lymphomas *are malignant tumors; they can also be round and bilateral, but sonographically they appear hypoechoic, not echogenic.* Fungal balls *are echogenic, nonshadowing, focal masses associated with fungal infections. Fungal balls are located within the drainage regions of the kidney, not within the renal cortex.* Rhabdomyomas *are the most common type of cardiac tumor in children; like angiomyolipomas, they have a strong association with tuberous sclerosis but are located in the heart, not the kidney.*

▸ de Bruyn R (ed): *Pediatric Ultrasound: How, Why and When*, 2nd edition (e-book). Philadelphia, Churchill Livingstone/Elsevier, 2010, pp 78, 80, 83.

▸ Rumack CM, Levine D (eds): *Diagnostic Ultrasound*, 5th edition. Philadelphia, Elsevier, 2018, pp 1816, 1822.

▸ Siegel MJ (ed): *Pediatric Sonography*, 4th edition. Philadelphia, Lippincott Williams & Wilkins, 2011, pp 239, 419, 423–424, 428.

320. D. Anterior.

The renal venous system runs parallel to the arterial system. The right renal vein lies anterior to the right renal artery within the renal hilum and drains directly into the inferior vena cava (IVC). The left renal vein is anterior to the left renal artery and travels posterior to the superior mesenteric artery (SMA) and anterior to the aorta as it approaches the IVC. The left renal vein is posterior to the splenic vein and the body of the pancreas. Since the IVC is farther away from the left kidney than the right, the left renal vein is approximately three times longer than the right renal vein. The left kidney is more commonly used for renal transplants due to the longer vessels.

See Color Plate 13, "The Abdominal Vasculature," on page xxxviii.

▶ Lazo DL: *Fundamentals of Sectional Anatomy: An Imaging Approach*, 2nd edition. Stamford, CT, Cengage Learning, 2015, p 212.
▶ Rumack CM, Levine D (eds): *Diagnostic Ultrasound*, 5th edition. Philadelphia, Elsevier, 2018, p 313.
▶ Siegel MJ (ed): *Pediatric Sonography*, 4th edition. Philadelphia, Lippincott Williams & Wilkins, 2011, p 387.

321. C. Metanephroi.

The metanephroi, *located in the inferior or caudal portion of the embryo, start to develop in the 5th conceptual week. They arise from the ureteric bud and intermediate mesoderm to become the permanent kidneys. The* pronephroi *are the rudimentary, nonfunctional tubes that appear early in the fourth conceptual week, located within the neck region of the embryo. The pronephroi disappear late in the fourth week and are replaced by the mesonephroi. The* mesonephroi *are located caudal to the pronephroi in the mid section of the embryo and develop into the mesonephric tubules and the mesonephric (wolffian) ducts. The mesonephroi perform kidney function for only a brief period, until replaced in week 5 by the metanephroi, which will develop into the permanent kidneys.*

▶ de Bruyn R (ed): *Pediatric Ultrasound: How, Why and When*, 2nd edition (e-book). Philadelphia, Churchill Livingstone/Elsevier, 2010, p 42.
▶ Moore KL, Persaud TVN, Torchia MG: *The Developing Human: Clinically Oriented Embryology*, 9th edition. Philadelphia, Elsevier Saunders, pp 247–250.
▶ Rumack CM, Levine D (eds): *Diagnostic Ultrasound*, 5th edition. Philadelphia, Elsevier, 2018, pp 1336–1338.

322. D. Multicystic dysplastic kidney (MCDK).

Multicystic dysplastic kidney (MCDK)—which may occur unilaterally or bilaterally—is the most commonly diagnosed unilateral cystic finding on prenatal ultrasound. Also known as Potter type 2, MCDK is a developmental anomaly, not an inherited genetic condition. The bilateral form of MCDK is incompatible with life. With unilateral disease one kidney appears with multiple randomly distributed cysts of varying sizes in place of a renal cortex. These cysts do not communicate with one another. Because the cystic kidney is nonfunctioning, the contralateral kidney will eventually show hypertrophy as it compensates and takes over the renal function. Autosomal dominant polycystic kidney disease (ADPKD) and autosomal recessive polycystic kidney disease (ARPKD) are both bilateral conditions and are genetic or hereditary. ADPKD is a systemic disease where cysts can develop in multiple organs and is more common than ARPKD. In neonatal ADPKD, cysts of varying sizes invade the entire kidney. Both kidneys will become enlarged and echogenic. In older children, kidneys can be of normal size, but cortical cysts are seen. In ARPKD, the medulla is most prominently involved. Numerous 1–2 mm cysts are seen within the renal medulla, causing the medullary pyramids to be more echogenic and showing less corticomedullary differentiation. In all ages, there is bilateral renal enlargement. The majority of patients with ARPKD have associated hepatic fibrosis and biliary ductal ectasia or Caroli's disease. Simple renal cysts occur in less than 1% of children, making them very uncommon, especially in utero.

▶ de Bruyn R (ed): *Pediatric Ultrasound: How, Why and When*, 2nd edition (e-book). Philadelphia, Churchill Livingstone/Elsevier, 2010, pp 32–33, 59, 72–74, 83.

▶ Rumack CM, Levine D (eds): *Diagnostic Ultrasound*, 5th edition. Philadelphia, Elsevier, 2018, pp 1346–1347, 1815.

▶ Siegel MJ (ed): *Pediatric Sonography*, 4th edition. Philadelphia, Lippincott Williams & Wilkins, 2011, pp 394–395, 405–408, 411–412.

323. A. Ureterocele.

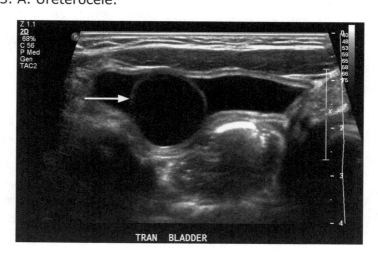

A ballooning or outpouching of the distal ureter into the bladder will create a cystic projection in the trigone known as a *ureterocele (arrow)*. Ureteroceles are most commonly caused by stenosis or obstruction but have also been associated with renal dysplasia. An *ectopic ureter* describes a ureter with an entry point into the bladder in an abnormal or ectopic location, such as the urethra or vagina. A *urachus* is a channel between the umbilicus and anterior bladder wall present during fetal development. It is not common for the channel to remain open past the fifth month of gestation. When each end of the channel closes, but the central portion remains open and traps fluid inside, a *urachal cyst* is formed. *Bladder diverticula* also appear as an outpouching of the bladder, but they are made up of the mucosal lining of the bladder, not the ureter. Sonographically, bladder diverticula appear as round or oval, anechoic fluid collections arising from the bladder and projecting outside (not within) the bladder lumen. Bladder diverticula appear more often in males.

▸ Rumack CM, Levine D (eds): *Diagnostic Ultrasound*, 5th edition. Philadelphia, Elsevier, 2018, pp 1359–1360, 1783–1784.

▸ Siegel MJ (ed): *Pediatric Sonography*, 4th edition. Philadelphia, Lippincott Williams & Wilkins, 2011, pp 400, 449–450.

324. **D. Parapelvic.**

Parapelvic cysts are located centrally within the renal sinus but do not communicate with the collecting system. If multiple parapelvic cysts are present, it is important to differentiate cysts from hydronephrosis. Communicating dilated calyces with a dilated renal pelvis can look similar to noncommunicating, multiple parapelvic cysts, and sonography can assist in making the differentiation. *Cortical* and *parenchymal cysts* are both located in the outer periphery of the kidney. An *extrarenal cyst* will not invade the renal tissue.

▸ Rumack CM, Levine D (eds): *Diagnostic Ultrasound*, 5th edition. Philadelphia, Elsevier, 2018, p 359.

325. **B. Persistent cloaca.**

A *persistent cloaca* is a congenital disorder in which the rectum, vagina, and urinary tract come together and fuse into a single channel. Cloaca is the Latin term for "sewer." Anomalies of the cloaca occur during fetal development. Persistent cloaca most often occurs in females, but it can occur in males without the vaginal component. A persistent cloaca is the most common cloacal defect. Clinical signs are only one perineal opening, an imperforate anus, and ambiguous genitalia. The urogenital sinus *is an anomaly comprising the urinary and reproductive systems, but it does not contain the rectum. The* urachus *is anterior to the peritoneum and extends from the anterior bladder dome to the umbilicus. A* patent urachus *occurs when the channel did not close before birth. A patent urachus is also a type of abdominal wall defect and may allow urine to leak through the umbilicus. A* megalourethra *is associated only with males and describes the severe dilatation of the penile urethra.*

▶ Rumack CM, Levine D (eds): *Diagnostic Ultrasound*, 5th edition. Philadelphia, Elsevier, 2018, p 1338.

▶ Siegel MJ (ed): *Pediatric Sonography*, 4th edition. Philadelphia, Lippincott Williams & Wilkins, 2011, pp 450–451.

326. C. 5 mm.

Because overdistention puts pressure on the bladder wall, the bladder is best imaged when it is moderately filled, not overdistended. The bladder wall is made up of mucosa, muscle, and subserosal layers. A normal bladder will demonstrate a nontrabeculated, smooth wall of the same thickness throughout. Whether a bladder is full or empty, a normal wall measurement should not exceed 5 mm.

▶ Rumack CM, Levine D (eds): *Diagnostic Ultrasound*, 5th edition. Philadelphia, Elsevier, 2018, p 1854.

▶ Siegel MJ (ed): *Pediatric Sonography*, 4th edition. Philadelphia, Lippincott Williams & Wilkins, 2011, p 448.

327. B. Crossed-fused ectopia.

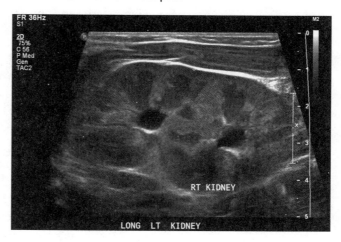

Crossed-fused ectopia *is a rare congenital anomaly where one kidney lies on the contralateral side of the body and is fused to the other kidney. The ureter of the misplaced kidney crosses back over the midline to its correct side and enters*

the bladder in its normal location. A pelvic kidney *is another congenital anomaly, where a kidney fails to ascend above the waist to its normal position within the renal fossa. An ectopic pelvic kidney remains on its normal side of the body. A* horseshoe kidney *is another congenital fusion anomaly; it occurs when two kidneys are fused at the lower poles. The two kidneys are connected by an isthmus located across the midline, but each kidney remains on its normal side of the body, making the shape of a horseshoe. Horseshoe kidneys are the most common congenital fusion anomaly and are not rare.* Duplex kidney *describes a kidney that contains two separate collecting systems; duplex kidneys usually are not in an ectopic location.*

▸ Rumack CM, Levine D (eds): *Diagnostic Ultrasound*, 5th edition. Philadelphia, Elsevier, 2018, pp 1784–1785.

▸ Siegel MJ (ed): *Pediatric Sonography*, 4th edition. Philadelphia, Lippincott Williams & Wilkins, 2011, pp 391–392.

328. **B. Left.**

    A donor kidney is usually taken from the left side. The left renal vein is almost three times longer than the right renal vein, and the vessel's extra length allows the renal pelvis of the transplant to be rotated anteriorly for easier access during surgery. In younger and smaller children, the transplant is placed intraperitoneally. The donor renal vein is anastomosed to the recipient external iliac vein. The donor renal artery is anastomosed to the recipient aorta. Transplants in older children are placed retroperitoneally. In this case, the renal arteries are instead anastomosed to the internal or external iliac artery, and the renal vein is anastomosed to the external iliac vein.

    ▸ de Bruyn R (ed): *Pediatric Ultrasound: How, Why and When,* 2nd edition (e-book). Philadelphia, Churchill Livingstone/Elsevier, 2010, pp 97–105.

    ▸ Siegel MJ (ed): *Pediatric Sonography*, 4th edition. Philadelphia, Lippincott Williams & Wilkins, 2011, pp 387, 440–441.

329. **A. Low velocity at the site of the stenosis.**

    When the lumen of the renal artery is narrowed by stenosis, the velocity of the flow through the narrowed portion will increase. Therefore, stenotic sites have a higher, not a lower, velocity. Aliasing can be seen within the area of stenosis with color Doppler. Significant stenosis of the main renal artery would be defined by a greater than 60% narrowing and a peak systolic velocity (PSV) of greater than 150 cm/sec at the stenotic site. Spectral Doppler may display a tardus parvus waveform distal to the stenosis showing a slower rise time and lower PSV. Renal size discrepancy, elevated RI proximal to the stenosis, and turbulence distal to the stenosis are all signs of renal artery stenosis.

▶ Rumack CM, Levine D (eds): *Diagnostic Ultrasound*, 5th edition. Philadelphia, Elsevier, 2018, p 1805.

▶ Siegel MJ (ed): *Pediatric Sonography*, 4th edition. Philadelphia, Lippincott Williams & Wilkins, 2011, pp 145–146, 432–433.

▶ Stavros AT, Parker SH, Yakes WF, et al: Segmental stenosis of the renal artery: pattern recognition of tardus and parvus abnormalities with duplex sonography. Radiology 184:479–485, 1992.

330. C. Wilms tumor.

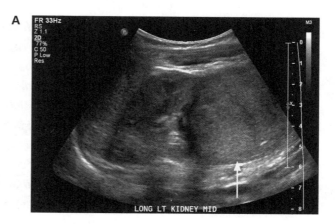

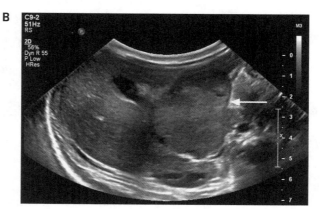

Wilms tumor (arrow), also known as nephroblastoma, is the most common pediatric renal malignancy (occurring in approximately 90% of renal malignancy cases in children). Image **A** demonstrates a tumor in the longitudinal plane, while image **B** was taken in the transverse plane. The average age of discovery is 3 years, and the majority are found before the age of 5. Clinical symptoms include abdominal distention, pain, and hematuria. Wilms tumors are solid masses, appearing echogenic and smooth-walled, and may contain venous lakes. Inferior vena cava (IVC) invasion with tumor thrombus can occur. Renal cell carcinoma *is rare under the age of 20 and accounts for only 2%–6% of pediatric renal malignancies.* Lymphomas *are not usually seen in children until after age 5. Because the kidneys don't contain lymphatic tissue, renal involvement is a late manifestation and not common. A* cystic nephroma *is another rare mass, but it is benign and more commonly occurs under the age of 2.*

▶ Rumack CM, Levine D (eds): *Diagnostic Ultrasound*, 5th edition. Philadelphia, Elsevier, 2018, pp 1818–1819.

▶ Siegel MJ (ed): *Pediatric Sonography*, 4th edition. Philadelphia, Lippincott Williams & Wilkins, 2011, pp 413, 418–419.

331. **D. Renal arteries with a higher resistance.**

Obstruction that reduces the venous outflow from the kidney will increase the interstitial pressure within the kidney, causing a sharp peak in the arterial flow. It is the higher systolic arterial peak and reduced diastolic flow that increase the resistive index (RI). Kidneys with normal function and perfusion have a low-resistance waveform. In all stages of renal vein thrombosis (RVT), the kidneys will have an increased echogenicity. Flow within the veins can be partially occluded around the thrombus or completely absent. There may be echogenic thrombus present within the vessel lumen. The corticomedullary junction is absent or indistinct throughout the stages of RVT due to the increased parenchymal echogenicity.

▶ Rumack CM, Levine D (eds): *Diagnostic Ultrasound*, 5th edition. Philadelphia, Elsevier, 2018, pp 1802–1805.

▶ Siegel MJ (ed): *Pediatric Sonography*, 4th edition. Philadelphia, Lippincott Williams & Wilkins, 2011, pp 435–436.

332. **B. Pyelonephritis.**

The most frequently visualized disorder of the urinary tract in children is infection. Bacterial pyelonephritis *is a common occurrence, resulting from an ascending infection due to vesicoureteral reflux (VUR) that eventually affects the renal tissue. Symptoms include fever and vomiting.* Escherichia coli *(E. coli) is the most common organism found with bacterial pyelonephritis. The kidneys can show overall or focal enlargement. Renal parenchyma may show areas of decreased or increased echogenicity. The walls of the renal pelvis or ureter may appear thickened. Hydronephrosis is not necessarily present.* Pyonephritis *is defined as purulent exudate seen within a hydronephrotic kidney and is also most commonly caused by* E. coli. Fungal balls *are nonshadowing focal areas of echogenicity within the collection system and are commonly caused by* Candida albicans. *Enlarged kidneys are seen with* glomerulonephritis, *but the clinical symptoms are usually hematuria and hypertension.*

▸ Rumack CM, Levine D (eds): *Diagnostic Ultrasound*, 5th edition. Philadelphia, Elsevier, 2018, pp 1792–1793.

▸ Siegel MJ (ed): *Pediatric Sonography*, 4th edition. Philadelphia, Lippincott Williams & Wilkins, 2011, pp 425–428, 430.

333. **D. Hypoechoic.**

Characteristically, Wilms tumors are large, solid, echogenic masses with well-defined, smooth capsules. Necrosis, fat, or hemorrhage may cause a more heterogeneous texture. Venous lakes may be present. If a Wilms tumor is suspected, a CT scan or MRI is usually performed to evaluate for tumor spread. Treatment for Wilms includes a radical nephrectomy, chemotherapy, and follow-up imaging.

▸ Rumack CM, Levine D (eds): *Diagnostic Ultrasound*, 5th edition. Philadelphia, Elsevier, 2018, pp 792–793.

▸ Siegel MJ (ed): *Pediatric Sonography*, 4th edition. Philadelphia, Lippincott Williams & Wilkins, 2011, pp 425–428, 430.

334. **C. Urinoma.**

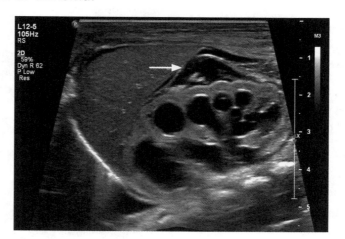

Due to high pressure resulting from obstruction or trauma, the fornix of a calyx can rupture and leak urine into the subcapsular or perirenal space, forming an anechoic urinoma (arrow). This rupture serves as a way of decompressing the collecting system. In this case the anechoic urine nicely marginates the fetal lobulation or scalloped renal cortical margin of this infant. Urinomas can also be found in transplanted kidneys when there is a defect at the site of ureteroneocystostomy, allowing urine leakage. In transplants, urinomas would almost always form within the first two weeks

of transplantation. If a urinoma remains and the urine doesn't eventually leak out into the retroperitoneal space, an abscess would be a delayed complication. Abscesses will appear more complex than urinomas and have thicker walls. A hematoma is often a result of trauma but is not a result of a ruptured calyx due to obstruction. Hematomas typically have internal echoes, making them appear more complex than a urinoma would.

▶ Rumack CM, Levine D (eds): *Diagnostic Ultrasound*, 5th edition. Philadelphia, Elsevier, 2018, pp 1358, 1809.

▶ Siegel MJ (ed): *Pediatric Sonography*, 4th edition. Philadelphia, Lippincott Williams & Wilkins, 2011, pp 402–403, 445–446.

▶ Titton R, Gervais, D, Hahn PF, et al: Urine leaks and urinomas: diagnosis and imaging-guided intervention. RadioGraphics 23:1133–1147, 2003.

335. A. Xanthogranulomatous pyelonephritis.

Xanthogranulomatous pyelonephritis *(XGP or XPN) is an unusual chronic kidney infection most commonly caused by* E. coli *and* Proteus *bacteria. The bacteria invade the renal parenchyma and diminish kidney function. Stones that take the shape of the renal pelvis and calyces, known as* staghorn calculi, *can be seen with this type of infection. XGP is unilateral in most cases, and treatment for focal disease is a partial or complete nephrectomy. Calculi are not usually associated with the other types of kidney infections.*

▶ de Bruyn R (ed): *Pediatric Ultrasound: How, Why and When*, 2nd edition (e-book). Philadelphia, Churchill Livingstone/Elsevier, 2010, pp 71–72, 87.

▶ Gupta S, Araya CE, Dharnidharka VR: Xanthogranulomatous pyelonephritis in pediatric patients: case report and review of literature. J Pediatr Urol 6:355–358, 2010.

▶ Rumack CM, Levine D (eds): *Diagnostic Ultrasound*, 5th edition. Philadelphia, Elsevier, 2018, pp 328, 1800.

▶ Siegel MJ (ed): *Pediatric Sonography*, 4th edition. Philadelphia, Lippincott Williams & Wilkins, 2011, pp 425–430.

336. D. Hyperechoic.

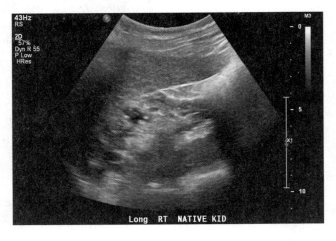

Chronic renal failure occurs when the remaining number of functioning nephrons is too low. This can lead to end-stage renal failure and eventually renal transplant. Causes of chronic renal failure include trauma, obstructive uropathy, renal dysplasia, reflex neuropathy, Alport syndrome, and autosomal recessive polycystic kidney disease (ARPKD). The kidneys will become smaller, have a thinned parenchyma, and appear hyperechoic. Symptoms of both acute and chronic renal failure include oliguria, anuria, and elevated blood urea nitrogen (BUN) and creatinine (CR) levels.

▶ Keough J: *Nursing Laboratory and Diagnostic Tests Demystified*, 2nd edition. New York, McGraw-Hill, 2017, pp 11, 36–38.

▶ Rumack CM, Levine D (eds): *Diagnostic Ultrasound*, 5th edition. Philadelphia, Elsevier, 2018, p 1795.

▶ Siegel MJ (ed): *Pediatric Sonography*, 4th edition. Philadelphia, Lippincott Williams & Wilkins, 2011, p 435.

337. B. Lymphocele.

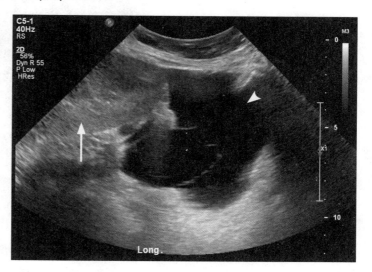

Complications following a renal transplant (arrow) include hypertension, lymphoceles, and arteriovenous fistulas. Seen postoperatively in approximately 20% of patients, lymphoceles are the most common. Identified as a perinephric fluid collection, a lymphocele (arrowhead) is made up of lymph that has seeped from severed lymph vessels in the transplant bed. Lymphoceles regularly appear hypoechoic but are complicated by internal septations. The borders are well defined. Most lymphoceles occur inferomedial to the transplant allograft. Hydronephrosis *due to obstruction in transplants most frequently occurs secondary to a distal ureter stenosis and would appear as fluid within the collecting system and ureter. A* urinoma *is not a common sequela of transplants and,*

if present, would occur within the first few weeks and appear anechoic. Hematomas are more commonly diagnosed in the period immediately after transplantation. Acute hemorrhages will appear echogenic, then change over time as the hematoma resolves.

▶ Akbar SA, Jafri SZH, Amendola MA, et al: Complications of renal transplantation. RadioGraphics 25:1335–1356, 2005. Available at https://pubs.rsna.org/doi/10.1148/rg.255045133.

▶ de Bruyn R (ed): *Pediatric Ultrasound: How, Why and When*, 2nd edition (e-book). Philadelphia, Churchill Livingstone/Elsevier, 2010, pp 99, 103–104.

▶ Rumack CM, Levine D (eds): *Diagnostic Ultrasound*, 5th edition. Philadelphia, Elsevier, 2018, p 1809.

▶ Siegel MJ (ed): *Pediatric Sonography*, 4th edition. Philadelphia, Lippincott Williams & Wilkins, 2011, pp 444–445.

338. **C. Hydronephrosis.**

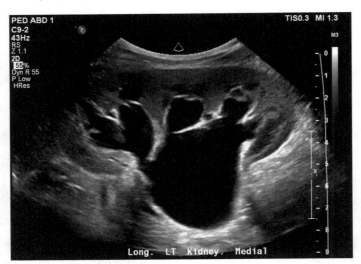

The dilatation or distention of the renal pelvis and calyces is known as hydronephrosis. *Visualizing fluid within the renal pelvis doesn't always mean there is an obstruction. Causes of hydronephrosis can be mechanical or functional. Untreated, urinary retention can lead to the destruction and atrophy of the renal parenchyma. Symptoms can include flank pain, urinary tract infection, hematuria, nausea, and vomiting. Reflux and posterior urethral valves (PUV) are mechanical causes of hydronephrosis. A* urinoma *is a fluid collection within the retroperitoneum due to a calyceal rupture.*

▶ Rumack CM, Levine D (eds): *Diagnostic Ultrasound*, 5th edition. Philadelphia, Elsevier, 2018, p 1785.

▶ Siegel MJ (ed): *Pediatric Sonography*, 4th edition. Philadelphia, Lippincott Williams & Wilkins, 2011, pp 393–402.

339. **A. Prone.**

Placing the patient in the prone position allows the kidney to be easily accessible from the back and gives better visualization of the lower pole, the preferred site of biopsy. The prone position also places the kidney closest to the skin so that the needle depth is as shallow as possible. Ultrasound guidance may be used and post-procedure imaging is performed to evaluate for hematoma. If the biopsy is done on a transplant, the patient would be placed in the supine position. Either decubitus position would not be an ideal position to stabilize the kidney for biopsy.

▶ Rumack CM, Levine D (eds): *Diagnostic Ultrasound*, 5th edition. Philadelphia, Elsevier, 2018, p 1846.

▶ Siegel MJ (ed): *Pediatric Sonography*, 4th edition. Philadelphia, Lippincott Williams & Wilkins, 2011, pp 683–684.

340. **C. Calyces.**

The renal hilum is the entrance to the renal sinus and contains the renal vein, renal artery, and ureter. Within the renal hilum the intrarenal artery branches into the segmental arteries. Prominent renal vessels within the hilum can mimic a dilated renal pelvis. The use of color Doppler imaging will distinguish blood from urine.

▶ Rumack CM, Levine D (eds): *Diagnostic Ultrasound*, 5th edition. Philadelphia, Elsevier, 2018, pp 313, 1783.

▶ Siegel MJ (ed): *Pediatric Sonography*, 4th edition. Philadelphia, Lippincott Williams & Wilkins, 2011, pp 386–387.

341. **A. Ear malformations.**

There is an association between ear malformations and structural renal anomalies. Because the ears and kidneys develop at different rates and times, it is not usually an isolated insult to the embryo, but a prolonged insult that can affect multiple areas during development over time. Hypotension is not an indication for renal sonography. Hypertension is an indication because it can damage the renal arteries, ultimately causing poor blood perfusion and altering the kidneys' appearance and performance. Isolated headaches without accompanying symptoms such as hypertension or abnormal lab values are not an indication for a renal sonogram. A sacral dimple is an indication for an ultrasound of the spine.

▶ Wang RY, Earl DL, Ruder RO, et al: Syndromic ear anomalies and renal ultrasounds. Pediatrics 108:E32, 2001.

342. D. Fetal lobulations.

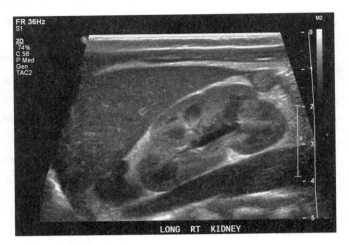

Fetal lobulations *appear as indented or scalloped margins around the kidney. Remnants of renunculi lobes that do not completely fuse cause the lobulations. Postnatally, the kidney margin will eventually become smoother. These lobulations are not to be confused with renal scarring. Junctional parenchymal defects also result from abnormal fusion of renunculi and are identified as prominent grooves that lead from the hilum to the cortex.* Junctional parenchymal defects, dromedary humps, and hypertrophied columns of Bertin *all interrupt the cortical region of the kidney and are solitary, not bilateral, variants.*

▶ de Bruyn R (ed): *Pediatric Ultrasound: How, Why and When*, 2nd edition (e-book). Philadelphia, Churchill Livingstone/Elsevier, 2010, pp 51, 68.
▶ Rumack CM, Levine D (eds): *Diagnostic Ultrasound*, 5th edition. Philadelphia, Elsevier, 2018, pp 1781–1782.
▶ Siegel MJ (ed): *Pediatric Sonography*, 4th edition. Philadelphia, Lippincott Williams & Wilkins, 2011, pp 389–390.

343. C. Relieve built-up pressure.

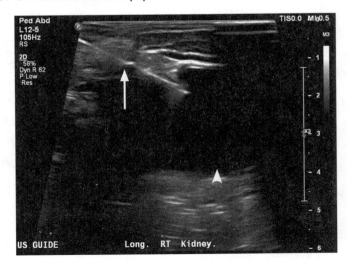

A percutaneous nephrostomy drainage is performed surgically to relieve built-up pressure caused by urine backed up in the kidney. A flexible plastic tube (arrow) is placed through the kidney and into the renal pelvis (arrowhead), exiting the body into a collecting bag. Urine drains into the bag, allowing the kidney to decompress. A nephrostolithotomy is the procedure that removes calculi from a kidney. Biopsies are surgical procedures performed to sample tissue, such as the renal cortex, to evaluate for disease. Urinary catheters are used in various instances to drain the bladder, not the kidney; the prefix nephro- refers to the kidney.

▶ Rumack CM, Levine D (eds): *Diagnostic Ultrasound: Pediatrics*, 4th edition. Philadelphia, Elsevier Mosby, 2018, pp 1864–1865.

▶ Siegel MJ (ed): *Pediatric Sonography*, 4th edition. Philadelphia, Lippincott Williams & Wilkins, 2011, pp 693–694.

344. B. Acoustic shadowing.

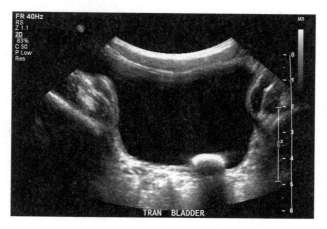

Acoustic shadowing occurs when the sound is absorbed or reflected by a structure of greater density or surrounding tissues. This prevents the sound wave from reaching the tissues deeper to the structure, thus causing a shadow. With bone or calculi, the sound beam is reflected by these dense materials and the shadow behind them appears anechoic. On the contrary, fluid-filled structures cause an increase of echoes posterior to them, known as posterior enhancement *or* increased through-transmission. *Posterior enhancement, reverberation, and ring-down artifacts are all echogenic artifacts and do not appear anechoic like acoustic shadowing.*

▶ de Bruyn R (ed): *Pediatric Ultrasound: How, Why and When*, 2nd edition (e-book). Philadelphia, Churchill Livingstone/Elsevier, 2010, pp 86–88.

▶ Rumack CM, Levine D (eds): *Diagnostic Ultrasound*, 5th edition. Philadelphia, Elsevier, 2018, p 21.

▶ Siegel MJ (ed): *Pediatric Sonography*, 4th edition. Philadelphia, Lippincott Williams & Wilkins, 2011, pp 25–27, 30–31.

345. **B. Fungal ball.**

The evidence of fungal balls is highly suggestive of a fungal infection. The most common fungal infection of the kidneys is caused by the Candida albicans organism. Fungal balls become evident in the later stages of the infection, are echogenic, and do not shadow. They can be located within the many areas of a dilated collecting system. Obstruction of the collecting system can occur if they are mobile and they can sometimes shift in location if the patient changes position. With nephrocalcinosis and medullary sponge kidney, the renal pyramids demonstrate an increased echogenicity that may or may not shadow, but both are present within the renal cortex. Angiomyolipomas are also nonshadowing and echogenic, but they occur within the cortex, not the collecting system.

▸ Rumack CM, Levine D (eds): *Diagnostic Ultrasound*, 5th edition. Philadelphia, Elsevier, 2018, pp 1794–1795.

▸ Siegel MJ (ed): *Pediatric Sonography*, 4th edition. Philadelphia, Lippincott Williams & Wilkins, 2011, pp 409–410, 423–424, 427–428, 437.

346. **A. Prune belly syndrome.**

A neurogenic bladder is dysfunctional and the result of impaired nerves that alter the bladder musculature. This is commonly seen with many conditions, including spinal anomalies and injuries. Sonographically, the bladder wall appears irregular or trabeculated and can be spastic with involuntary contractions. Patients with neurogenic bladders usually suffer from incontinence. Prune belly syndrome, also known as Eagle-Barrett syndrome, affects the abdominal wall muscles; with this syndrome the muscles are underdeveloped or absent. The bladder will be thin-walled and enlarged, with accompanying urinary tract dilatation.

▸ Rumack CM, Levine D (eds): *Diagnostic Ultrasound*, 5th edition. Philadelphia, Elsevier, 2018, pp 1361–1362, 1788, 1906.

▸ Siegel MJ (ed): *Pediatric Sonography*, 4th edition. Philadelphia, Lippincott Williams & Wilkins, 2011, pp 403–405, 451–452.

347. **D. Space of Retzius.**

The space of Retzius is an extraperitoneal, retropubic space located posterior to the symphysis pubis and anterior to the bladder. Morison's pouch, the pouch of Douglas, and the anterior cul-de-sac all lie intraperitoneal. Morison's pouch is the hepatorenal recess that separates the right kidney and the liver. The pouch of Douglas *lies between the uterus and the rectum. The* anterior cul-de-sac *is the space between the uterus and the bladder.*

▸ Hagen-Ansert SL: *Textbook of Diagnostic Ultrasonography*, 6th edition. S. Louis, Elsevier Mosby, 2006, pp 854, 872.
▸ Rumack CM, Levine D (eds): *Diagnostic Ultrasound*, 5th edition. Philadelphia, Elsevier, 2018, p 566.
▸ Siegel MJ (ed): *Pediatric Sonography*, 4th edition. Philadelphia, Lippincott Williams & Wilkins, 2011, pp 325, 450.

348. B. Renal cell carcinoma.

Most pediatric renal malignancies occur before 5 years of age. Rare under the age of 20, renal cell carcinoma, *when it occurs in children, is diagnosed at a mean age of 10 years and affects males twice as often as it does females.* Nephroblastomas (Wilms tumors) *and* rhabdoid tumors *both occur most commonly under the age of 3.* Nephroblastomatosis *is a precursor to nephroblastoma and occurs at an even younger age or during infancy.*

▸ Rumack CM, Levine D (eds): *Diagnostic Ultrasound*, 5th edition. Philadelphia, Elsevier, 2018, pp 1820–1821.
▸ Siegel MJ (ed): *Pediatric Sonography*, 4th edition. Philadelphia, Lippincott Williams & Wilkins, 2011, pp 413–421.

349. C. Renal hypoplasia.

Renal hypoplasia *is defined as a kidney or kidneys measuring more than 2 standard deviations below the expected mean for age. Unilateral cases are usually asymptomatic and an incidental finding. The affected kidney appears normal, just smaller in size than expected. The contralateral kidney can become hypertrophic from compensating for the decreased function of the hypoplastic kidney. Bilateral renal hypoplasia is associated with renal insufficiency.* Renal hyperplasia *would be an enlargement of the kidney.* Renal agenesis *is the absence of one or both kidneys; bilateral renal agenesis is incompatible with life.* Renal ectopia *is the abnormal location of the kidney.*

▸ Finn LS, Husain AN: The kidney and the lower urinary tract. In Husain AN, Stocker JT, Dehner LP (eds): *Pediatric Pathology*, 4th edition. Philadelphia, Wolters Kluwer, 2016, pp 800–864.
▸ Rumack CM, Levine D (eds): *Diagnostic Ultrasound*, 5th edition. Philadelphia, Elsevier, 2018, p 1776.
▸ Siegel MJ (ed): *Pediatric Sonography*, 4th edition. Philadelphia, Lippincott Williams & Wilkins, 2011, p 391.

350. **D. Von Hippel–Lindau disease.**

Von Hippel–Lindau disease *is an autosomal dominant inherited disease associated with tumors and cysts in multiple organs. Renal cysts of varying sizes are seen in approximately 60% of patients. The catecholamine-secreting tumor known as* pheochromocytoma *is associated with von Hippel–Lindau disease and can cause life-threatening hypertension. Patients with this disease also have an increased risk for renal cell carcinoma.* Autosomal recessive polycystic kidney disease (ARPKD) *is an inherited disease that is also a multisystem condition but is associated with periportal hepatic fibrosis and biliary ductal ectasia, known as Caroli disease.* Multicystic dysplastic kidney disease *(MCDK) and* glomerulocystic disease *are not inherited diseases.*

▶ Rumack CM, Levine D (eds): *Diagnostic Ultrasound*, 5th edition. Philadelphia, Elsevier, 2018, p 1816.

▶ Siegel MJ (ed): *Pediatric Sonography*, 4th edition. Philadelphia, Lippincott Williams & Wilkins, 2011, pp 405–412.

351. **B. Creatinine (CR).**

Muscle activity produces a waste product called creatinine (CR) *that is normally removed from the blood by the kidneys. When kidney function slows down or is compromised, serum CR levels rise.* Blood urea nitrogen (BUN) *is also a waste product in the blood, coming from the breakdown of protein foods and the body's metabolism. When kidney function is impaired or slows, both BUN levels and CR levels will rise.* Glomerular filtration rate *(GFR) measures how much kidney function is present. This level will fall, not rise, when kidney function is decreased.*

▶ Keough J: *Nursing Laboratory and Diagnostic Tests Demystified*, 2nd edition. New York, McGraw-Hill, 2017, pp 11, 36–38, 54–55.

▶ National Kidney Foundation: Know your kidney numbers: two simple tests. Available at https://www.kidney.org/atoz/content/know-your-kidney-numbers-two-simple-tests.

352. D. Mesoblastic nephroma.

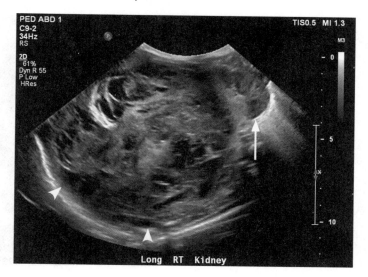

Mesoblastic nephroma *has many names—fetal renal hamartoma, mesenchymal hamartoma of infancy, and leiomyomatous hamartoma. Usually apparent before an infant reaches 6 months old, a mesoblastic nephroma (arrowheads) is the most common benign tumor of the infant kidney (arrow). Sonographically, it is large and echogenic and may demonstrate a whorled appearance. When there are areas of necrosis or hemorrhage within, the echotexture becomes more heterogeneous. The most common clinical sign is an abdominal mass, but hypertension may also be present. Treatment is heminephrectomy or nephrectomy. Wilms tumor, renal cell carcinoma, and lymphoma are malignant masses more commonly diagnosed after infancy.*

▸ de Bruyn R (ed): *Pediatric Ultrasound: How, Why and When*, 2nd edition (e-book). Philadelphia, Churchill Livingstone/Elsevier, 2010, pp 105–106, 109–110.

▸ Khashu M, Osiovich H, Sargent MA: Congenital mesoblastic nephroma presenting with neonatal hypertension. J Perinatol 25:433–435, 2005.

▸ Rumack CM, Levine D (eds): *Diagnostic Ultrasound*, 5th edition. Philadelphia, Elsevier, 2018, pp 1818–1820.

▸ Siegel MJ (ed): *Pediatric Sonography*, 4th edition. Philadelphia, Lippincott Williams & Wilkins, 2011, pp 413, 418–419, 422–423.

353. B. Nephrocalcinosis.

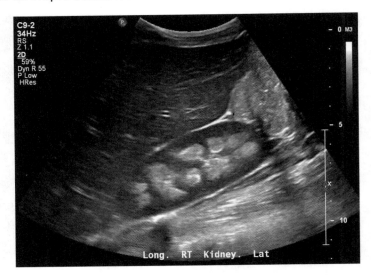

Nephrocalcinosis *is the term used for calcifications within the tubules or interstitial tissues of the kidney and varies in severity. Causes include metabolic disorders such as acute tubular necrosis (ATN), structural abnormalities, syndromes, infection, corticosteroids, and diuretic therapy. Calcium and mineral removal done by normal lymphatic flow will collect within the kidneys and present as microscopic or macroscopic nephrocalcinosis. Typically, the sonographic appearance is bilateral, echogenic renal pyramids with or without shadowing. Nephrocalcinosis may be found in the cortex, but not as commonly.* Staghorn calculi *are macroscopic calcifications that take on the shape of the renal pelvis.* Urolithiasis *and* nephrolithiasis *refer to one or more focal renal calculi or stones.*

▸ de Bruyn R (ed): *Pediatric Ultrasound: How, Why and When*, 2nd edition (e-book). Philadelphia, Churchill Livingstone/Elsevier, 2010, pp 86–92.

▸ Milliner DS: Calculi. In Kaplan BS, Meyers KEC (eds): *Pediatric Nephrology and Urology: The Requisites in Pediatrics*. Philadelphia, Elsevier Mosby, 2004, pp 361–374.

▸ Rumack CM, Levine D (eds): *Diagnostic Ultrasound*, 5th edition. Philadelphia, Elsevier, 2018, pp 1798, 1800, 2743, 2750.

▸ Siegel MJ (ed): *Pediatric Sonography*, 4th edition. Philadelphia, Lippincott Williams & Wilkins, 2011, pp 431, 437.

354. A. Stones.

See Color Plate 9 on page xxxvi.

Acoustic shadowing is more likely to appear during visualization of stones greater than 5 mm in diameter. The use of high-scale color Doppler can assist in diagnosing renal calculi when a twinkling artifact *is observed. This color phenomenon occurs as noise behind a highly reflective object and can be* used to indicate calculi. The "twinkle" is demonstrated as a random mixture of red and blue pixels in the high-frequency shift spectrum. Twinkle artifacts can be used to help identify gallstones as well as kidney stones.

▸ Kamaya A, Tuthill T, Rubin JM: Twinkling artifact on color Doppler sonography: dependence on machine parameters and underlying cause. Am J Roentgenol 180:215–222, 2003.

▸ Rumack CM, Levine D (eds): *Diagnostic Ultrasound*, 5th edition. Philadelphia, Elsevier, 2018, pp 1799, 1801.

▸ Siegel MJ (ed): *Pediatric Sonography*, 4th edition. Philadelphia, Lippincott Williams & Wilkins, 2011, p 39.

355. B. Glomerulonephritis.

Glomerulonephritis *is found most commonly in patients 6–7 years old. In the acute stage, kidneys can be normal in size or show bilateral enlargement with increased cortical echogenicity. In the chronic stage kidneys become smaller and more echogenic, and they lose their corticomedullary differentiation. In* xanthogranulomatous pyelonephritis *(XGP) the kidneys are also enlarged, but the renal cortex demonstrates hypoechoic masses that may represent dilated calyces or parenchymal destruction. With* nephrocalcinosis *calcification is more common in the medulla than in the cortex. The renal cortex is usually not discernible in* multicystic dysplastic kidney *(MCDK), as multiple cysts of varying sizes invade the entire kidney. MCDK is most often detected prenatally and seen on only one side. However, it can occur bilaterally.*

▸ Rumack CM, Levine D (eds): *Diagnostic Ultrasound*, 5th edition. Philadelphia, Elsevier, 2018, pp 370–371, 1796–1798.

▸ Siegel MJ (ed): *Pediatric Sonography*, 4th edition. Philadelphia, Lippincott Williams & Wilkins, 2011, pp 411–412, 429–430.

356. A. Computed tomography (CT).

Computed tomography (CT) is the preferred study of choice in patients with suspected blunt force abdominal trauma. Sonography is useful in identifying hematomas and vascular integrity, but CT is better at categorizing and revealing the extent of the injury. CT is a faster modality than magnetic resonance imaging (MRI) and better for unstable patients. Sonography is more commonly used for following the course of the renal injury or as hematomas resolve. Nuclear medicine is not used in cases of acute renal trauma, but it could be helpful in assessing remaining function several months later.

▸ de Bruyn R (ed): *Pediatric Ultrasound: How, Why and When*, 2nd edition (e-book). Philadelphia, Churchill Livingstone/Elsevier, 2010, pp 97, 170, 202.

▸ Rumack CM, Levine D (eds): *Diagnostic Ultrasound*, 5th edition. Philadelphia, Elsevier, 2018, p 1801.

▸ Siegel MJ (ed): *Pediatric Sonography*, 4th edition. Philadelphia, Lippincott Williams & Wilkins, 2011, pp 438–440.

357. C. Lymphoma.

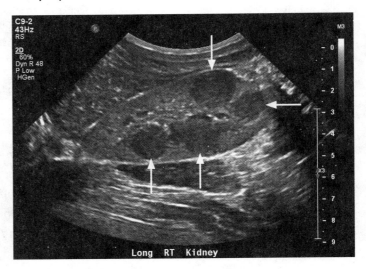

Multiple homogeneous and hypoechoic cortical masses (arrows) can be seen in patients with non-Hodgkin lymphoma. The symptoms include fever, abdominal pain, and lymphadenopathy. Lymphomas are seen in adolescents more often than in children. *The primary B-cell lymphoma that arises from the mediastinum is more commonly found in the kidneys.* Neuroblastomas *and* cystic nephromas *usually occur at a much younger age, are usually contained to one tumor, and are both heterogeneous.* Angiomyolipomas *can be multiple in number and located within the renal cortex, but they are hyperechoic, not hypoechoic.*

▸ National Cancer Institute: Childhood non-Hodgkin lymphoma treatment. Available at https://www.cancer.gov/types/lymphoma/patient/child-nhl-treatment-pdq.

▸ Rumack CM, Levine D (eds): *Diagnostic Ultrasound*, 5th edition. Philadelphia, Elsevier, 2018, pp 1820, 1823.

▸ Siegel MJ (ed): *Pediatric Sonography*, 4th edition. Philadelphia, Lippincott Williams & Wilkins, 2011, pp 419–420.

358. A. 10 mm.

The neonatal renal pelvis should measure less than 10 mm and is not usually associated with calyceal dilatation. An anteroposterior (AP) diameter greater than 10 mm is more likely suggestive of obstructive uropathy. Color Doppler can help differentiate between renal vessels and the renal pelvis. The renal pelvis diameter can change in certain positions and often will increase in the prone position. For this reason, the optimal position for measuring the renal pelvis would be supine.

▶ Bouzada MC, Oliveira EA, Pereira AK, et al: Diagnostic accuracy of postnatal renal pelvic diameter as a predictor of uropathy: a prospective study. Pediatr Radiol 34:798–804, 2004.

▶ de Bruyn R (ed): *Pediatric Ultrasound: How, Why and When*, 2nd edition (e-book). Philadelphia, Churchill Livingstone/Elsevier, 2010, pp 30–31.

▶ Siegel MJ (ed): *Pediatric Sonography*, 4th edition. Philadelphia, Lippincott Williams & Wilkins, 2011, p 386.

359. C. Dilated posterior urethra.

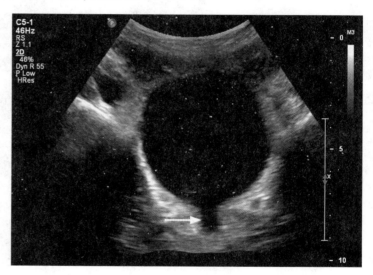

A dilated posterior urethra *(arrow)* is seen in this image of the bladder, giving the bladder a "keyhole" appearance. This is typically seen in cases of posterior urethral valves (PUV), which is the most common cause of urethral obstruction in boys. Accompanying sonographic findings of PUV would include bilateral hydronephrosis and hydroureter, renal parenchymal thinning, a dilated, thick-walled bladder, and a dilated posterior urethra. Due to its central and inferior position in the bladder, this image is most consistent with a dilated posterior urethra.

▶ Rumack CM, Levine D (eds): *Diagnostic Ultrasound*, 5th edition. Philadelphia, Elsevier, 2018, p 1362.

▶ Siegel MJ (ed): *Pediatric Sonography*, 4th edition. Philadelphia, Lippincott Williams & Wilkins, 2011, pp 400–404.

360. B. Bladder.

A Hutch diverticulum *(also known as a periureteral diverticulum) is a herniation of mucosa through a weak point in the bladder detrusor muscles near the ureterovesical junction (UVJ). Bladder diverticula can be congenital or acquired. Congenital or primary diverticula, such as Hutch diverticula, are usually solitary and larger than acquired diverticula. Secondary or acquired diverticula can be due to obstruction, reflux, or a neurogenic bladder and are more often multiple in number. Most diverticula are asymptomatic, but larger ones can cause obstruction or reflux.*

▶ Boechat MI, Lebowitz RL: Diverticula of the bladder in children. Pediatr Radiol 10:22–28, 1978.

▶ Rumack CM, Levine D (eds): *Diagnostic Ultrasound*, 5th edition. Philadelphia, Elsevier, 2018, p 310.

▶ Siegel MJ (ed): *Pediatric Sonography*, 4th edition. Philadelphia, Lippincott Williams & Wilkins, 2011, p 449.

361. A. Bilateral renal agenesis.

Prune belly syndrome, *also known as* Eagle-Barrett syndrome, *is so named for the appearance of the associated absence or underdevelopment of the abdominal muscles, which allows the abdomen to bulge out and gives the skin the wrinkled appearance of a prune. Patients with prune belly syndrome have a triad of conditions that include hypoplastic or absent abdominal wall muscles, urinary tract anomalies, and cryptorchidism (undescended testes). The urinary system usually consists of a large bladder, dilated and tortuous ureters, and megalourethra. Prune belly is most commonly diagnosed in the neonatal period and occurs almost entirely in males, although up to 4% of cases are in females. Other associations include intestinal malrotation or atresia, imperforate anus, and urachal abnormalities. If pulmonary hypoplasia occurs, Potter's syndrome and death may result.* Bilateral renal agenesis *is a fatal condition and is not found with prune belly syndrome.*

▶ Rumack CM, Levine D (eds): *Diagnostic Ultrasound*, 5th edition. Philadelphia, Elsevier, 2018, pp 1361–1362, 1788, 1906.

▶ Siegel MJ (ed): *Pediatric Sonography*, 4th edition. Philadelphia, Lippincott Williams & Wilkins, 2011, pp 403–405.

362. D. Patent urachus.

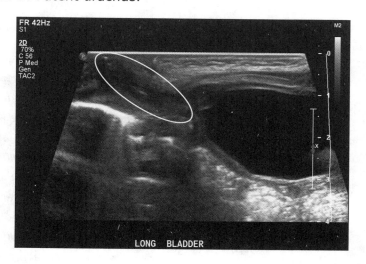

During fetal development, the urachus (circled) is a tubular channel connecting the umbilicus and the anterior fetal bladder wall. The urachus usually closes by the fifth month of gestation. When a urachus remains patent, the neonate or infant patient will present with an inflamed umbilical region that stays wet. Patent urachal abnormalities are associated with urinary tract obstruction and ventral wall defects, where urine can leak through the umbilicus. A urachal cyst occurs when the umbilical and bladder ends close but leave fluid trapped in the center of the channel. A urachal cyst does not communicate with the outside umbilicus or inner bladder. A persistent cloaca is a single perineal opening defect of the urethra, vagina, and rectum for the outlet of all urine, genital secretions, and fecal material. An umbilical hernia is a bulging of abdominal layers or tissue into the umbilicus.

▶ Rumack CM, Levine D (eds): *Diagnostic Ultrasound*, 5th edition. Philadelphia, Elsevier, 2018, pp 1337, 1791–1792, 1907–1909.

▶ Siegel MJ (ed): *Pediatric Sonography*, 4th edition. Philadelphia, Lippincott Williams & Wilkins, 2011, pp 450–451.

363. **C. Arcuate arteries.**

A pseudoaneurysm can occur after a localized rupture of an artery and is typically contained by soft tissues. The majority of pseudoaneurysms are extrarenal and involve transplant allografts. Intrarenal pseudoaneurysms are a possible complication of percutaneous renal biopsy and typically involve the arcuate arteries due to the biopsy location within the outer cortex. These are often best seen by dialing down the scale on color Doppler images until the turbulent flow in the aneurysm is more apparent. Most pseudoaneurysms are asymptomatic, but if there is a rupture into the collecting system, hematuria can occur. Pseudoaneurysms generally resolve on their own. When the patient is prone, the main renal and segmental arteries are usually deeper than the biopsy depth. Interlobar *(cortical radiate)* arteries *run along the corticomedullary junction and give rise to the* arcuate arteries, *making the interlobar arteries deeper than the normal biopsy depth as well.*

▶ de Bruyn R (ed): *Pediatric Ultrasound: How, Why and When,* 2nd edition (e-book). Philadelphia, Churchill Livingstone/Elsevier, 2010, p 104.
▶ Oh S, Bashir O, et al: Renal artery. Available from Radiopaedia at https://radiopaedia.org/articles/renal-artery.
▶ Rumack CM, Levine D (eds): *Diagnostic Ultrasound,* 5th edition. Philadelphia, Elsevier, 2018, pp 664, 669–670, 1809, 1811.
▶ Siegel MJ (ed): *Pediatric Sonography,* 4th edition. Philadelphia, Lippincott Williams & Wilkins, 2011, p 444.

364. **D. Megacystis.**

An abnormally large, distended, and smooth-walled bladder is termed megacystis. *This rare condition is usually congenital and can be seen in syndromes such as megacystis-microcolon-intestinal hypoperistalsis syndrome (MMIHS) and megacystis-megaureter syndrome. Reflux and urinary tract infections are associated with megacystis. Bladder exstrophy is caused by an abnormal closure of the abdominal wall during fetal development, resulting in a small bladder exposed to the outside of the body. A neurogenic bladder is usually large but typically has a thickened, trabeculated wall.*

▶ Rumack CM, Levine D (eds): *Diagnostic Ultrasound,* 5th edition. Philadelphia, Elsevier, 2018, pp 1360, 1362, 1788–1791.
▶ Siegel MJ (ed): *Pediatric Sonography,* 4th edition. Philadelphia, Lippincott Williams & Wilkins, 2011, pp 449, 451.

365. B. Pyonephrosis.

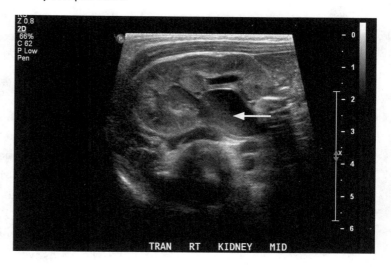

When urine remains stagnant within the collecting system, bacteria can develop, most commonly E. coli. Purulent exudate seen within the hydronephrotic collecting system (arrow), referred to as pyonephritis, *appears sonographically as mobile, internal echoes or a fluid-debris level. Pyonephritis can lead to symptomatic* pyonephrosis, *infection of the renal collecting system. Pyonephrosis is an urgent scenario that requires immediate treatment with percutaneous or surgical drainage. Symptoms of pyonephrosis include fever, chills, and flank pain. Untreated pyonephrosis can lead to bacteremia, septic shock, and parenchymal destruction. Destruction of the parenchyma can result in a loss of renal function.* Pyelonephritis *is infectious interstitial nephritis with similar symptoms and bacterial origin, but it primarily affects the renal tissue, may not demonstrate hydronephrosis, and is not a medical emergency. Pyelonephritis is treated with antibiotics.* Fungal balls *are also an infectious process but appear as echogenic, round structures within the collecting system.* Cystitis *is bladder inflammation.*

▶ Medscape: Pyonephrosis. Available at https://emedicine.medscape.com/article/440548-overview.

▶ Rumack CM, Levine D (eds): *Diagnostic Ultrasound*, 5th edition. Philadelphia, Elsevier, 2018, pp 1793–1794.

▶ Sharma R, Weerakkody Y, et al: Pyonephrosis. Available from Radiopaedia at https://radiopaedia.org/articles/pyonephrosis.

▶ Siegel MJ (ed): *Pediatric Sonography*, 4th edition. Philadelphia, Lippincott Williams & Wilkins, 2011, pp 425, 427–428.

366. **A. Bilateral renal agenesis.**

Bilateral renal agenesis is a rare congenital anomaly that is incompatible with life because there is a complete absence of renal tissue. Most patients have pulmonary hypoplasia due to oligohydramnios in utero, in which case it is secondary to classic Potter sequence. Sonographically, the kidneys and renal arteries are absent and the bladder is either absent or small. The adrenal glands are usually present but will appear elongated. Unilateral renal agenesis *is more common and is compatible with life.* Autosomal recessive polycystic kidney disease *(ARPKD),* autosomal dominant polycystic kidney disease *(ADPKD), and* Eagle-Barrett syndrome *(prune belly syndrome) are all compatible with life, although there are many associations with ARPKD and ADPKD that complicate other organ systems and impair overall health.*

▶ Rumack CM, Levine D (eds): *Diagnostic Ultrasound*, 5th edition. Philadelphia, Elsevier, 2018, pp 1342–1344.

▶ Siegel MJ (ed): *Pediatric Sonography*, 4th edition. Philadelphia, Lippincott Williams & Wilkins, 2011, pp 390, 403–408.

367. **B. Isthmus.**

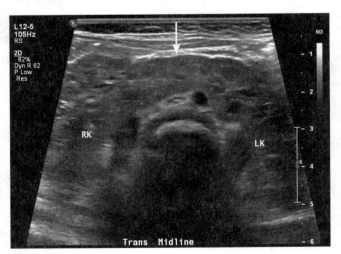

The central band of tissue that fuses together the two kidney segments of a horseshoe kidney is known as the isthmus *(arrow). It may consist of functioning renal parenchyma or a fibrous band. The site of fusion in a horseshoe kidney usually occurs at the lower poles. A* moiety *is defined as a part, section, or portion and is the term used to describe the upper or lower pole of a kidney.* Renunculi *are small, fetal renal*

segments that fuse into lobes to form lobulations seen in fetal and infant kidneys. Bridge *suggests a connection but simply is not the medical term used to describe the tissue that connects the two kidneys.*

▶ Rumack CM, Levine D (eds): *Diagnostic Ultrasound*, 5th edition. Philadelphia, Elsevier, 2018, pp 1345, 1784.

▶ Siegel MJ (ed): *Pediatric Sonography*, 4th edition. Philadelphia, Lippincott Williams & Wilkins, 2011, pp 389, 392–393.

368. **D. Tuberous sclerosis.**

Tuberous sclerosis *is a multisystem disorder that is autosomal dominant and inherited. This uncommon condition causes multisystemic lesions (cystic and solid). Adolescents and adults more frequently have hyperechoic angiomyolipomas. Other systemic tumors include rhabdomyomas, hamartomas, and astrocytomas.* Eagle-Barrett syndrome *results in a dilated and distended urinary tract due to the lack of abdominal muscles, also known as prune belly syndrome.* Henoch-Schönlein purpura *is a disease that includes vasculitis within the walls of the small vessels of the kidneys, resulting in echogenic renal parenchyma and elevated resistive indices.* Von Hippel–Lindau syndrome *is also an inherited autosomal dominant, multisystem disease, but it is more commonly associated with renal cysts.*

▶ Rumack CM, Levine D (eds): *Diagnostic Ultrasound*, 5th edition. Philadelphia, Elsevier, 2018, p 1816.

▶ Siegel MJ (ed): *Pediatric Sonography*, 4th edition. Philadelphia, Lippincott Williams & Wilkins, 2011, pp 403, 410, 431.

369. **C. Autosomal recessive polycystic kidney disease (ARPKD).**

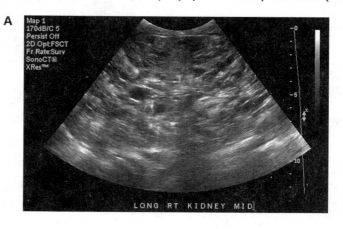

(figure continues . . .)

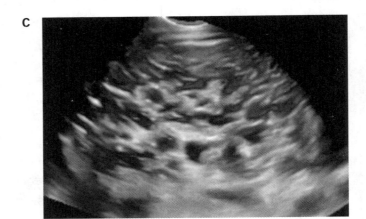

See Color Plate 22 on page xlii.

In the past, autosomal recessive polycystic kidney disease (ARPKD) has been known as infantile polycystic kidney disease and Potter type 1. ARPKD is an inherited disease of varying severity. The majority of patients have accompanying hepatic abnormalities. Renal disease and hepatic fibrosis will vary inversely, meaning the more severe the renal disease, the less severe the hepatic disease and vice versa. Dilated collecting tubules form multiple small cysts that are radially arranged and extend from the medulla to the outer cortex, as seen in cases from different patients in images **A**, **B**, and **C**. Neonates will have bilateral, markedly enlarged, and echogenic kidneys, lack of corticomedullary differentiation, and dilated bile ducts. The kidneys in older children can be normal in size or enlarged. The renal pyramids will appear hyperechoic, and small cysts within the medulla may be seen. Cirrhosis and portal hypertension may cause dilated bile ducts. Caroli syndrome *is characterized by cystic dilatation or ectasia of the bile ducts. In* autosomal dominant polycystic kidney disease (ADPKD) *there are also multiple cysts of varying sizes throughout the bilateral kidneys, but ADPKD is not associated with periportal hepatic fibrosis or Caroli syndrome.*

Medullary cystic disease *is bilateral, but the kidneys will appear smaller than normal.* Multicystic dysplastic kidney *(MCDK) is predominantly unilateral but can be bilateral; if bilateral, MCDK is incompatible with life.*

▶ de Bruyn R (ed): *Pediatric Ultrasound: How, Why and When*, 2nd edition (e-book). Philadelphia, Churchill Livingstone/Elsevier, 2010, pp 34, 74–76.

▶ Dell KM: Polysystic disease. In Kaplan BS, Meyers KEC (eds): *Pediatric Nephrology and Urology: The Requisites in Pediatrics*. Philadelphia, Elsevier Mosby, 2004, pp 214–222.

▶ Osathanondh V, Potter E: Pathogenesis of polycystic kidneys. Arch Pathol 77:458–512, 1964.

▶ Rumack CM, Levine D (eds): *Diagnostic Ultrasound*, 5th edition. Philadelphia, Elsevier, 2018, pp 1348–1350, 1814–1815.

▶ Siegel MJ (ed): *Pediatric Sonography*, 4th edition. Philadelphia, Lippincott Williams & Wilkins, 2011, pp 405–411.

370. 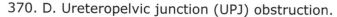 D. Ureteropelvic junction (UPJ) obstruction.

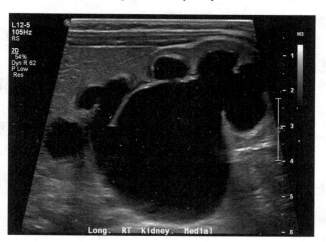

Ureteropelvic junction *(UPJ)* obstruction *occurs when the area between the renal pelvis and the ureter is blocked, causing urine to build up within the collecting system of the kidney. It is usually diagnosed by prenatal ultrasound and caused by some sort of stricture or crossing vessel. Sonographically, a larger cystic area represents a dilated renal pelvis and smaller communicating cystic areas represent the dilated calyces. The renal parenchyma is thinned and there is no dilated ureter seen. UPJ obstruction is the most frequent cause of urinary obstruction in children. Chronic UPJ obstruction can cause significant kidney damage. UPJ obstruction can also be caused by stones, scarring, or infection.* Vesicoureteral reflux *(VUR),* ureterovesical junction *(UVJ), and* posterior urethral valves *(PUV) all demonstrate a dilated ureter, whereas UPJ does not.*

▶ Finn LS, Husain AN: The kidney and lower urinary tract. In Husain AN, Stocker JT, Dehner LP (eds): *Pediatric Pathology*, 4th edition. Philadelphia, Wolters Kluwer, 2016, pp 800–864.

▶ Rumack CM, Levine D (eds): *Diagnostic Ultrasound*, 5th edition. Philadelphia, Elsevier, 2018, pp 1354–1358, 1786–1787.

▶ Siegel MJ (ed): *Pediatric Sonography*, 4th edition. Philadelphia, Lippincott Williams & Wilkins, 2011, pp 394–400.

▶ Washington University School of Medicine in St. Louis, Urologic Surgery: Ureteropelvic junction (UPJ) obstruction in children. Available at https://urology.wustl.edu/en/Patient-Care/Pediatric-Urology/UPJ-Obstruction-in-Children.

371. **B. Dromedary hump.**

A dromedary hump appears as a bulge along the lateral margin of the middle of the left kidney. Like the hypertrophied column of Bertin, junctional parenchymal defect, and fetal lobulations, it is a normal variant, but the dromedary hump is found only on the left side.

▶ Siegel MJ (ed): *Pediatric Sonography*, 4th edition. Philadelphia, Lippincott Williams & Wilkins, 2011, p 390.

372. **A. 12 MHz.**

Whether it is a linear or curved array, the highest possible transducer frequency that will adequately penetrate the area of interest should be utilized. Most of the time, the linear 12 MHz transducer provides optimal resolution of early infant kidneys.

▶ Rumack CM, Levine D (eds): *Diagnostic Ultrasound*, 5th edition. Philadelphia, Elsevier, 2018, p 1776.

▶ Siegel MJ (ed): *Pediatric Sonography*, 4th edition. Philadelphia, Lippincott Williams & Wilkins, 2011, pp 384–385.

373. **C. Megaureter.**

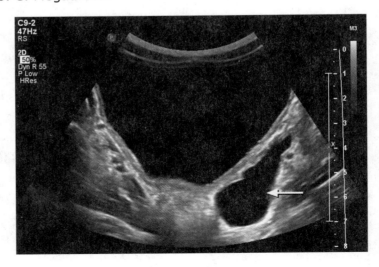

A dilated ureter is known as a megaureter *(arrow). Megaureters may be caused by congenital or primary obstruction, but they also result from reflux. The distal portion of the ureter, prior to its insertion into the bladder, is usually the affected region.* Bladder diverticula *occur congenitally as pouches within the bladder wall.* Ureteroceles *are seen projecting into the bladder.* Hydronephrosis *defines a dilated renal pelvis and calyces and is visualized at the kidney level.*

▶ de Bruyn R (ed): *Pediatric Ultrasound: How, Why and When*, 2nd edition (e-book). Philadelphia, Churchill Livingstone/Elsevier, 2010, pp 46, 59.

▶ Meyer JS, Lebowitz RL: Primary megaureter in infants and children: a review. Urol Radiol 14:296–305, 1992.

▶ Rumack CM, Levine D (eds): *Diagnostic Ultrasound*, 5th edition. Philadelphia, Elsevier, 2018, pp 1358–359, 1786–1788.

▶ Siegel MJ (ed): *Pediatric Sonography*, 4th edition. Philadelphia, Lippincott Williams & Wilkins, 2011, pp 395–398.

374. **D. There is no routine exam preparation.**

There is no routine preparation for a renal ultrasound exam. Ideally, patients should be somewhat hydrated for bladder imaging, but 32 ounces of water would be excessive. In younger children, the timing of bladder fullness may be difficult to predict. Certain specific conditions and imaging scenarios may require pre- and post-void bladder imaging, but ultrasound of the kidneys alone does not require patient preparation.

▶ Rumack CM, Levine D (eds): *Diagnostic Ultrasound*, 5th edition. Philadelphia, Elsevier, 2018, p 1776.

▶ Siegel MJ (ed): *Pediatric Sonography*, 4th edition. Philadelphia, Lippincott Williams & Wilkins, 2011, p 384.

375. **C. Blood urea nitrogen (BUN).**

Blood urea nitrogen *(BUN) is the end product of the breakdown of protein foods and metabolism. Normal kidney function releases BUN out of the kidney and into the bloodstream. BUN can be elevated in situations where the kidney function is impaired, such as medical renal disease, obstruction, and tumors.* Creatinine *(CR) is the end product of the conversion of creatine phosphate after skeletal muscle exertion. Once creatine converts to CR, it is carried through the blood to the kidneys for filtering and excretion in urine.*

▶ Keough J: *Nursing Laboratory and Diagnostic Tests Demystified*, 2nd edition. New York, McGraw-Hill, 2017, pp 11, 36–38, 54–55.

376. **A. Medullary sponge kidney.**

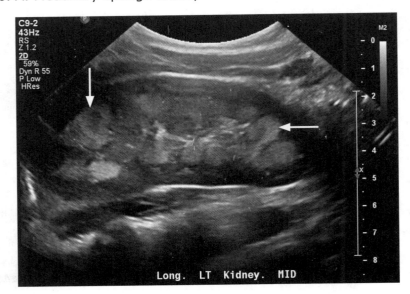

Medullary sponge kidney *(arrows)*, also known as *medullary tubular ectasia,* is a type of medullary cystic disease. It is not inherited but occurs sporadically. The collecting tubules become dilated within the renal pyramids. Often deposits of calcium occur at the site of the dilated tubules, causing nephrocalcinosis. The renal pyramids appear echogenic and the outflow of urine can be reduced. *Urolithiasis refers to a more focal renal calculus or stone.* Multicystic dysplastic kidney *(MCDK) demonstrates multiple cysts within a single kidney.* Nephroblastomatosis *presents as renal enlargement with a hypoechoic rind and multiple masses.*

▸ de Bruyn R (ed): *Pediatric Ultrasound: How, Why and When*, 2nd edition (e-book). Philadelphia, Churchill Livingstone/Elsevier, 2010, pp 81–82.
▸ Rumack CM, Levine D (eds): *Diagnostic Ultrasound*, 5th edition. Philadelphia, Elsevier, 2018, pp 339–340, 359, 1012, 1799.
▸ Siegel MJ (ed): *Pediatric Sonography*, 4th edition. Philadelphia, Lippincott Williams & Wilkins, 2011, pp 409–412, 417–418, 437.
▸ Wood BP: Renal cystic disease in infants and children. Urol Radiol 14:284–295, 1992.

377. **B. Large, edematous kidneys.**

Acute renal failure has a sudden onset and can be reversible. Many factors can cause acute failure, including deceased blood flow, obstruction, infection, medicine toxicity, glomerulonephritis, and other medical renal diseases. Kidneys will initially appear large and edematous with an increased echogenicity. When renal failure is chronic, the kidneys are small and echogenic, with a thinned parenchyma.

In both acute and chronic renal failure, there are elevated blood urea nitrogen (BUN) and creatinine (CR) levels due to the decrease in the kidneys' ability to eliminate waste into the bloodstream. Lab values would not be a sonographic characteristic.

▶ Rumack CM, Levine D (eds): *Diagnostic Ultrasound*, 5th edition. Philadelphia, Elsevier, 2018, pp 1795–1796.

▶ Siegel MJ (ed): *Pediatric Sonography*, 4th edition. Philadelphia, Lippincott Williams & Wilkins, 2011, pp 430, 435.

378. **D. Duplex kidney.**

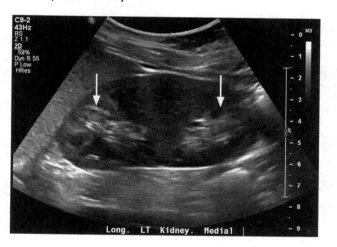

Of all the congenital anomalies of the urinary tract, a duplex kidney (arrows) is the most common. It can be partial (bifid renal pelvis to a Y-shaped ureter) or complete (two separate renal pelves and ureters that enter the bladder in separate orifices). Of all duplication anomalies, 95% are partial. Complete duplications are less common in boys. Sonography of duplex kidneys will show two echogenic renal sinuses divided by normal renal parenchyma. A hypertrophied column of Bertin is a thickened layer of cortex that splays the renal pyramids and projects into the renal sinus. It will appear isoechoic to the renal cortex and can mimic a mass. A cortical fusion defect presents as an echogenic, linear fusion line in the upper or middle third of one kidney. A horseshoe kidney consists of both kidneys fused together by a connecting isthmus.

▶ de Bruyn R (ed): *Pediatric Ultrasound: How, Why and When*, 2nd edition (e-book). Philadelphia, Churchill Livingstone/Elsevier, 2010, pp 31–32, 46, 62–67.

▶ Rumack CM, Levine D (eds): *Diagnostic Ultrasound*, 5th edition. Philadelphia, Elsevier, 2018, pp 1783–1784.

▶ Siegel MJ (ed): *Pediatric Sonography*, 4th edition. Philadelphia, Lippincott Williams & Wilkins, 2011, pp 389, 392–393, 39.

379. **A. Bladder exstrophy.**

When the infraumbilical abdominal wall fails to close in the midline, the anterior wall of the bladder may be exposed to the outside. This is known as bladder exstrophy. Depending on the severity of the defect, the bladder neck and urethra may also be exposed. Bladder exstrophy requires surgery to close the abdominal wall, and a bladder augmentation is usually performed. Patent urachus *is the result of the urachus not closing before birth, leaving a tubular opening between the bladder and the umbilicus.* Bladder diverticula *occur congenitally as pouches within the bladder wall.* Megacystis *is usually caused by a distal stenosis and can be seen on ultrasound as early as the first trimester screening.*

▶ Rumack CM, Levine D (eds): *Diagnostic Ultrasound*, 5th edition. Philadelphia, Elsevier, 2018, p 1791.

▶ Siegel MJ (ed): *Pediatric Sonography*, 4th edition. Philadelphia, Lippincott Williams & Wilkins, 2011, pp 449–450.

380. **B. Avulsion.**

The classification of renal injuries is typically divided into four groups:

(1) *Minor lesions: hematomas, contusions, or small corticomedullary lacerations not extending into the collecting system*

(2) *Major injuries: lacerations that extend into the collecting system and fractures that separate the kidney into two parts*

(3) *Catastrophic injuries: shattered kidneys, injuries to the vascular pedicle, and arterial occlusion*

(4) *Avulsion: laceration of the ureteropelvic junction or renal pelvis*

Computed tomography (CT) is the preferred modality for revealing the extent of renal injury, but ultrasound is commonly used for follow-up.

▶ de Bruyn R (ed): *Pediatric Ultrasound: How, Why and When*, 2nd edition (e-book). Philadelphia, Churchill Livingstone/Elsevier, 2010, p 97.

▶ Rumack CM, Levine D (eds): *Diagnostic Ultrasound*, 5th edition. Philadelphia, Elsevier, 2018, p 365.

▶ Siegel MJ (ed): *Pediatric Sonography*, 4th edition. Philadelphia, Lippincott Williams & Wilkins, 2011, pp 438–440.

381. D. Nephroblastomatosis.

In the fetus, nephroblastomatosis *is diagnosed by the presence of fetal renal blastoma or nephrogenic rests after 26 weeks of gestation. The embryonal remnants, or rests, are the precursor to Wilms tumor. These rests can be intralobar, perilobar (most common), or both. The type with a documented higher incidence of Wilms tumor is intralobar. Sonographically, the kidneys are bilaterally enlarged but maintain their shape. Nephroblastomatosis can present with hypoechoic masses occurring focally, multifocally, or diffusely. Treatment is usually the same chemotherapy that would be used in stage 1 of Wilms tumor, also known as* nephroblastoma. Neuroblastoma *is a malignant tumor originating from the adrenal glands or along the paraspinal sympathetic ganglia.* Mesoblastic nephroma *is a benign tumor commonly seen in the first few months of life.*

▶ de Bruyn R (ed): *Pediatric Ultrasound: How, Why and When*, 2nd edition (e-book). Philadelphia, Churchill Livingstone/Elsevier, 2010, pp 87, 111.

▶ Finn LS, Husain AN: The kidney and lower urinary tract. In Husain AN, Stocker JT, Dehner LP (eds): *Pediatric Pathology*, 4th edition. Philadelphia, Wolters Kluwer, 2016, pp 800–864.

▶ Rohrschneider WK, Weirich A, Rieden K, et al: US, CT and MR imaging characteristics of nephroblastomatosis. Pediatr Radiol 28:435–443, 1998.

▶ Rumack CM, Levine D (eds): *Diagnostic Ultrasound*, 5th edition. Philadelphia, Elsevier, 2018, p 1818.

▶ Siegel MJ (ed): *Pediatric Sonography*, 4th edition. Philadelphia, Lippincott Williams & Wilkins, 2011, pp 417–418.

382. B. Multicystic dysplastic kidney (MCDK).

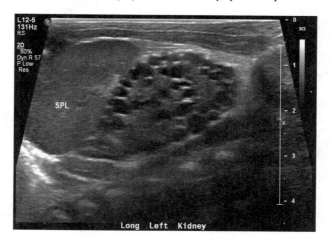

Multicystic dysplastic kidney *(MCDK) is nonhereditary and is most often unilateral. On occasion, it may be bilateral. There are two types of unilateral MCDK, simple and complicated.* Simple MCDK *has a contralateral normal kidney.* Complicated

MCDK *has contralateral renal abnormalities. The MCDK kidney is nonfunctioning and will eventually atrophy. Bilateral MCDK is not compatible with life, as both kidneys will be nonfunctioning. Most cases are diagnosed prenatally. Sonographically, the cysts do not communicate, there is no discernible renal pelvis or sinus, and renal parenchyma is absent.* Autosomal recessive polycystic kidney disease (ARPKD), *autosomal dominant polycystic kidney disease* (ADPKD), *and* glomerulocystic disease *are all bilateral renal diseases.*

▶ de Bruyn R (ed): *Pediatric Ultrasound: How, Why and When*, 2nd edition (e-book). Philadelphia, Churchill Livingstone/Elsevier, 2010, pp 32, 33, 59, 72–74.

▶ Rumack CM, Levine D (eds): *Diagnostic Ultrasound*, 5th edition. Philadelphia, Elsevier, 2018, pp 1346–1347, 1815–1816.

▶ Siegel MJ (ed): *Pediatric Sonography*, 4th edition. Philadelphia, Lippincott Williams & Wilkins, 2011, pp 405–412.

383. **D. Acute tubular necrosis (ATN).**

Acute tubular necrosis *(ATN) occurs when the renal tubules experience a nephrotoxic or ischemic injury severe enough to cause renal failure. If the cause of ATN is ischemia, the kidneys usually remain normal in appearance. ATN due to nephrotoxicity (from antibiotics, nonsteroidal anti-inflammatories, or chemotherapy) can cause an increase in renal size, renal pyramid enlargement, and increased echogenicity of the kidneys.* Glomerulonephritis *is an acutely inflamed kidney brought on by an immune response.* Xanthogranulomatous pyelonephritis *(XGP) follows a recurrent bacterial urinary tract infection.* Henoch-Schönlein purpura *is associated most commonly with upper respiratory infections and is demonstrated within the kidneys as vasculitis of the renal arteries.*

▶ Rumack CM, Levine D (eds): *Diagnostic Ultrasound*, 5th edition. Philadelphia, Elsevier, 2018, pp 370, 1795–1797.

▶ Siegel MJ (ed): *Pediatric Sonography*, 4th edition. Philadelphia, Lippincott Williams & Wilkins, 2011, pp 429–431.

384. **B. Ectopic.**

Ectopic ureters *are usually seen draining the upper pole moiety of complete ureteropelvic duplication anomalies. The lower pole moiety most commonly has the normal ureter insertion into the posterior bladder wall. In females, sites of ectopic insertions include the bladder neck, vestibule, vagina,* urethra, uterus, cervix, or rectum. In males, the ectopic ureter can insert into the bladder neck, inferomedial to the normal location (Weigert-Meyer rule), urethra, genital structures, or the rectum. The Weigert-Meyer rule states that with duplex kidney and complete ureteral duplication, upper and lower moieties have their own ureters with their own orifices into the bladder (or elsewhere).

▶ Glassberg KI, Braren V, Duckett JW, et al: Suggested terminology for duplex systems, ectopic ureters and ureteroceles. J Urol 132:1153–1154, 1984.

▶ Pierre-Hugues V, Augdal TA, Avni FE, et al: Standardization of pediatric uroradiological terms: a multidisciplinary European glossary. Pediatr Radiol 48:291–303, 2018. Available at https://link.springer.com/article/10.1007%2Fs00247-017-4006-7.

▶ Rumack CM, Levine D (eds): *Diagnostic Ultrasound*, 5th edition. Philadelphia, Elsevier, 2018, pp 1904–1905.

▶ Siegel MJ (ed): *Pediatric Sonography*, 4th edition. Philadelphia, Lippincott Williams & Wilkins, 2011, pp 399–400.

385. C. Rhabdoid tumor.

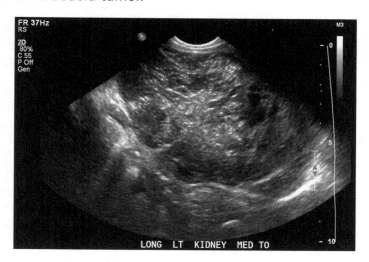

Rhabdoid tumors *(arrow) and* clear cell tumors *are both rare, highly aggressive, malignant medullary tumors. The sonographic features for both are large, heterogeneous masses with indistinct margins that arise from within the kidney. Rhabdoid tumors typically occur in infants and children under the age of 2. Most often unilateral, they have a poor prognosis. Clinical signs are abdominal mass, hematuria, fever, hypertension, and hypercalcemia. The lungs, liver, brain, and lymph nodes may show metastatic spread with rhabdoid tumors, but with clear cell tumors, the diagnostic difference is medullary infiltration and bone metastases.*

Wilms, lymphoma, and renal cell carcinoma *occur more commonly in older children or adults.* Lymphomas *are small, hypoechoic masses within the cortex.* Wilms tumors *are also cortical masses.* Renal cell carcinoma *is medullary but rare under the age of 20.*

▶ de Bruyn R (ed): *Pediatric Ultrasound: How, Why and When*, 2nd edition (e-book). Philadelphia, Churchill Livingstone/Elsevier, 2010, pp 106, 111.

▶ Siegel MJ (ed): *Pediatric Sonography*, 4th edition. Philadelphia, Lippincott Williams & Wilkins, 2011, pp 413–421.

386. **A. Junctional parenchymal defect.**

Cortical fusion defects, *or* junctional parenchymal defects, *of the kidney are identified as an echogenic triangular focus or line extending from the defect to the renal hilum or medulla. The fusion defects occur during the embryologic fusion of the renunculi. These defects usually are found within the upper or middle third of the kidney, most commonly on the right side. Junctional parenchymal defects should not be confused with parenchymal scarring. Scars are associated with parenchymal thinning, while cortical fusion defects are not.* Fetal lobulations *are echogenic indentations lying between the pyramids or calyces, causing the kidney to appear to have a scalloped border.* Dromedary humps *and* hypertrophied columns of Bertin *are similar in echogenicity to the renal cortex; they do not display the increased echogenicity seen with junctional parenchymal defects.*

▶ Rumack CM, Levine D (eds): *Diagnostic Ultrasound*, 5th edition. Philadelphia, Elsevier, 2018, p 1781.

▶ Siegel MJ (ed): *Pediatric Sonography*, 4th edition. Philadelphia, Lippincott Williams & Wilkins, 2011, pp 389–390.

387. **B. Vesicoureteral reflux (VUR).**

Vesicoureteral reflux *(VUR) is the reversed flow of urine from the bladder upward and into the ureters or collecting system. Under fluoroscopy, contrast is administered through a bladder catheter to fill the bladder, and reflux can be observed. Currently, some facilities are using ultrasound voiding cystography (USVC), done with contrast-enhanced ultrasound and microbubbles instead of contrast and radiation.* Primary VUR *is caused by an abnormal angle where the distal ureter inserts into the bladder.* Secondary VUR *is VUR secondary to another condition and may be caused* by multiple factors, such as bladder outlet obstruction, voiding dysfunction, neurogenic disease, and prune belly syndrome. Ureteral jets, ureteropelvic junction (UPJ) obstruction, and hydronephrosis can all be diagnosed by ultrasound and do not require radiography.

▶ Novljan G, Leart TK, Ključevšek D, et al: Ultrasound detection of vesicoureteral reflux in children. J Urol 184:319–324, 2010. Available at https://www.jurology.com/article/S0022-5347(10)00144-8/fulltext.

▶ Rumack CM, Levine D (eds): *Diagnostic Ultrasound*, 5th edition. Philadelphia, Elsevier, 2018, pp 1360, 1906–1907

▶ Siegel MJ (ed): *Pediatric Sonography*, 4th edition. Philadelphia, Lippincott Williams & Wilkins, 2011, pp 394, 397–398.

388. D. Cystic nephroma.

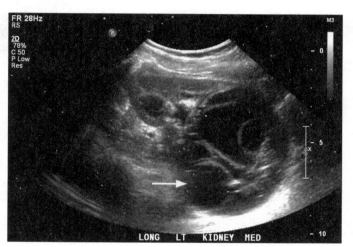

Cystic nephromas *(arrow) or multilocular cystic nephromas are nonhereditary, benign cystic masses. They can occur at any age. Sonographically, they appear as well circumscribed and multicystic, sometimes containing echogenic septations or mucoid material. Treatment is heminephrectomy or nephrectomy.* Nephroblastoma *(*Wilms tumor*) and* rhabdoid tumors *are malignant masses.* Angiomyolipomas *are benign but appear as small, echogenic masses and are usually multiple in number.*

▶ de Bruyn R (ed): *Pediatric Ultrasound: How, Why and When*, 2nd edition (e-book). Philadelphia, Churchill Livingstone/Elsevier, 2010, p 81.

▶ Rumack CM, Levine D (eds): *Diagnostic Ultrasound*, 5th edition. Philadelphia, Elsevier, 2018, pp 1820, 1822.

▶ Siegel MJ (ed): *Pediatric Sonography*, 4th edition. Philadelphia, Lippincott Williams & Wilkins, 2011, pp 412–416, 420, 423–424.

389. B. Interlobar.

Vasculature of the Kidney

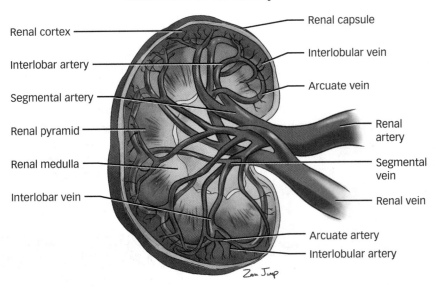

See Color Plate 23 on page xlii.

The main renal artery divides within the hilum to form several pairs of segmental arteries. Segmental arteries *course through the medulla toward the pyramids. The segmental arteries divide into the interlobar arteries.* The interlobar arteries *follow the periphery of the pyramids, coursing between them. At the outer edge of the pyramids, the interlobar arteries give rise to the arcuate arteries.* Arcuate arteries *trace the outer edge of the pyramids, branching into interlobular arteries.* Interlobular arteries *are located within the renal cortex, coursing in a direction similar to that of the interlobar arteries, but are an extension of the arcuate arteries that reach out toward the kidney border.*

▶ Siegel MJ (ed): *Pediatric Sonography*, 4th edition. Philadelphia, Lippincott Williams & Wilkins, 2011, pp 386–387.

390. C. Tardus parvus.

See Color Plate 3 on page xxxiv.

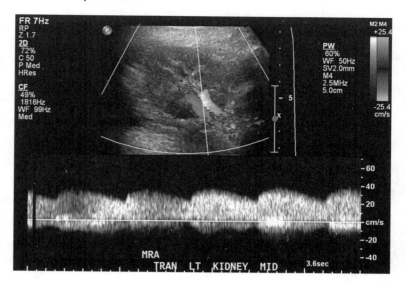

A tardus parvus *waveform demonstrates a rounded, more flattened appearance due to the slow rise or delayed, dampened upstroke to peak systolic velocity. This type of waveform is diagnostic of renal artery stenosis (RAS). A normal renal artery has a sharp, steep upstroke to peak systolic velocity and in pediatric patients will normally show an early peak systolic notch.* Early systole *occurs before peak systolic velocity and* late systole *would occur afterward.* Acceleration time *defines the time elapsed between the start of the systolic upstroke and the first or early peak.*

▶ de Bruyn R (ed): *Pediatric Ultrasound: How, Why and When*, 2nd edition (e-book). Philadelphia, Churchill Livingstone/Elsevier, 2010, pp 94–95.

▶ Goldberg B, McGahan J: *Atlas of Ultrasound Measurements*, 2nd edition. Philadelphia, Elsevier Mosby, 2006, pp 396–397.

▶ Rumack CM, Levine D (eds): *Diagnostic Ultrasound*, 5th edition. Philadelphia, Elsevier, 2018, pp 387, 1805.

▶ Siegel MJ (ed): *Pediatric Sonography*, 4th edition. Philadelphia, Lippincott Williams & Wilkins, 2011, pp 145–146, 432–433.

PART 10

Adrenal Glands

391. **C. Catecholamines.**

Catecholamines (dopamine, epinephrine, and norepinephrine) are a group of hormones produced by the adrenal medulla. Catecholamines affect blood pressure, the contraction of smooth muscle, and the body's ability to regulate metabolic rate and temperature. Of patients with neuroblastomas, 90% show increased catecholamines in serum or urine levels. Pheochromocytomas are a type of adrenal tumor also known to secrete catecholamines. Cortisol *is a steroid hormone produced by the adrenal cortex.* Adrenocorticotropic hormone (ACTH) *is secreted by the pituitary gland to stimulate the adrenal gland to produce androgens (estrogen and testosterone), glucocorticoids (cortisol and cortisone), and mineralocorticoids (aldosterone and corticosterone).* Creatinine (CR) *is a waste product of muscle activity and is normally removed from the blood by the kidneys.*

▶ Keough J: *Nursing Laboratory and Diagnostic Tests Demystified*, 2nd edition. New York, McGraw-Hill, 2017, pp 54–55.

▶ Siegel MJ (ed): *Pediatric Sonography*, 4th edition. Philadelphia, Lippincott Williams & Wilkins, 2011, pp 462, 465.

392. **B. Anteromedial.**

The left adrenal gland lies anteromedial to the upper pole of the left kidney. The left adrenal gland is positioned lateral to the aorta and left diaphragmatic crus. It is medial to the spleen but posterior to the splenic vessels and pancreatic tail. The right adrenal gland lies anterosuperior to the right kidney, lateral to the diaphragmatic crus, medial to the right lobe of the liver, and posterior to the inferior vena cava.

▶ de Bruyn R (ed): *Pediatric Ultrasound: How, Why and When*, 2nd edition (e-book). Philadelphia, Churchill Livingstone/Elsevier, 2010, p 115.

▶ Rumack CM, Levine D (eds): *Diagnostic Ultrasound*, 5th edition. Philadelphia, Elsevier, 2018, pp 1820–1822.

▶ Siegel MJ (ed): *Pediatric Sonography*, 4th edition. Philadelphia, Lippincott Williams & Wilkins, 2011, p 462.

393. A. Neuroblastoma.

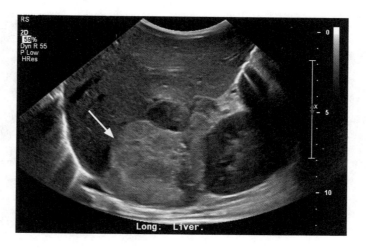

The solid malignant tumor that occurs the most in children extracranially is a neuroblastoma. Neuroblastomas comprise 8%–10% of all childhood cancers. The majority will occur between the ages of 1 and 5, with a median age of diagnosis at 22 months. This image demonstrates a mass (arrow) located between the liver and the right kidney. On ultrasound, neuroblastomas appear solid and lobulated, with varying echogenicity. Microcalcifications may be present. Wilms tumors, also known as nephroblastomas, occur in the same age range but are the most common renal malignancy. Hepatoblastomas occur in children under the age of 3 but are echogenic liver cancers with well-circumscribed smooth borders.

▶ Brodeur GM, Hogarty MG, Bagatell R, et al: Neuroblastoma. In Pizzo PA, Poplack DG (eds): *Principles and Practice of Pediatric Oncology*, 7th edition. Philadelphia, Wolters Kluwer, 2016, pp 771–796.

▶ Gurney JG, Davis S, Severson RK, et al: Trends in cancer incidence among children in the U.S. Cancer 78:532–541, 1996.

▶ Rumack CM, Levine D (eds): *Diagnostic Ultrasound*, 5th edition. Philadelphia, Elsevier, 2018, pp 1825–1826.

▶ Siegel MJ (ed): *Pediatric Sonography*, 4th edition. Philadelphia, Lippincott Williams & Wilkins, 2011, pp 413, 465, 470.

394. D. Absorbing calcium.

Cortisol, *a steroid hormone, is produced by the adrenal cortex. It is released in response to stress and low blood sugar levels. Roles of cortisol are to increase blood sugar levels, suppress the immune system, aid in regulation of blood pressure during and after stress, and assist with metabolism. The absorption of calcium is controlled by the parathyroid hormone (PTH).*

▶ Keough J: *Nursing Laboratory and Diagnostic Tests Demystified*, 2nd edition. New York, McGraw-Hill, 2017, pp 212, 221, 231.

395. **D. Hyperechoic.**

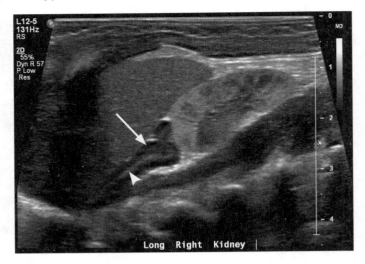

In newborns, the medulla *(arrowhead) of the adrenal gland typically appears thin and hyperechoic. The medulla is surrounded by a thicker, hypoechoic area known as the* cortex *(arrow). As the patient ages and the adrenal gland atrophies, there is less differentiation between the cortex and the medulla.*

▸ de Bruyn R (ed): *Pediatric Ultrasound: How, Why and When*, 2nd edition (e-book). Philadelphia, Churchill Livingstone/Elsevier, 2010, p 115.
▸ Rumack CM, Levine D (eds): *Diagnostic Ultrasound*, 5th edition. Philadelphia, Elsevier, 2018, pp 1820–1822.
▸ Siegel MJ (ed): *Pediatric Sonography*, 4th edition. Philadelphia, Lippincott Williams & Wilkins, 2011, pp 462–463.

396. **B. Inferior vena cava (IVC).**

The right adrenal gland *lies posterior and lateral to the* inferior vena cava (IVC). *The* quadratus lumborum *muscle lies posterior and lateral to the right adrenal gland. The* pancreatic tail *is on the left side of the body, making the right adrenal gland medial to it. Each adrenal gland lies within the perirenal fascia, superior to the kidneys. The right adrenal gland is anterosuperior to the upper pole of the right kidney. The left adrenal gland is anteromedial to the upper pole of the left kidney.*

▸ de Bruyn R (ed): *Pediatric Ultrasound: How, Why and When*, 2nd edition (e-book). Philadelphia, Churchill Livingstone/Elsevier, 2010, pp 114–115.
▸ Rumack CM, Levine D (eds): *Diagnostic Ultrasound*, 5th edition. Philadelphia, Elsevier, 2018, pp 1820–1822.
▸ Siegel MJ (ed): *Pediatric Sonography*, 4th edition. Philadelphia, Lippincott Williams & Wilkins, 2011, pp 462–463.

397. **A. Hypokalemia.**

The overproduction of the mineralocorticoid aldosterone can cause decreased levels of potassium, known as hypokalemia. Causes of aldosterone overproduction include aldosteronoma, adrenal hyperplasia, and adrenal cancer. Aldosterone release from the adrenal cortex is triggered by the hormone renin from the kidneys. Aldosterone controls the fluid and electrolyte balance in the body by facilitating the retention of fluid and sodium.

▶ Keough J: *Nursing Laboratory and Diagnostic Tests Demystified*, 2nd edition. New York, McGraw-Hill, 2017, pp 218–219.

▶ Siegel MJ (ed): *Pediatric Sonography*, 4th edition. Philadelphia, Lippincott Williams & Wilkins, 2011, p 473.

398. **C. Adrenal hemorrhage.**

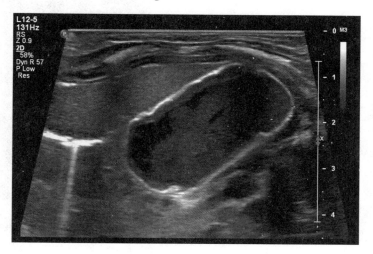

Although adrenal hemorrhage can occur antenatally, it is more commonly associated with birth trauma and perinatal anoxia, and it is seen more often in infants born of diabetic mothers. Adrenal hemorrhage can also be caused by shock, septicemia, and anticoagulation therapy. Hemorrhages can be unilateral or bilateral and have a higher incidence on the right side. On ultrasound, the adrenal gland is replaced by a suprarenal mass that appears round, oval (as seen in the center of this image), or triangular in shape. Acute hemorrhage may appear isoechoic or hyperechoic to the kidney and over time will become hypoechoic or cyst-like as the clot liquefies. These hemorrhages usually decrease in size within 1–2 weeks. Their sonographic appearance may be confused with neuroblastoma, but patient age and clinical history will help

differentiate between the two. Utilizing color Doppler can also aid in the differentation of tumor from hemorrhage. Adrenal hemorrhages typically occur in newborns, whereas neuroblastomas typically occur in children between the ages of 1 and 5.

▶ de Bruyn R (ed): *Pediatric Ultrasound: How, Why and When*, 2nd edition (e-book). Philadelphia, Churchill Livingstone/Elsevier, 2010, pp 117–118.

▶ Lee W, Cornstock CH, Jurcak-Zaleski S: Prenatal diagnosis of adrenal hemorrhage by ultrasonography. J Ultrasound Med 11:369–371, 1992.

▶ Siegel MJ (ed): *Pediatric Sonography*, 4th edition. Philadelphia, Lippincott Williams & Wilkins, 2011, pp 473–475.

399. **A. Congenital adrenal hyperplasia (CAH).**

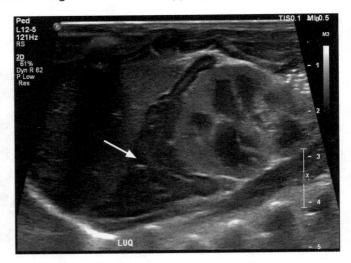

Congenital adrenal hyperplasia *(arrow)*, also known as CAH, is a recessively inherited condition causing adrenal insufficiency. Genetically female infants will present with ambiguous genitalia—a condition (to use older terminology) referred to as pseudohermaphroditism. In most patients, CAH is caused by a 21-hydroxylase (enzyme) deficiency. Adolescents showing a late onset of CAH have symptoms that include premature adrenarche, hirsutism, and/or menstrual irregularity. *Wolman disease affects lipid metabolism and is associated with enlarged adrenal glands. Adrenocortical tumors are not associated with ambiguous genitalia in infants.*

▶ de Bruyn R (ed): *Pediatric Ultrasound: How, Why and When*, 2nd edition (e-book). Philadelphia, Churchill Livingstone/Elsevier, 2010, pp 117, 219.

▶ Henwood MJ, Katz LEL: Disorders of the adrenal gland. In Moshang T (ed): *Pediatric Endocrinology: The Requisites in Pediatrics*. St. Louis, Elsevier Mosby, 2005, pp 193–213.

▶ Rumack CM, Levine D (eds): *Diagnostic Ultrasound*, 5th edition. Philadelphia, Elsevier, 2018, pp 1822–1824, 1900–1901.

▶ Siegel MJ (ed): *Pediatric Sonography*, 4th edition. Philadelphia, Lippincott Williams & Wilkins, 2011, p 476.

400. D. Aldosterone.

Renin, a hormone released by the kidneys, is responsible for signaling the adrenal glands to release aldosterone. Aldosterone is the main mineralocorticoid and a steroid hormone produced by the cortex of the adrenal gland. Aldosterone regulates blood pressure by balancing the water and sodium absorption in the body. Sodium *regulates osmotic pressure in the cells and fluids.* Adrenaline *is a hormone released from the adrenal glands to assist the body in a stressful "fight or flight" situation by preparing the heart and muscles for increased activity.* Creatinine phosphate *provides energy to skeletal muscles.* Creatinine (CR) *is filtered from the blood through the kidneys and excreted into urine. CR levels can be evaluated for dehydration and kidney function.*

▶ Keough J: *Nursing Laboratory and Diagnostic Tests Demystified,* 2nd edition. New York, McGraw-Hill, 2017, pp 54–55.

401. C. Venous lakes.

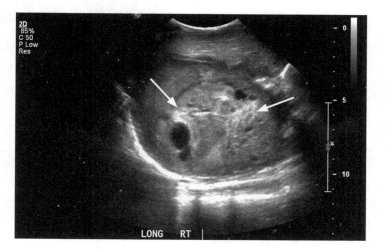

Patients with neuroblastoma usually present with multiple symptoms. Abdominal mass, unexplained weight loss, irritability, malaise, anemia, and bone pain are common. The majority of neuroblastomas occur between the ages of 1 and 5, with an average age of 22 months. Sonographically, neuroblastomas are solid with lobulated borders. They may have areas of hemorrhage or microcalcifications (arrows). Surrounding abdominal vasculature may be displaced by the mass. Lymphadenopathy may also be visualized. Venous lakes *are a common feature found within Wilms tumors and are* not *a typical finding with neuroblastoma.*

▶ de Bruyn R (ed): *Pediatric Ultrasound: How, Why and When,* 2nd edition (e-book). Philadelphia, Churchill Livingstone/Elsevier, 2010, pp 106, 108, 118, 119, 120–125.

- Rumack CM, Levine D (eds): *Diagnostic Ultrasound*, 5th edition. Philadelphia, Elsevier, 2018, pp 1818–1820.
- Siegel MJ (ed): *Pediatric Sonography*, 4th edition. Philadelphia, Lippincott Williams & Wilkins, 2011, pp 465–470.

402. **D. C-shaped.**

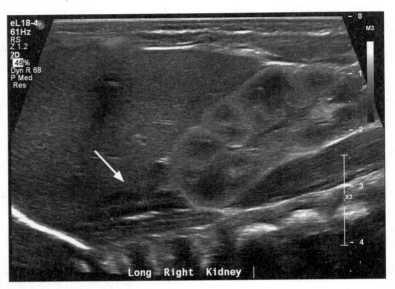

The adrenal glands (arrow) overlie the kidneys. They have been described as having a wishbone appearance, a V shape, or a Y shape. The adrenal glands form a cap over the upper pole of the kidneys.

- de Bruyn R (ed): *Pediatric Ultrasound: How, Why and When*, 2nd edition (e-book). Philadelphia, Churchill Livingstone/Elsevier, 2010, pp 115–116.
- Rumack CM, Levine D (eds): *Diagnostic Ultrasound*, 5th edition. Philadelphia, Elsevier, 2018, pp 1820–1822.
- Siegel MJ (ed): *Pediatric Sonography*, 4th edition. Philadelphia, Lippincott Williams & Wilkins, 2011, p 462.

403. **B. Medullaris.**

The cortex of the adrenal gland is separated into three zones:

(1) Glomerulosa: the outermost layer, which secretes aldosterone

(2) Zona fasciculata: the middle and widest layer, responsible for the synthesis of glucocorticoids (cortisol)

(3) Zona reticularis: the innermost layer, which produces androgens

The synthesis of the adrenal cortical steroid hormones requires the hypothalamic-pituitary-adrenal relationship to be functioning properly. By secreting a corticotropin-releasing hormone, the hypothalamus stimulates the pituitary to release adrenocorticotropic hormone (ACTH). ACTH then stimulates the layers of the adrenal gland to produce their respective hormones.

▶ Rumack CM, Levine D (eds): *Diagnostic Ultrasound*, 5th edition. Philadelphia, Elsevier, 2018, p 417.

▶ Siegel MJ (ed): *Pediatric Sonography*, 4th edition. Philadelphia, Lippincott Williams & Wilkins, 2011, p 462.

404. **C. Cortisol.**

Cortisol *is produced by the adrenal cortex and aids in elevating blood pressure or glucose when needed, as well as reducing the immune response. Catecholamines such as epinephrine (adrenaline), norepinephrine, and dopamine are synthesized and stored in the adrenal medulla. Epinephrine/adrenaline helps prepare the body for "fight or flight," the stress response, which affects the nervous system, cardiovascular system, metabolic rate, temperature, and smooth muscles. Norepinephrine is a vasoconstrictor. Dopamine is a vasodilator.*

▶ Keough J: *Nursing Laboratory and Diagnostic Tests Demystified*, 2nd edition. New York, McGraw-Hill, 2017, p 212.

405. **C. Lymphadenopathy.**

Both neuroblastomas and Wilms tumors are well-defined, solid masses, and both invade or displace adjacent vessels. However, there are a few characteristics that separate them on ultrasound. Lymphadenopathy is not usually a feature of the Wilms tumor, but it is a feature of neuroblastoma. Neuroblastomas are more commonly associated with anterior displacement of the aorta, inferior vena cava (IVC), and renal veins, as well as encasement of the IVC, superior mesenteric artery (SMA), and superior mesenteric vein (SMV). Wilms tumors more commonly invade the IVC and renal veins with tumor thrombus, making Doppler essential in the sonographic evaluation of these masses.

▶ de Bruyn R (ed): *Pediatric Ultrasound: How, Why and When*, 2nd edition (e-book). Philadelphia, Churchill Livingstone/Elsevier, 2010, pp 120–123, 125.

▶ Rumack CM, Levine D (eds): *Diagnostic Ultrasound*, 5th edition. Philadelphia, Elsevier, 2018, pp 1818–1820, 1825–1826.

▶ Siegel MJ (ed): *Pediatric Sonography*, 4th edition. Philadelphia, Lippincott Williams & Wilkins, 2011, pp 413–416, 465–470.

406. B. Adrenal hemorrhage.

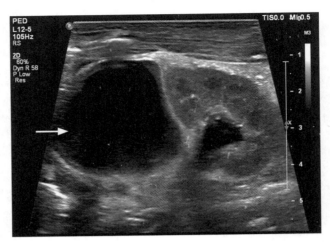

Adrenal hemorrhages *(arrow) are seen most often in term neonates as a result of birth trauma or perinatal anoxia. Clinical symptoms include a palpable abdominal mass, anemia, and jaundice. Adrenal hemorrhages are usually isoechoic or hyperechoic on ultrasound; then, as the clot liquefies in the later stages, they will appear hypoechoic or cyst-like, as seen in this image. Adrenal cysts can be pseudocysts secondary to a prior adrenal hemorrhage. Cysts can occur from infection, most commonly from echinococcal disease. Adrenal cysts are also associated with Beckwith-Wiedemann syndrome. Adrenocortical adenomas are cortisol-producing masses that appear homogeneous and are associated with Cushing syndrome. Adrenal hypertrophy can occur with renal agenesis. The ipsilateral adrenal gland will elongate and thicken.*

▸ de Bruyn R (ed): *Pediatric Ultrasound: How, Why and When*, 2nd edition (e-book). Philadelphia, Churchill Livingstone/Elsevier, 2010, pp 117–119.
▸ Rumack CM, Levine D (eds): *Diagnostic Ultrasound*, 5th edition. Philadelphia, Elsevier, 2018, pp 1822–1825.
▸ Siegel MJ (ed): *Pediatric Sonography*, 4th edition. Philadelphia, Lippincott Williams & Wilkins, 2011, pp 464, 473–475.

407. A. Wolman.

Both Wolman and Addison are diseases that calcify the adrenal glands. Wolman disease is recessively inherited, presenting in the first few weeks of life, and it is usually fatal. Addison disease is a long-term disease affecting all age groups and occurs due to adrenal insufficiency of hormone production. With Wolman disease, newborns present with clinical symptoms such as hepatosplenomegaly, vomiting, diarrhea, steatorrhea, and anemia. The adrenal cortex enlarges with fatty cells, then calcifies in areas of necrosis. Cushing and Beckwith-Wiedemann are syndromes, both associated with adrenocortical tumors and adenomas.

▶ de Bruyn R (ed): *Pediatric Ultrasound: How, Why and When*, 2nd edition (e-book). Philadelphia, Churchill Livingstone/Elsevier, 2010, p 127.
▶ Siegel MJ (ed): *Pediatric Sonography*, 4th edition. Philadelphia, Lippincott Williams & Wilkins, 2011, pp 472–473, 477.

408. B. Hypoechoic.

In newborns, the hyperechoic thinner adrenal medulla is surrounded by a hypoechoic thicker area known as the cortex. The adrenal cortex secretes aldosterone and synthesizes glucocorticoids (cortisol) and androgens. The medulla produces catecholamines (epinephrine, norepinephrine, and dopamine).

▶ de Bruyn R (ed): *Pediatric Ultrasound: How, Why and When*, 2nd edition (e-book). Philadelphia, Churchill Livingstone/Elsevier, 2010, pp 115–116.
▶ Rumack CM, Levine D (eds): *Diagnostic Ultrasound*, 5th edition. Philadelphia, Elsevier, 2018, pp 1820–1822.
▶ Siegel MJ (ed): *Pediatric Sonography*, 4th edition. Philadelphia, Lippincott Williams & Wilkins, 2011, pp 462–463.

409. C. Encasement of the inferior vena cava (IVC).

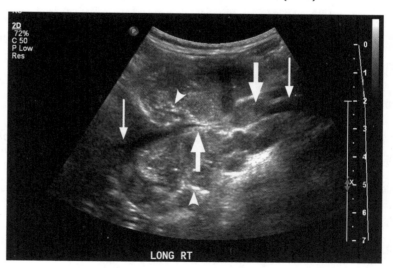

Unlike Wilms tumors, neuroblastomas do not infiltrate and invade abdominal vessels, but instead encase and displace them (thick arrows). This image shows the tumor surrounding and compressing the inferior vena cava (thin arrows). When an abdominal mass is found, Doppler examination is important

to evaluate for proper perfusion of surrounding vessels. Neuroblastomas are known to have lobulated borders and microcalcifications within the tumor, as seen in this image (arrowheads). Since most neuroblastomas are advanced at the time of discovery, a majority will already have evidence of metastatic disease.

▸ Brodeur GM, Hogarty MG, Bagatell R, et al: Neuroblastoma. In Pizzo PA, Poplack DG (eds): *Principles and Practice of Pediatric Oncology*, 7th edition. Philadelphia, Wolters Kluwer, 2016, pp 771–796.

▸ de Bruyn R (ed): *Pediatric Ultrasound: How, Why and When*, 2nd edition (e-book). Philadelphia, Churchill Livingstone/Elsevier, 2010, pp 106, 120–125.

▸ Rumack CM, Levine D (eds): *Diagnostic Ultrasound*, 5th edition. Philadelphia, Elsevier, 2018, pp 1825–1826.

▸ Siegel MJ (ed): *Pediatric Sonography*, 4th edition. Philadelphia, Lippincott Williams & Wilkins, 2011, pp 465–470.

410. **D. Cushing.**

Adrenocorticotropic hormone *(ACTH) is produced in the pituitary gland but regulates cortisol levels. An increase in ACTH production can result in an increase in cortisol production. In older children,* Cushing syndrome *is often due to an excess of ACTH production, resulting in excess cortisol. Cushing syndrome that occurs in children under the age of 10 is usually ACTH-independent and more likely caused by a cortical adenoma or adrenal carcinoma. Symptoms include generalized truncal obesity, hirsutism, hypertension, muscle wasting, and abdominal striae (stretch marks).* Beckwith-Wiedemann *is a syndrome consisting of macrosomia, macroglossia, hemihypertrophy, visceromegaly, and umbilical hernia or omphalocele.* Wolman *and* Addison *are diseases.* Wolman disease *is a lipid disorder and* Addison disease *is adrenal insufficiency.*

▸ Siegel MJ (ed): *Pediatric Sonography*, 4th edition. Philadelphia, Lippincott Williams & Wilkins, 2011, pp 156, 226, 472–473, 477.

411. **B. Pheochromocytoma.**

Usually benign, up to 70% of pheochromocytomas *originate from the adrenal medulla. Of all cases of pheochromcytoma, 95% occur in adults; it is uncommon in children. Clinical symptoms can include catecholamines present in the blood or urine, hypertension, paroxysmal headache, tachycardia, palpitations, diaphoresis, and palor. On ultrasound* pheochromocytomas appear as large, solid masses with sharp margins. Smaller tumors tend to appear more homogeneous than larger tumors. Areas of necrosis, hemorrhage, and calcifications can be seen in larger pheochromocytomas, making them more heterogeneous. In patients with multiple endocrine neoplasia (MEN) type 2 there is an increased incidence of pheochromocytomas. Adenomas are benign masses associated with the overproduction of cortisol. Neuroblastoma and ganglioneuroblastoma are both malignant tumors. Catecholamines may be found in the urine of patients with neuroblastoma, but hypertension and paroxysmal headaches are not typical clinical symptoms of a neuroblastoma.

▶ de Bruyn R (ed): *Pediatric Ultrasound: How, Why and When*, 2nd edition (e-book). Philadelphia, Churchill Livingstone/Elsevier, 2010, pp 94, 95–97, 127, 129.
▶ Rumack CM, Levine D (eds): *Diagnostic Ultrasound*, 5th edition. Philadelphia, Elsevier, 2018, pp 1826–1827.
▶ Siegel MJ (ed): *Pediatric Sonography*, 4th edition. Philadelphia, Lippincott Williams & Wilkins, 2011, pp 470–471.

412. **B. Complex.**

Although adrenal cysts are uncommon in children, their typical sonographic appearance is well circumscribed, round, and complex because adrenal cysts are usually secondary to hemorrhage or infection. Septations, fluid levels, and wall calcifications may be seen. True simple (i.e., purely cystic) adrenal cysts are rare. Adrenal cysts are associated with Beckwith-Wiedemann syndrome and can be large and multilocular.

▶ de Bruyn R (ed): *Pediatric Ultrasound: How, Why and When*, 2nd edition (e-book). Philadelphia, Churchill Livingstone/Elsevier, 2010, pp 118–119.
▶ Siegel MJ (ed): *Pediatric Sonography*, 4th edition. Philadelphia, Lippincott Williams & Wilkins, 2011, p 475.

413. **C. Adrenal abscess.**

Although rare, adrenal abscess may be a cause of a neonatal suprarenal mass. Escherichia coli (E. coli) is the most common cause, but Staphylococcus aureus (S. aureus) and Group B Streptococcus have also been present. Adrenal abscesses are usually unilateral, predominantly thick-walled, and hypoechoic. They may contain gravity-dependent echogenic *debris. Differential diagnosis may require clinical correlation and often a biopsy or aspiration. Fever and leukocytosis are not usually clinical findings with hemorrhage, adenoma, or adrenal hyperplasia.*

▸ de Bruyn R (ed): *Pediatric Ultrasound: How, Why and When*, 2nd edition (e-book). Philadelphia, Churchill Livingstone/Elsevier, 2010, p 118.

▸ Siegel MJ (ed): *Pediatric Sonography*, 4th edition. Philadelphia, Lippincott Williams & Wilkins, 2011, pp 470, 473–476.

414. A. 4S neuroblastoma.

A 4S neuroblastoma, also known as NBL-2, is a special form of neuroblastoma occurring in the neonatal period (birth to 1 year of age). 4S neuroblastomas usually take a more benign course and have a better prognosis than neuroblastomas occurring in older children. Infants will present with an enlarged liver that may become large enough to cause respiratory difficulty. On ultrasound, the liver is described as having a speckled, "pepper pot" heterogeneous texture. Dark purple or blue lesions may be present on the skin of patients with 4S neuroblastoma, which is commonly described as a "blueberry muffin" appearance. 4S neuroblastomas have even been discovered in the fetal period. Treatment is usually not required for 4S neuroblastoma, as tumor regression occurs in most cases. Pheochromocytomas, ganglioneuroblastomas, and adenomas are not associated with skin discolorations.

▸ Rumack CM, Levine D (eds): *Diagnostic Ultrasound*, 5th edition. Philadelphia, Elsevier, 2018, pp 1825–1826.

▸ Siegel MJ (ed): *Pediatric Sonography*, 4th edition. Philadelphia, Lippincott Williams & Wilkins, 2011, pp 465–467.

415. D. Heterogeneous.

Cortisol-producing adenomas are adrenocortical tumors. They are round or oval, homogeneous, and echogenic masses. They range in size from 2 to 5 cm in diameter. If color Doppler is applied, peripheral or central vascularity may be visible. The amount of adipose tissue within the tumor will affect the echogenicity of the adenoma.

▸ Rumack CM, Levine D (eds): *Diagnostic Ultrasound*, 5th edition. Philadelphia, Elsevier, 2018, p 1827.

▸ Siegel MJ (ed): *Pediatric Sonography*, 4th edition. Philadelphia, Lippincott Williams & Wilkins, 2011, pp 472–473.

416. **A. Ganglioneuroblastoma.**

Ganglioneuroblastoma *is a malignant neural crest tumor composed of primitive and differentiated ganglia cells and nerve tissue. Ganglioneuroblastomas most often occur at age 7 or later. When they are adrenal in location, a well-defined solid, homogeneous or heterogeneous mass is present, with 60% exhibiting fine, speckled calcifications. The most common location is the adrenal gland, but other locations include the mediastinum, retroperitoneum, head, neck, and pelvis. Clinical symptoms are similar to neuroblastoma.* Adrenal myelolipomas, adenomas, *and* hemangioendotheliomas *are confined to the region of the adrenal glands.*

▶ de Bruyn R (ed): *Pediatric Ultrasound: How, Why and When*, 2nd edition (e-book). Philadelphia, Churchill Livingstone/Elsevier, 2010, pp 119, 125.

▶ Siegel MJ (ed): *Pediatric Sonography*, 4th edition. Philadelphia, Lippincott Williams & Wilkins, 2011, p 470.

PART 11

GI Tract and Mesentery

417. D. Gastroesophageal junction.

The esophagus is a tube that connects the pharynx (superiorly) to the stomach (inferiorly). The esophagus can be divided into cervical, thoracic, and abdominal portions. Evaluation of the esophagus is limited in the cervical and thoracic portions because the lungs do not allow transmission of the ultrasound beam. The abdominal portion (gastroesophageal junction) can be more easily assessed with sonography. Gastroesophageal reflux and hiatal hernias are conditions that can be detected with ultrasound. To evaluate the abdominal portion of the esophagus, place the transducer midline using the subxiphoid area as a scanning window. In the sagittal plane, the esophagus appears as a hypoechoic tubular structure that connects to the stomach, and in a transverse plane it appears as a target sign. Because esophageal evaluation is limited with ultrasound, fluoroscopy and endoscopy are the modalities of choice.

▶ Rumack CM, Levine D (eds): *Diagnostic Ultrasound*, 5th edition. Philadelphia, Elsevier, 2018, p 1834.

▶ Siegel MJ (ed): *Pediatric Sonography*, 4th edition. Philadelphia, Lippincott Williams & Wilkins, 2011, p 339.

418. A. Transient small-bowel intussusception.

A transient small-bowel intussusception (SBI) is a common finding in young children. Symptoms include abdominal pain, vomiting, and diarrhea. Characteristics of a transient SBI are a peristalsing structure that resembles a target and resolves with continuous monitoring. The location and size of the intussusception can help differentiate a small-bowel intussusception from a large-bowel (ileocolic) intussusception. SBIs measure about 1.5 cm in the short axis while large-bowel intussusceptions usually exceed 3 cm. Transient SBIs are most commonly located in the left upper quadrant and paraumbilical region, whereas ileocolic intussusceptions are frequently in the right lower quadrant. Appendicitis also appears as a target sign structure, but it is usually located in the right lower quadrant and peristalsis is not seen. Children with Crohn disease *are typically diagnosed after 10 years of age, and the ultrasound appearance is an inflamed bowel wall measuring more than 3 mm.*

▸ de Bruyn R (ed): *Pediatric Ultrasound: How, Why and When*, 2nd edition (e-book). Philadelphia, Churchill Livingstone/Elsevier, 2010, pp 192–193.
▸ Rumack CM, Levine D (eds): *Diagnostic Ultrasound*, 5th edition. Philadelphia, Elsevier, 2018, pp 1845, 1853.
▸ Siegel MJ (ed): *Pediatric Sonography*, 4th edition. Philadelphia, Lippincott Williams & Wilkins, 2011, pp 358–360.

419. **C. Crohn disease.**

See Color Plate 4 on page xxxiv.

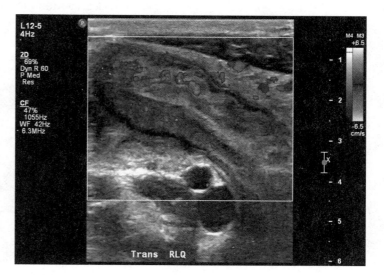

In children, Crohn disease *is the most common chronic inflammatory disease involving the small bowel. It is diagnosed most frequently in adolescents and young adults. Some of the clinical symptoms include chronic abdominal pain, nausea, vomiting, diarrhea (with or without blood), fever, anorexia, and weight loss. Children with Crohn disease can present with growth restriction, bone weakness, and delayed puberty. Crohn disease usually affects the terminal ileum (located in the right lower quadrant), but it can be seen in any portion of the gastrointestinal tract. Sonographic findings of Crohn disease include segmental bowel wall inflammation (with a wall thickness that measures greater than 3 mm), noncompressible bowel segments, decreased peristalsis, and hyperemia in the affected bowel. Symptoms of* appendicitis *include acute (not chronic) periumbilical or right lower quadrant pain, fever, and leukocytosis. Appendicitis is an acute process and is not associated with weight loss*

or anorexia. An ileus *appears as dilated fluid-filled bowel loops and is not associated with fever, anorexia, or chronic abdominal pain.* Intussusception *is uncommon in patients over 4 years of age.*

▶ Rumack CM, Levine D (eds): *Diagnostic Ultrasound*, 5th edition. Philadelphia, Elsevier, 2018, pp 1853, 1855–1857.

▶ Siegel MJ (ed): *Pediatric Sonography*, 4th edition. Philadelphia, Lippincott Williams & Wilkins, 2011, pp 359–360, 366.

420. **B. Ileum.**

See Color Plate 24 on page xliii.

A The Gastrointestinal Tract

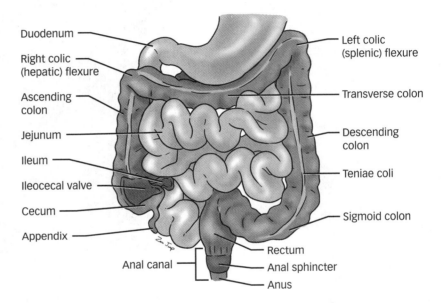

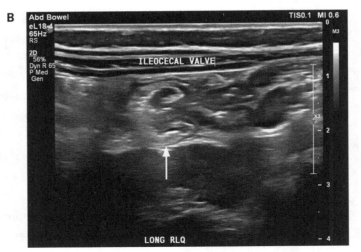

A *Diagram of the gastrointestinal tract. The most distal portion of the small bowel is the ileum, the last segment of the small bowel. The duodenum is the most proximal portion of the small intestine and connects the stomach with*

the jejunum. The jejunum, or middle portion, connects the duodenum and the ileum. The cecum is the first portion of the large bowel and connects the ileum to the colon. **B** The ileocecal valve (arrow) appears on ultrasound as an inverted 3-shaped structure and connects the ileum and the cecum.

▶ Healthline: Small intestine. Available at https://www.healthline.com/human-body-maps/small-intestine.

421. C. Ascending colon.

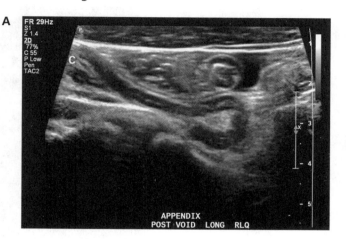

See Color Plate 25 on page xliii.

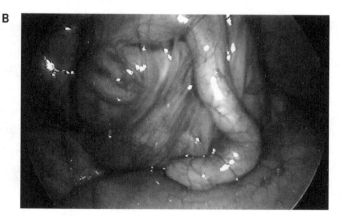

These two images show **A** an ultrasound image of the normal appendix, and **B** a correlative photo of gross anatomy of the normal appendix during surgery. For the ultrasound evaluation of the appendix, a helpful landmark is the ascending colon. By scanning laterally, following the ascending colon inferiorly, you can identify the cecum and terminal ileum. The appendix is attached to the cecum (C), about 1 to 2 cm below the ileocecal valve. The appendix is often seen coursing anterior to the iliac vessels (transverse view) and then posteriorly or retrocecally. A retrocecal appendix can be difficult to visualize, and the use of a low-frequency transducer may be helpful.

The lower pole of the right kidney, the psoas muscle, and the right lobe of the liver are not usually used as landmarks for evaluating the appendix.

▸ Rumack CM, Levine D (eds): *Diagnostic Ultrasound*, 5th edition. Philadelphia, Elsevier, 2018, p 1857.

▸ Siegel MJ (ed): *Pediatric Sonography*, 4th edition. Philadelphia, Lippincott Williams & Wilkins, 2011, pp 366–369.

422. **D. Hypertrophic pyloric stenosis.**

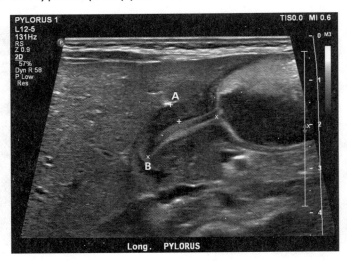

Hypertrophic pyloric stenosis is a progressive disorder in which the muscular portion of the pylorus is thickened, causing obstruction of the pyloric channel. Patients with pyloric stenosis normally present between the ages of 2 and 12 weeks old and commonly have a history of nonbilious projectile vomiting and weight loss. On ultrasound, the pyloric muscle appears thickened, measuring 3 mm or more (A), and the pyloric channel is elongated, measuring 17 mm or more (B). The stomach can be filled with fluid, but the fluid will not be seen passing through the pyloric channel. Midgut malrotation *and* gastroesophageal reflux *are differential diagnoses for pyloric stenosis, but this image shows only the abnormal pylorus and not the gastroesophageal junction or an inversion of the mesenteric vessels seen in malrotation. In duodenal atresia the "double bubble" sign can be seen with a fluid-filled proximal duodenum and stomach.*

▸ de Bruyn R (ed): *Pediatric Ultrasound: How, Why and When*, 2nd edition (e-book). Philadelphia, Churchill Livingstone/Elsevier, 2010, pp 184–185.

▸ Rumack CM, Levine D (eds): *Diagnostic Ultrasound*, 5th edition. Philadelphia, Elsevier, 2018, pp 1835, 1841.

▸ Siegel MJ (ed): *Pediatric Sonography*, 4th edition. Philadelphia, Lippincott Williams & Wilkins, 2011, pp 342–344.

423. **B. Hirschsprung disease.**

Hirschsprung disease is a congenital condition in which there is lack of peristaltic bowel movement. In Hirschsprung disease, some of the nerves that produce peristalsis in the bowel are absent, and this leads to intestinal obstruction due to the lack of peristalsis. *Henoch-Schönlein purpura* is a condition that involves the small vessels in multiple body systems and is associated with intramural intestinal hemorrhage and intussusception in children. *Cystic fibrosis* and *Kawasaki disease* are conditions that are associated with small-bowel wall thickness and not with large-bowel obstruction.

▸ MedlinePlus: Hirschsprung disease. Available at https://medlineplus.gov/ency/article/001140.htm.

▸ Rumack CM, Levine D (eds): *Diagnostic Ultrasound*, 5th edition. Philadelphia, Elsevier, 2018, p 1853.

▸ Siegel MJ (ed): *Pediatric Sonography*, 4th edition. Philadelphia, Lippincott Williams & Wilkins, 2011, pp 362–363.

424. **A. Mucosal layer.**

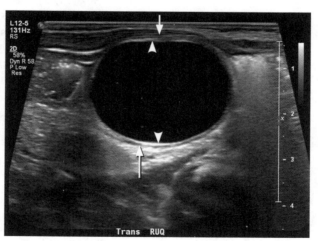

Gastrointestinal duplication cysts are unilocular cystic structures that are typically lined with intestinal mucosa and can arise from any portion of the gastrointestinal tract. Duplication cysts have well-defined borders and commonly a double-layered wall, as seen in this image. The most internal echogenic layer represents the mucosa (arrowheads), and the hypoechoic outer layer represents the muscular wall (arrows). These sonographic findings help to differentiate duplication cysts from other cystic abnormalities in the abdomen. Serosal layers of duplication cysts are not visible on ultrasound, and they do not contain a fibrinous layer.

▸ de Bruyn R (ed): *Pediatric Ultrasound: How, Why and When*, 2nd edition (e-book). Philadelphia, Churchill Livingstone/Elsevier, 2010, pp 191–192.

▸ Rumack CM, Levine D (eds): *Diagnostic Ultrasound*, 5th edition. Philadelphia, Elsevier, 2018, p 1860.

▸ Siegel MJ (ed): *Pediatric Sonography*, 4th edition. Philadelphia, Lippincott Williams & Wilkins, 2011, p 346.

425. **C. Distend the stomach with clear fluid.**

The stomach can be evaluated with ultrasound when its lumen is filled with fluid. This helps with the visualization of the stomach layers and allows evaluation for reflux and gastric emptying. The antrum and pyloric area can be evaluated using the liver as a scanning window, and usually the patient is scanned in a supine or right lateral decubitus position, not in a left lateral decubitus or erect position. Maintaining the patient fasting for 3 hours will increase the amount of air within the stomach, making the ultrasound examination difficult. Although ultrasound can be helpful in the evaluation of some stomach pathologies, radiography of the upper GI tract is the imaging modality of choice.

▸ de Bruyn R (ed): *Pediatric Ultrasound: How, Why and When*, 2nd edition (e-book). Philadelphia, Churchill Livingstone/Elsevier, 2010, pp 183–184.

▸ Rumack CM, Levine D (eds): *Diagnostic Ultrasound*, 5th edition. Philadelphia, Elsevier, 2018, pp 1834–1835.

▸ Siegel MJ (ed): *Pediatric Sonography*, 4th edition. Philadelphia, Lippincott Williams & Wilkins, 2011, p 341.

426. **C. Meckel diverticulum.**

Meckel diverticulum is a congenital abnormality that occurs when there is a remnant of the omphalomesenteric duct (the duct that connects the ileum to the yolk sac during early gestation). Meckel diverticulum is fairly common and asymptomatic. When a Meckel diverticulum is complicated, it usually presents in early childhood. It is important to know that a Meckel diverticulum arises from the ileum and not from the cecum, because cases of inflamed Meckel diverticulum can be mistaken for appendicitis (which arises from the cecum). Crohn disease is an abnormality in which the intestinal walls are inflamed, causing a narrowing of the bowel lumen. An inflamed portion of the bowel will not appear blind-ending. In many patients Meckel diverticulum is the leading cause of intussusception.

▸ Rumack CM, Levine D (eds): *Diagnostic Ultrasound*, 5th edition. Philadelphia, Elsevier, 2018, p 1860.

▸ Siegel MJ (ed): *Pediatric Sonography*, 4th edition. Philadelphia, Lippincott Williams & Wilkins, 2011, p 373.

427. A. Midgut volvulus.

See Color Plate 26 on page xliv.

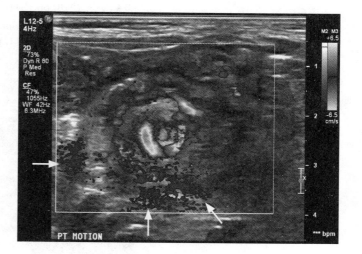

A midgut volvulus *refers to a duodenal obstruction caused by intestinal malrotation. Malrotation has varying rotational abnormalities but may cause the superior mesenteric artery (SMA) and vein (SMV) to be reversed in relative position. Normally the SMV is anterior and to the right of the SMA. With malrotation, the SMV is positioned to the left of the SMA. Intestinal malrotation is the cause of volvulus. If midgut volvulus occurs, the proximal duodenum (C-loop) becomes fluid-filled and dilated. The mesentery and SMV twist clockwise around the SMA, resulting in the "whirpool sign" seen in this image. This finding is characteristic of midgut volvulus. (Note also the noise, appearing as blue speckles [arrows]—a common finding when using color Doppler on infants and children due to crying and motion.) Patients with a volvulus usually present within the first month of life with bilious vomiting, and contrast fluoroscopy of the upper gastrointestinal (UGI) tract is best for the diagnosis. Treatment is a Ladd procedure.*

Duodenal atresia, *in which there is a complete closure of the duodenum, is the most common cause of congenital duodenal obstruction.* An annular pancreas *is a congenital abnormality in which pancreatic tissue completely encircles the second portion of the duodenum. This abnormality may also cause a duodenal obstruction.* Pyloric stenosis *refers to the hypertrophy of the muscular layers of the pylorus, which causes an obstruction of the gastric outlet.*

▸ Chandler C, Fisher KL: Sonographic findings of midgut malrotation with volvulus: a case of upper intestinal obstruction in a neonate. J Diagn Med Sonogr 34:385–389, 2018.

▸ de Bruyn R (ed): *Pediatric Ultrasound: How, Why and When*, 2nd edition (e-book). Philadelphia, Churchill Livingstone/Elsevier, 2010, pp 189–190.

▶ Rumack CM, Levine D (eds): *Diagnostic Ultrasound*, 5th edition. Philadelphia, Elsevier, 2018, pp 1841–1842.

▶ Siegel MJ (ed): *Pediatric Sonography*, 4th edition. Philadelphia, Lippincott Williams & Wilkins, 2011, pp 350, 352–355.

428. B. Intussusception.

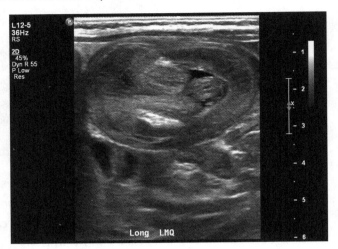

This image demonstrates the classic doughnut, target, or "cinnamon bun" sign associated with intussusception. The word intussusception *is from the Latin* intus, *meaning "within," plus* suscipere, *meaning "to take up." An intussusception occurs when a proximal portion of the intestine telescopes or invaginates into a more distal segment of bowel. Intussusceptions are the most common type of acute bowel obstruction in children between the ages of 3 months and 4 years, occurring more often in males. The cause of an intussusception is most frequently idiopathic. Clinical symptoms of intussusception are intermittent abdominal pain, vomiting, and bloody, "currant jelly" stools. The ultrasound appearance of an intussusception is of a complex mass with a targeted appearance in an axial plane, which represents the multiple mucosal and muscular layers of bowel. An echogenic center may be seen (as appears in this image), indicating the presence of mesentery within the intussusception. In a longitudinal plane, the mass can appear similar to a kidney, known as the "pseudokidney" sign. The most common location of intussusception is ileocecal, and this is seen in the right abdomen, measuring approximately 3 cm.* Appendicitis *and* Crohn disease *are more common in older children, and an* ileus *will demonstrate a fluid-filled, nonperistalsing segment of bowel.*

▶ de Bruyn R (ed): *Pediatric Ultrasound: How, Why and When*, 2nd edition (e-book). Philadelphia, Churchill Livingstone/Elsevier, 2010, pp 192–193.

▶ Kang P, Peters A: Intussusception. Appl Radiol 43:42–43, 2014.

▶ Poole E, Penny SM: Pediatric intussusception: the cinnamon bun sign. J Diagn Med Sonogr 34:275–280, 2018.

▶ Rumack CM, Levine D (eds): *Diagnostic Ultrasound*, 5th edition. Philadelphia, Elsevier, 2018, pp 1843–1847.

▶ Siegel MJ (ed): *Pediatric Sonography*, 4th edition. Philadelphia, Lippincott Williams & Wilkins, 2011, pp 355–358.

429. D. Appendicitis.

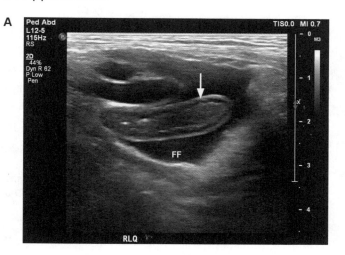

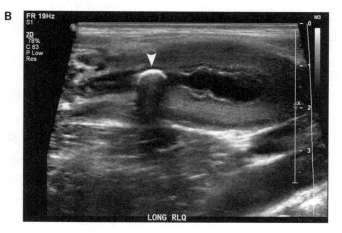

Appendicitis *is an acute process in which the appendix becomes inflamed and is the most common cause of emergency surgery in older children and adolescents. The typical clinical presentation for appendicitis is acute periumbilical pain that migrates and focuses in the right lower quadrant, accompanied by fever and leukocytosis (elevated white blood cell count or WBC). Although in some cases the clinical diagnosis of appendicitis can easily be made, ultrasound has become a very helpful tool for a more precise diagnosis.*

A *Appendicitis is visualized on ultrasound as a noncompressible appendix (arrow) measuring 6 mm or more, with increased echogenicity of the periappendiceal fat and hyperemia. Some* *free fluid (FF) may be seen adjacent to the appendix or in the cul-de-sac.* **B** *An appendicolith—a calcified deposit in the appendix (arrowhead)—may be present as well.* The ability to correlate the focal point of tenderness with the location of the appendix gives ultrasound a diagnostic advantage over other imaging modalities. Intussusception is an uncommon finding in older children. Crohn disease and ileus are pathologies that clinically can resemble acute appendicitis (ileus usually presents with diffuse abdominal pain instead), but the imaging findings are different from those seen in these images (A and B) of the inflamed appendix. Sonographically, with Crohn disease the bowel wall appears thickened and hyperemic, but the intestinal portion affected is not blind-ending like the appendix. The ultrasound appearance of an ileus is a distended fluid-filled bowel loop with no peristalsis.

▶ de Bruyn R (ed): *Pediatric Ultrasound: How, Why and When*, 2nd edition (e-book). Philadelphia, Churchill Livingstone/Elsevier, 2010, pp 193–194, 196.

▶ Rumack CM, Levine D (eds): *Diagnostic Ultrasound*, 5th edition. Philadelphia, Elsevier, 2018, pp 1855–1857.

▶ Siegel MJ (ed): *Pediatric Sonography*, 4th edition. Philadelphia, Lippincott Williams & Wilkins, 2011, pp 366–372.

430. D. Lesser omentum.

The *omentum is a peritoneal fold that supports the stomach and the intestines. The omentum is divided into the lesser and greater omentum. The* lesser omentum *extends along the lesser curvature of the stomach and connects it to the liver. The* greater omentum *connects the greater curvature of the stomach to the colon and splenic hilum. The* mesentery *is a peritoneal fold that that connects the intestines to the posterior abdominal wall.* Morison's pouch *is a space in the abdomen that separates the liver and the right kidney.*

▶ de Bruyn R (ed): *Pediatric Ultrasound: How, Why and When*, 2nd edition (e-book). Philadelphia, Churchill Livingstone/Elsevier, 2010, pp 202–204.

431. C. Trichobezoar.

A bezoar *is an undigested mass in the gastrointestinal tract that can cause an obstruction. Among the different types of bezoars, the most common in older children are trichobezoars. Trichobezoars are composed of ingested hair. On ultrasound a trichobezoar appears as a curved linear structure in the* anterior portion of the mass that obscures the posterior apect of the same mass due to lack of penetration through the hair. (It is important to recognize that the mass is mostly obscured, except for the anterior curved linear portion.) Trichobezoars can lead to Rapunzel syndrome, which refers to the extension of the hair into the duodenum. Phytobezoars are bezoars composed of indigestible plant material (fiber, skins, and seeds). Lactobezoars are composed of milk and mucus and are the most common type of bezoars in infants, frequently caused by the incorrect preparation of powdered milk and water. A foreign-body bezoar is a bezoar that may be composed of any type of foreign material, such as paper or plastic.

▸ Rumack CM, Levine D (eds): *Diagnostic Ultrasound*, 5th edition. Philadelphia, Elsevier, 2018, p 1840.

▸ Siegel MJ (ed): *Pediatric Sonography*, 4th edition. Philadelphia, Lippincott Williams & Wilkins, 2011, p 348.

432. **A. Duodenal diverticulum.**

Double bubble sign is the term used to describe the presence of a dilated proximal duodenum and the stomach, as classically seen with duodenal atresia. Duodenal atresia, severe duodenal stenosis, and duodenal diaphragms *(webs) are congenital conditions in which there is a severe obstruction of the duodenum that leads to distention of its proximal portion. Although the diagnosis of these conditions is usually made with plain radiography, when there is an associated tracheoesophageal fistula (due to esophageal atresia) there is no air within the stomach, making the diagnosis difficult with radiography and easier with ultrasound. These types of conditions are usually seen prenatally, and if not detected prenatally may result in the patient presenting with bilious vomiting within the first 24 hours of life. A* duodenal diverticulum *is a pouch that arises from the duodenum and is* not *associated with a double bubble sign.*

▸ Rumack CM, Levine D (eds): *Diagnostic Ultrasound*, 5th edition. Philadelphia, Elsevier, 2018, pp 1841–1842.

▸ Siegel MJ (ed): *Pediatric Sonography*, 4th edition. Philadelphia, Lippincott Williams & Wilkins, 2011, p 350.

433. B. Muscle thickness of 3 mm.

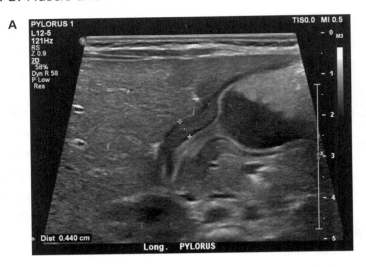

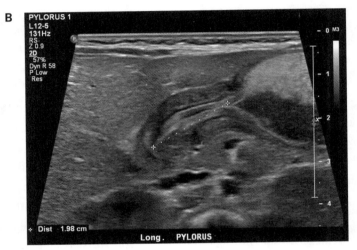

A *A measurement of the pyloric muscle thickness that is equal to or greater than 3 mm is considered abnormal.* ***B*** *An abnormal length for the pyloric channel is considered to be equal to or greater than 17 mm. These measurements are characteristic for the diagnosis of a hypertrophic pylorus. Premature infants with hypertrophic pyloric stenosis may present with a muscle wall thickness equal to or greater than 2.5 mm and a pyloric channel length equal to or greater than 14 mm. Standard measurements for premature infants with pyloric stenosis or even for patients presenting before 2 weeks of age are not established, but it is known that the size of the hypertrophic pylorus in these patients is relatively smaller.*

▶ Rumack CM, Levine D (eds): *Diagnostic Ultrasound*, 5th edition. Philadelphia, Elsevier, 2018, pp 1835–1836.

▶ Siegel MJ (ed): *Pediatric Sonography*, 4th edition. Philadelphia, Lippincott Williams & Wilkins, 2011, p 342.

434. A. Ileus.

There are two types of bowel obstruction, mechanical and functional. A mechanical obstruction *occurs when the intestinal tract is physically blocked by something. A* functional obstruction *occurs when there is failure of the intestine to move normally, causing an obstruction.* Intussusception, volvulus, *and* duplication cysts *are pathologies that can block the intestinal tract, leading to a mechanical obstruction. Usually with a mechanical obstruction, the bowel appears fluid-filled and there is hyperperistalsis proximal to the obstruction. An* ileus *is a functional obstruction caused by lack of peristalsis of the intestine. It can be the result of nervous system disorders or infections.*

▶ Healthline: Intestinal obstructions. Available at https://www.healthline.com/health/intestinal-obstructions#causes.

▶ Rumack CM, Levine D (eds): *Diagnostic Ultrasound*, 5th edition. Philadelphia, Elsevier, 2018, pp 1842–1843.

▶ Siegel MJ (ed): *Pediatric Sonography*, 4th edition. Philadelphia, Lippincott Williams & Wilkins, 2011, pp 358–359.

435. A. Non-Hodgkin lymphoma.

Lymphomas *are the most common malignant tumor affecting the small intestine in childhood.* Non-Hodgkin lymphomas *are more common than* Hodgkin lymphomas *in the small bowel. The ileum is the most frequent site of involvement.* Leiomyosarcomas *and* adenocarcinomas *are rare malignancies of the small bowel in childhood.*

▶ Rumack CM, Levine D (eds): *Diagnostic Ultrasound*, 5th edition. Philadelphia, Elsevier, 2018, p 1862.

▶ Siegel MJ (ed): *Pediatric Sonography*, 4th edition. Philadelphia, Lippincott Williams & Wilkins, 2011, p 365.

436. C. Air reduction enema.

The most common treatment for intussusception is an air reduction enema *under fluoroscopic guidance. This procedure is performed by inserting a catheter into the patient's rectum and pushing air in to reduce the intussusception.* Hydrostatic reductions *are similar but use water-soluble contrast instead of air. This method is not performed as much but provides an option in which fluoroscopy is not needed because ultrasound can help with guidance.* Surgical reductions *of intussusceptions are rarely used in younger children and are performed only when there is a leading cause of the intussusception or when the patient is older than the normal age range for idiopathic* intussusception (6 months to 4 years). Surgical resection of the intussuscepted bowel is performed only when the intestine is necrotic and not viable or if air reduction is unsuccessful. To assess for bowel perfusion in an intussusception, color Doppler flow may be useful to demonstrate patent vascularity.

▶ de Bruyn R (ed): *Pediatric Ultrasound: How, Why and When*, 2nd edition (e-book). Philadelphia, Churchill Livingstone/Elsevier, 2010, pp 193, 195.
▶ Rumack CM, Levine D (eds): *Diagnostic Ultrasound*, 5th edition. Philadelphia, Elsevier, 2018, pp 1844–1845.
▶ Siegel MJ (ed): *Pediatric Sonography*, 4th edition. Philadelphia, Lippincott Williams & Wilkins, 2011, p 356.

437. C. Midgut malrotation.

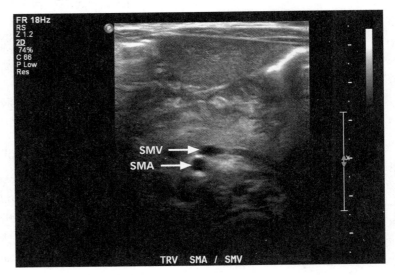

Infants presenting with bilious vomiting should be assessed for midgut malrotation. The presence of bilious vomiting and the inversion of the superior mesenteric vein (SMV) and superior mesenteric artery (SMA) on ultrasound, accompanied by a dilated proximal duodenum, are characteristics of midgut malrotation with volvulus. In normal anatomy, the SMV lies to the right of the SMA. When there is an abnormal rotation of the bowel during fetal development (malrotation), the position of the mesenteric vessels can be reversed. The presence of a fluid-filled proximal duodenum and bilious vomiting should rule out pyloric stenosis because in this condition passage of fluid through the pyloric channel to the duodenum is minimal or absent. An annular pancreas—a ring-shaped pancreas that encircles the duodenum—is an uncommon cause of congenital duodenal obstruction. This can lead to duodenal obstruction and a distended proximal duodenum can be seen, but the position of the mesenteric vessels should not be affected. A duodenal web is a condition in which there is a membrane (diaphragm)

within the duodenum at the level of the ampulla of Vater, which causes duodenal obstruction. With a duodenal web the mesenteric vessels also remain in their normal positions.

▶ Bell DJ, Gaillard F, et al: Intestinal malrotation. Available from Radiopaedia at https://radiopaedia.org/articles/intestinal-malrotation.

▶ Chandler C, Fisher KL: Sonographic findings of midgut malrotation with volvulus: a case of upper intestinal obstruction in a neonate. J Diagn Med Sonogr 34:385–389, 2018.

▶ de Bruyn R (ed): *Pediatric Ultrasound: How, Why and When*, 2nd edition (e-book). Philadelphia, Churchill Livingstone/Elsevier, 2010, p 189.

▶ Dufour D, Delaet MH, Dassonville M, et al: Midgut malrotation, the reliability of sonographic diagnosis. Pediatr Radiol 22:21–23. Available at https://www.ncbi.nlm.nih.gov/pubmed/1594305

▶ Rumack CM, Levine D (eds): *Diagnostic Ultrasound*, 5th edition. Philadelphia, Elsevier, 2018, pp 1841–1842.

▶ Siegel MJ (ed): *Pediatric Sonography*, 4th edition. Philadelphia, Lippincott Williams & Wilkins, 2011, pp 350, 352–355.

438. **B. Mesentery.**

The *mesentery is a double peritoneal fold that connects the intestines to the posterior abdominal wall. The mesentery keeps the intestines in place, but at the same time it also allows movement. Evaluating the mesentery can be helpful during inflammatory processes such as Crohn disease and appendicitis, because it becomes echogenic and therefore easy to differentiate from other structures. The* visceral peritoneum *is the layer of peritoneum that covers the abdominal organs. The* greater *and* lesser omenta *are peritoneal folds that extend along the stomach, connecting it to the liver, colon, and spleen.*

▶ de Bruyn R (ed): *Pediatric Ultrasound: How, Why and When*, 2nd edition (e-book). Philadelphia, Churchill Livingstone/Elsevier, 2010, p 201.

439. **D. Pyloric stenosis.**

Nonbilious projectile vomiting and a positive "olive sign" are classic symptoms characteristic of hypertrophic pyloric stenosis. *Infants with pyloric stenosis usually present between the ages of 2 and 12 weeks of life. The* olive sign *is a palpable olive-shaped mass in the epigastrium or slightly to its right that represents the enlarged pylorus. Patients with* volvulus, duodenal atresia, *and* midgut malrotation *usually present with bilious vomiting and not with a positive olive sign.*

▶ de Bruyn R (ed): *Pediatric Ultrasound: How, Why and When*, 2nd edition (e-book). Philadelphia, Churchill Livingstone/Elsevier, 2010, pp 184–185.

▶ Rumack CM, Levine D (eds): *Diagnostic Ultrasound*, 5th edition. Philadelphia, Elsevier, 2018, p 1835.

▶ Siegel MJ (ed): *Pediatric Sonography*, 4th edition. Philadelphia, Lippincott Williams & Wilkins, 2011, p 342.

440. A. Imperforate anus.

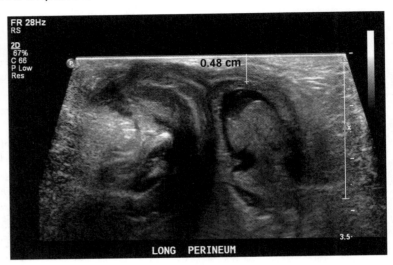

An imperforate anus *or* anorectal malformation *is a congenital abnormality in which the posterior opening of the digestive tract (the anus) is not formed. This condition can be classified depending on the distance of the rectal termination (rectal pouch) from the perineum. Ultrasound has proved to be an accurate tool for defining the type of anorectal malformation by allowing measurement of the distance between the rectal pouch and the perineum, as seen in this image. The most accurate measurements are obtained in the longitudinal plane with a high-frequency transducer using a transperineal approach. A rectal pouch–to–perineal distance of 10 mm ± 4 mm suggests a low lesion, and a distance greater than 15 mm indicates a diagnosis of a high lesion. Identifying the nature of the lesion (low or high in relation to the levator ani muscle) is important because it determines patient management and treatment. Note in this image that the rectal pouch–to–perineal distance is 0.48 cm (4.8 mm), considered low.* Rectovaginal fistulas *and* cloacae *are abnormalities that can be seen in conjunction with an imperforate anus, but the measurement of the distance between the rectal pouch and the perineum is specific only for the management of imperforate anus and is not useful for other conditions.*

▸ Rumack CM, Levine D (eds): *Diagnostic Ultrasound*, 5th edition. Philadelphia, Elsevier, 2018, pp 1847–1848.
▸ Siegel MJ (ed): *Pediatric Sonography*, 4th edition. Philadelphia, Lippincott Williams & Wilkins, 2011, pp 373–374.

441. **B. Pylorospasm.**

Pylorospasm *or* antral dyskinesia *occurs when the pylorus becomes mildly thickened and inconsistently elongated. The sonographic appearance of a pylorospasm is similar to that of hypertrophic pyloric stenosis, but usually the muscle wall thickness does not reach 3 mm. Also, during prolonged observation the pylorus can be seen relaxing, becoming normal in appearance, and fluid can be seen passing through the channel to the duodenum. With* hypertrophic pyloric stenosis *resolution of the abnormal pyloric appearance will not occur and the muscle wall thickness is 3 mm or greater. With* gastroesophageal reflux *the size and appearance of the pylorus are not affected. An* anisotropic effect *is an artifact caused by the perpendicular insonation of sound waves between the ultrasound beam and the muscle fibers. This artifact causes the muscular wall to appear echogenic instead of hypoechoic.*

▶ Rumack CM, Levine D (eds): *Diagnostic Ultrasound*, 5th edition. Philadelphia, Elsevier, 2018, pp 1836–1838.

▶ Siegel MJ (ed): *Pediatric Sonography*, 4th edition. Philadelphia, Lippincott Williams & Wilkins, 2011, pp 344–355.

442. **C. Necrotizing enterocolitis.**

Necrotizing enterocolitis *(NEC) is a disease in which bowel ischemia occurs, leading to necrosis of the intestine. NEC most commonly affects premature infants and can be caused by infection of the bowel or hypoxia. Ultrasound findings of NEC include portal vein gas, distended loops of intestine, and thick-walled bowel.* Intussusception *is extremely uncommon in premature infants.* Pseudomembranous colitis *is an infectious disease that occurs in patients on antibiotic therapy.* Imperforate anus *is a congenital malformation and the gestational age at birth plays no role in its occurrence.*

▶ MedlinePlus: Necrotizing enterocolitis. Available at https://medlineplus.gov/ency/article/001148.htm.

▶ Rumack CM, Levine D (eds): *Diagnostic Ultrasound*, 5th edition. Philadelphia, Elsevier, 2018, p 1854.

▶ Siegel MJ (ed): *Pediatric Sonography*, 4th edition. Philadelphia, Lippincott Williams & Wilkins, 2011, pp 373–375.

443. D. 350 cm/sec or greater.

See Color Plate 27 on page xliv.

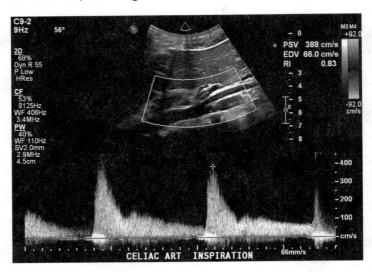

Median arcuate ligament syndrome *(MALS) is also known as celiac artery compression syndrome or Dunbar syndrome. It occurs when the median arcuate ligament is positioned too low, causing compression of the celiac artery during expiration. Patients with MALS typically present with chronic abdominal pain in the supine position, especially postrandially, and weight loss. The sonographic evaluation consists of obtaining Doppler velocities of the celiac artery during expiration and measuring the peak systolic velocity (PSV). In the pediatric population, a PSV greater than 350 cm/sec during expiration and an aorta/celiac artery deflection angle (DA) over 50 degrees are the standard. The finding in this image of a PSV of 388 cm/sec indicates compression of the celiac artery, helping to confirm the diagnosis of MALS. Although ultrasound is an effective alternative method of evaluating for MALS, computed tomography (CT) and angiography are the main modalities used for the diagnosis.*

▶ Gruber H, Loizides A, Peer S, et al: Ultrasound of the median arcuate ligament syndrome: a new approach to diagnosis. Med Ultrason 14:5–9, 2012. Available at https://www.ncbi.nlm.nih.gov/m/pubmed/22396932/.

▶ Kallus SJ, Singhal P, Palese C, et al: Median arcuate ligament syndrome: an unusual cause of chronic abdominal pain. Available at https://pdfs.semanticscholar.org/0a2b/c88f078b90b641f447d3d0a0c58dfb2235fe.pdf.

444. D. Polyp.

Polyps are the most common primary benign tumor of the bowel in childhood, occurring in the small bowel and colon. Polyps appear as hyperechoic masses that can be seen protruding into fluid-filled bowel. Although ultrasound is not the modality of choice for diagnosis of intestinal polyps, ultrasound *is useful in identifying polyps as a cause of intussusception.* Duplication cysts *are congenital anomalies more commonly seen in the small intestine rather than in the colon and are less common than polyps.* Lymphomas *are malignant lesions, not benign.* Hemangiomas *rarely involve the intestines.*

▶ Rumack CM, Levine D (eds): *Diagnostic Ultrasound*, 5th edition. Philadelphia, Elsevier, 2018, p 1862.

▶ Siegel MJ (ed): *Pediatric Sonography*, 4th edition. Philadelphia, Lippincott Williams & Wilkins, 2011, pp 365, 377–378.

445. **C. Ileus.**

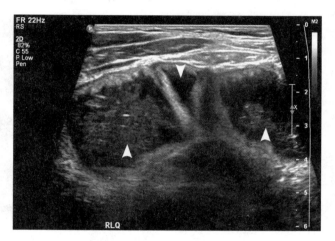

Ileus *is a nonmechanical obstruction, or functional disorder, of the bowel in which normal peristalsis is absent. On ultrasound, fluid-filled bowel loops (arrowheads) can be seen without peristalsis. Some common causes of ileus include abdominal or pelvic surgery, appendicitis, Hirschsprung disease, and abuse of narcotics (which is typically not seen in the pediatric population and may just be a side effect of the constipation associated with narcotics).* Appendicitis *normally presents with periumbilical or right lower quadrant pain (not diffuse). Although appendicitis may cause ileus, the diagnosis cannot be made based only on the previously mentioned findings.* Crohn disease *may cause diffuse abdominal pain, but the ultrasound appearance is of a thickened intestinal wall with decreased intraluminal space.* Intussusception *is a type of mechanical obstruction and a target sign is typically present with ultrasound.*

▶ MedlinePlus: Intestinal obstruction. Available at https://medlineplus.gov/ency/article/000260.htm.

▶ Siegel MJ (ed): *Pediatric Sonography*, 4th edition. Philadelphia, Lippincott Williams & Wilkins, 2011, pp 358–359.

446. **A. Ascending colon.**

See Color Plate 24, "The Gastrointestinal Tract," on page xliii.

The cecum is the connection between the ileum (small intestine) and the ascending colon (large intestine). The large intestine (or colon) is located laterally in the abdomen. On the right side, the ascending colon travels upward to meet the hepatic flexure, which connects it to the transverse colon. The transverse colon is in the epigastric region and is slightly curved downward in the middle. The transverse colon connects to the left-sided splenic flexure. From the splenic flexure, traveling downward and laterally, the descending colon leads to the sigmoid colon inferiorly and then to the rectum. Evaluation of the colon with ultrasound is limited due to the presence of gas and fecal material. The large intestine shows minimal peristalsis and a multilayered wall that can be seen with ultrasound.

▶ Rumack CM, Levine D (eds): *Diagnostic Ultrasound*, 5th edition. Philadelphia, Elsevier, 2018, p 1847.

▶ Siegel MJ (ed): *Pediatric Sonography*, 4th edition. Philadelphia, Lippincott Williams & Wilkins, 2011, p 373.

PART 12

Pediatric Hip

447. B. Coronal.

See Color Plate 28 on page xlv.

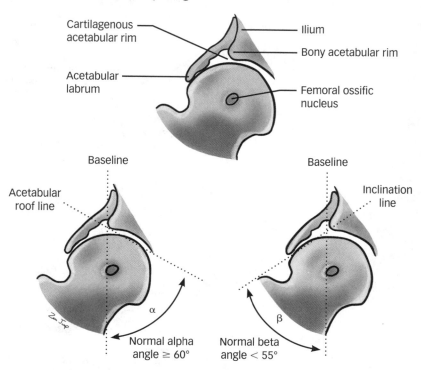

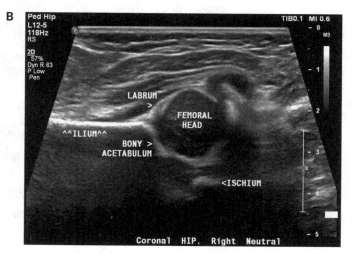

A Diagram of pediatric hip angle measurements. For evaluation for developmental dysplasia of the hip (DDH), a diagnostic hip ultrasound should include both coronal and transverse planes. However, it is the coronal plane (image **B**) where measurements are taken. The mid portion of the bony acetabulum, straight iliac line, a portion of the labrum, and the ischium should be evident in the coronal image. To perform measurements, angles are drawn and femoral head coverage is calculated. Dynamic imaging can be performed to include measurements in neutral, flexed, and stressed positions. Alpha angles (α) are measured from the lateral or posterolateral aspect of the hip in the coronal plane. If beta angles (β) are obtained, they are also measured in the coronal plane.

▶ de Bruyn R (ed): *Pediatric Ultrasound: How, Why and When*, 2nd edition (e-book). Philadelphia, Churchill Livingstone/Elsevier, 2010, p 322.
▶ Rumack CM, Levine D (eds): *Diagnostic Ultrasound*, 5th edition. Philadelphia, Elsevier, 2018, pp 1923–1924.
▶ Siegel MJ (ed): *Pediatric Sonography*, 4th edition. Philadelphia, Lippincott Williams & Wilkins, 2011, pp 607–611.

448. **D. Hip effusion.**

Hip effusion *is associated with hip pain or a limp in children under the age of 10. Children may present with hip pain, not wanting to place weight on that hip, and/or fever. Hip effusion can be caused by infection, transient synovitis, or septic arthritis. Hip dysplasia and dislocation are most commonly diagnosed in infancy. A hip sprain may cause pain and limping but would not be accompanied by a fever.*

▶ de Bruyn R (ed): *Pediatric Ultrasound: How, Why and When*, 2nd edition (e-book). Philadelphia, Churchill Livingstone/Elsevier, 2010, pp 331–337.
▶ Rumack CM, Levine D (eds): *Diagnostic Ultrasound*, 5th edition. Philadelphia, Elsevier, 2018, pp 1930–1931.
▶ Siegel MJ (ed): *Pediatric Sonography*, 4th edition. Philadelphia, Lippincott Williams & Wilkins, 2011, pp 624–626.

449. **C. Pavlik.**

Known as the Pavlik *harness, this method for treating developmental dysplasia of the hip (DDH) was originally introduced by Arnold Pavlik, a Czech orthopedic surgeon in the 1950s. Currently, the Pavlik harness is the standard of care. A Pavlik harness holds the legs in a flexed abduction so the femoral heads are positioned within the acetabula. If an infant is wearing a harness, the order may specify a static hip ultrasound with the harness left in place so the infant can be evaluated as the hip joint is being treated; during such a study you should also check the placement of the femoral head within the joint. No flexion or stress maneuvers are done with the harness on.* Ortolani *and* Barlow *are the names of* the maneuvers a pediatrician routinely performs on infants to screen for hip dysplasia. Reinhard Graf is the Austrian orthopedic surgeon who developed the initial measurement technique for the diagnosis of developmental hip dysplasia.

▶ de Bruyn R (ed): *Pediatric Ultrasound: How, Why and When*, 2nd edition (e-book). Philadelphia, Churchill Livingstone/Elsevier, 2010, pp 321, 326–327, 329–330.

▶ Knipe H, Gaillard F, et al: Ultrasound classification of developmental dysplasia of the hip. Available from Radiopaedia at http://radiopaedia.org/articles/ultrasound-classification-of-developmental-dysplasia-of-the-hip-1.

▶ Rumack CM, Levine D (eds): *Diagnostic Ultrasound*, 5th edition. Philadelphia, Elsevier, 2018, p 1929.

▶ Siegel MJ (ed): *Pediatric Sonography*, 4th edition. Philadelphia, Lippincott Williams & Wilkins, 2011, pp 607, 611.

450. **C. Hypoechoic.**

Ossified structures of the hip joint such as the ilium and the acetabulum are echogenic and highly reflective. The fibrocartilaginous labrum will appear hyperechoic in comparison to the less dense femoral head cartilage. Ossification of the femoral head develops between 2 and 8 months and will appear as a focal, echogenic ossification within the center of the femoral head.

▶ Rumack CM, Levine D (eds): *Diagnostic Ultrasound*, 5th edition. Philadelphia, Elsevier, 2018, p 1923.

▶ Siegel MJ (ed): *Pediatric Sonography*, 4th edition. Philadelphia, Lippincott Williams & Wilkins, 2011, p 605.

451. **D. 60 degrees.**

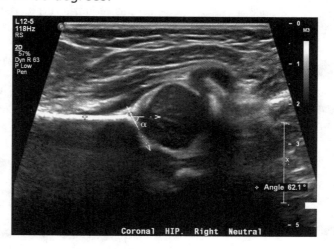

See also the answer to question 455.

Refer to the image here as well as the image and diagram with answer 447 above: Described as the "bony roof" angle, the alpha angle (α), is the angle between the straight edge of the iliac bone and the bony acetabular roof. The first line is drawn on the horizontal, echogenic iliac bone. The second line is drawn along the acetabulum. The angle between these two lines is the alpha angle. The normal alpha angle is 60 degrees or greater.

▶ de Bruyn R (ed): *Pediatric Ultrasound: How, Why and When*, 2nd edition (e-book). Philadelphia, Churchill Livingstone/Elsevier, 2010, pp 322–326.
▶ Rumack CM, Levine D (eds): *Diagnostic Ultrasound*, 5th edition. Philadelphia, Elsevier, 2018, pp 1924–1926.
▶ Siegel MJ (ed): *Pediatric Sonography*, 4th edition. Philadelphia, Lippincott Williams & Wilkins, 2011, p 611.

452. C. 50%.

Femoral head coverage by the acetabulum is figured by the acetabular depth in relation to the diameter of the femoral head. Coverage should be at least 50%. Coverage less than 50% indicates laxity, subluxation, or dislocation.

▶ de Bruyn R (ed): *Pediatric Ultrasound: How, Why and When*, 2nd edition (e-book). Philadelphia, Churchill Livingstone/Elsevier, 2010, pp 327–329.
▶ Rumack CM, Levine D (eds): *Diagnostic Ultrasound*, 5th edition. Philadelphia, Elsevier, 2018, p 1924.

453. A. Pulvinar.

Pulvinar *is intra-articular fibrofatty tissue. On ultrasound, it will appear echogenic but not as bright as bone. Pulvinar thickness can fill the acetabulum and be an obstacle to the reduction of a dysplastic hip. The* hip capsule *is a space within the synovial linings of the joint. The* triradiate cartilage, *like pulvinar, lies medial to the femoral head but is hypoechoic on ultrasound. The* iliopsoas tendon *is located anterior to the femoral head and acetabulum.*

▶ Rumack CM, Levine D (eds): *Diagnostic Ultrasound*, 5th edition. Philadelphia, Elsevier, 2018, p 1924.
▶ Siegel MJ (ed): *Pediatric Sonography*, 4th edition. Philadelphia, Lippincott Williams & Wilkins, 2011, pp 611, 625–626.

454. D. Hip effusion.

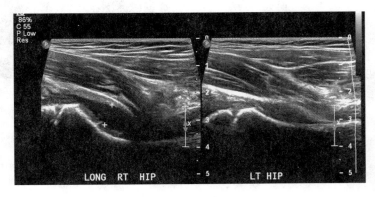

To evaluate for hip effusion, have the patient lie supine with the leg in a neutral, extended position. An anterior approach is used in the sagittal plane, with the transducer parallel to the long axis of the femoral neck. A high-frequency linear transducer is optimal. Anterior to the echogenic femur (seen posterior to the calipers), the joint capsule is composed of anterior and posterior layers. Fluid within the joint appears anechoic and the capsule is distended and bulges anteriorly. The hip joint capsule normally extends inferiorly and anterior to the femoral neck. To measure the width of the capsule, place the calipers anterior to the femoral neck. Comparison views should always be obtained for capsule symmetry. When comparing the symptomatic (painful) and asymptomatic sides, be sure the leg positions are the same bilaterally. The child might be splinting the painful hip and holding it in the least painful posture (usually slightly abducted). Be sure to match that position on the comparison normal side. When you compare the affected limb to the unaffected limb, the difference in capsule width should not exceed 2 mm. Hip dysplasia *is the abnormal positioning of the femur within the acetabulum. A* popliteal cyst *occurs posterior to the knee.* Cellulitis *is soft tissue inflammation and does not usually involve a fluid collection.*

▶ de Bruyn R (ed): *Pediatric Ultrasound: How, Why and When*, 2nd edition (e-book). Philadelphia, Churchill Livingstone/Elsevier, 2010, pp 332–334.
▶ Rumack CM, Levine D (eds): *Diagnostic Ultrasound*, 5th edition. Philadelphia, Elsevier, 2018, pp 1930–1931.
▶ Siegel MJ (ed): *Pediatric Sonography*, 4th edition. Philadelphia, Lippincott Williams & Wilkins, 2011, pp 624–626.

455. **B. Graf.**

See also the answer to question 447.

Reinhard Graf, an Austrian orthopedic surgeon, created the European approach to measuring the hip joint for dysplasia. His technique is based on the coronal scan plane and angles placed along the cartilage component of the roof of the acetabulum. The scale developed by Graf describes the depth and shape of the acetabulum. In the Graf classification of DDH, a type I hip is normal, with an alpha angle greater than or equal to 60 degrees. A type II DDH hip has an alpha angle ranging from 43 to 59 degrees. If the alpha angle is less than 43 degrees it is classified as type III DDH. Type IV DDH is diagnosed in the presence of gross dislocation and the inability to measure an alpha angle (which will be less than

43 degrees). The primary American method of classifying DDH, developed by H. Ted Harcke, MD, is more of a dynamic approach and shows the relationship of the femoral head movement within the acetabulum.

▶ Clarke NMP, Harcke HT, McHugh P, et al: Real-time ultrasound as an aid to the diagnosis and treatment of congenital hip dislocation and dysplasia in the infant. J Bone Joint Surg 67-B:406–412, 1985.
▶ de Bruyn R (ed): *Pediatric Ultrasound: How, Why and When*, 2nd edition (e-book). Philadelphia, Churchill Livingstone/Elsevier, 2010, pp 320, 322–327, 329.
▶ Rumack CM, Levine D (eds): *Diagnostic Ultrasound*, 5th edition. Philadelphia, Elsevier, 2018, p 1922.
▶ Siegel MJ (ed): *Pediatric Sonography*, 4th edition. Philadelphia, Lippincott Williams & Wilkins, 2011, p 611.
▶ Stephenson SR, Dahiya N: *Musculoskeletal Sonography Review: A Q&A Review for the ARDMS Musculoskeletal Sonographer Exam*. Pasadena, CA, Davies Publishing, 2019, pp 247–248.

456. **A. Ortolani.**

The Ortolani maneuver *assesses whether a dislocated hip can be reduced. By flexing the hip 90 degrees and abducting it into a frog-leg position, the pediatrician should be able to move the femoral head back into the acetabulum. If the femoral head passes over the posterior labrum and back into place, a palpable "clunk" can be felt. The* Barlow maneuver *is the opposite of the Ortolani maneuver; the hip is adducted rather than abducted. Graf developed the initial measurement technique used to diagnose hip dysplasia. Pavlik developed the harness treatment for hip dysplasia.*

▶ de Bruyn R (ed): *Pediatric Ultrasound: How, Why and When*, 2nd edition (e-book). Philadelphia, Churchill Livingstone/Elsevier, 2010, pp 321, 326.
▶ Rumack CM, Levine D (eds): *Diagnostic Ultrasound*, 5th edition. Philadelphia, Elsevier, 2018, p 1923.
▶ Siegel MJ (ed): *Pediatric Sonography*, 4th edition. Philadelphia, Lippincott Williams & Wilkins, 2011, p 607.

457. **A. Flexed and abducted.**

Normal development of the hip requires contact between the femoral head and the acetabulum. Flexing and abducting the leg 90 degrees will move the femoral head back within the hip socket by external rotation. This will push the femoral head toward the triradiate cartilage and stimulate development of the acetabulum. Pediatric orthopedic surgeons are aware of the critical safe zone (how much flexion, how much abduction) for setting the straps on the Pavlik harness to safely promote reduction while avoiding the complication of ischemic necrosis. The acetabulum–to–femoral head coverage usually becomes normal within 6–8 weeks of harness treatment. If an infant is wearing a harness during a follow-up ultrasound examination, the ordering physician usually prefers the exam to be done while the patient remains in the harness.

▶ de Bruyn R (ed): *Pediatric Ultrasound: How, Why and When*, 2nd edition (e-book). Philadelphia, Churchill Livingstone/Elsevier, 2010, p 330.
▶ Rosendahl K, Toma P: Ultrasound in the diagnosis of developmental dysplasia of the hip in newborns—the European approach: a review of methods, accuracy and clinical validity. Eur Radiol 17:1960–1967, 2007.
▶ Rumack CM, Levine D (eds): *Diagnostic Ultrasound*, 5th edition. Philadelphia, Elsevier, 2018, p 1929.
▶ Siegel MJ (ed): *Pediatric Sonography*, 4th edition. Philadelphia, Lippincott Williams & Wilkins, 2011, pp 607, 611–612.

458. **D. Anterior.**

Sonography is the method of choice to evaluate for hip effusion because with this condition hip radiographs can often appear normal. The patient is placed supine, allowing the legs to fall into a neutral position. Scanning is performed from an anterior approach. The transducer is positioned in a sagittal plane, parallel to the long axis of the femoral neck. If present, a fluid-filled joint capsule will have a bulging, convex anterior margin. Alternate transverse views can be obtained and may be helpful in identifying fluid in areas not seen in the sagittal plane.

▶ de Bruyn R (ed): *Pediatric Ultrasound: How, Why and When*, 2nd edition (e-book). Philadelphia, Churchill Livingstone/Elsevier, 2010, pp 332–334.
▶ Rumack CM, Levine D (eds): *Diagnostic Ultrasound*, 5th edition. Philadelphia, Elsevier, 2018, pp 1930–1931.
▶ Siegel MJ (ed): *Pediatric Sonography*, 4th edition. Philadelphia, Lippincott Williams & Wilkins, 2011, pp 625–626.

459. **A. Family history.**

Normal hip development requires early detection and treatment of developmental dysplasia of the hip (DDH). If DDH goes undiscovered, it can result in problems when children are at the walking age. There are many congenital risk factors for DDH—family history, female infant, firstborn child, breech presentation in utero, hip clunk on exam, skull deformities, foot deformities, congenital torticollis, and oligohydramnios in utero. Polyhydramnios in utero is not a risk factor due to the increased range of motion made possible by excess amniotic fluid, versus the decreased range of motion with oligohydramnios.

▶ de Bruyn R (ed): *Pediatric Ultrasound: How, Why and When*, 2nd edition (e-book). Philadelphia, Churchill Livingstone/Elsevier, 2010, p 321.

▶ Rumack CM, Levine D (eds): *Diagnostic Ultrasound*, 5th edition. Philadelphia, Elsevier, 2018, pp 1921–1922.

▶ Siegel MJ (ed): *Pediatric Sonography*, 4th edition. Philadelphia, Lippincott Williams & Wilkins, 2011, p 607.

460. **B. Barlow.**

The Barlow maneuver *is performed by a physician in an attempt to dislocate the femoral head. The doctor flexes the hip, adducts the leg, and then pushes the knee posteriorly and superiorly. This movement allows the leg to function like a piston. If the femoral head moves over the posterior labrum as it exits the socket, a palpable vibration or "clunk" can be felt. A clunk or click is an indication of instability and posterior displacement.*

▶ de Bruyn R (ed): *Pediatric Ultrasound: How, Why and When*, 2nd edition (e-book). Philadelphia, Churchill Livingstone/Elsevier, 2010, pp 320–321, 326–327.

▶ Rumack CM, Levine D (eds): *Diagnostic Ultrasound*, 5th edition. Philadelphia, Elsevier, 2018, p 1923.

▶ Siegel MJ (ed): *Pediatric Sonography*, 4th edition. Philadelphia, Lippincott Williams & Wilkins, 2011, p 607.

461. **C. Swelling.**

Occurring in the metaphyses of long bones, osteomyelitis *is most often a blood-borne infection, commonly from Staphylococcus aureus. Two of the common sites are the distal femur and the proximal tibia. Patients with sickle cell anemia are at a higher risk of developing osteomyelitis. Clinically the signs and symptoms of osteomyelitis and transient synovitis are similar, but symptoms for osteomyelitis tend to be more severe and include a hot, erythematous swollen area. The earliest ultrasound sign of osteomyelitis is subperiosteal effusion. When scanning, it is important to observe the overlying tissue layers and muscle for evidence of myositis, which can accompany the infection. Hot, erythematous swelling can also be seen in cases of cellulitis.*

▶ de Bruyn R (ed): *Pediatric Ultrasound: How, Why and When*, 2nd edition (e-book). Philadelphia, Churchill Livingstone/Elsevier, 2010, pp 330–331.

▶ Rumack CM, Levine D (eds): *Diagnostic Ultrasound*, 5th edition. Philadelphia, Elsevier, 2018, pp 1930, 1936–1938.

▶ Siegel MJ (ed): *Pediatric Sonography*, 4th edition. Philadelphia, Lippincott Williams & Wilkins, 2011, p 625.

462. **D. 12 weeks of age.**

Late diagnosis of developmental hip dysplasia (DDH) can result in a poor patient outcome because the tissues are more flexible and respond to treatment better at an earlier age. "Late" diagnosis refers to a diagnosis that is made after 12 weeks of age. The examination is best performed in the newborn period, when an infant is 4–6 weeks old. By this age most immature hips have stabilized. After early infancy, muscles tighten and may not respond as well to treatment. The ossification of the femoral head between ages 2 and 8 months can make hip sonography more difficult by impairing visualization of the acetabulum. After 6 months of age, it is usually easier to obtain a radiograph.

▸ de Bruyn R (ed): *Pediatric Ultrasound: How, Why and When*, 2nd edition (e-book). Philadelphia, Churchill Livingstone/Elsevier, 2010, p 320.
▸ Rumack CM, Levine D (eds): *Diagnostic Ultrasound*, 5th edition. Philadelphia, Elsevier, 2018, p 1921.
▸ Siegel MJ (ed): *Pediatric Sonography*, 4th edition. Philadelphia, Lippincott Williams & Wilkins, 2011, p 607.

463. A. Dislocated.

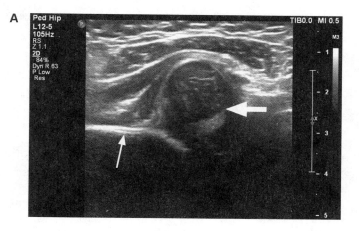

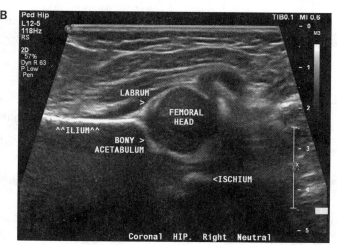

In image **A**, the femoral head (thick arrow) is displaced out of the acetabulum both superiorly and laterally and up above the ilium (thin arrow). There is no coverage or contact with the acetabulum, which appears to have a more flattened angle.

A normal femoral head (image **B**) would be seated in the center of the acetabulum and have contact. Subluxation describes the partial dislocation of the femur within the acetabulum.

▶ de Bruyn R (ed): *Pediatric Ultrasound: How, Why and When*, 2nd edition (e-book). Philadelphia, Churchill Livingstone/Elsevier, 2010, pp 322–327.
▶ Rumack CM, Levine D (eds): *Diagnostic Ultrasound*, 5th edition. Philadelphia, Elsevier, 2018, p 1924.
▶ Siegel MJ (ed): *Pediatric Sonography*, 4th edition. Philadelphia, Lippincott Williams & Wilkins, 2011, pp 610–611.

464. **C. Children.**

Transient synovitis *(aseptic effusion), also called* irritable hip, *is most common in children 5–10 years old. Symptoms are hip pain during movement, limping, decreased range of motion (particularly external rotation), and joint effusion. Patients may be afebrile or have a low-grade fever, and transient synovitis often follows a viral infection. If the patient develops pain during rest, an elevated white blood cell count, and a high fever, septic arthritis should be considered. Treatment for transient synovitis is usually rest, and the symptoms tend to resolve within 48 hours. Arthrocentesis or joint aspiration may be necessary if there are signs of sepsis, a more critical condition requiring urgent attention. Hip pain with or without reduced range of motion could be secondary to psoas pathology (abscess), a reason to scan "north" along the psoas.*

▶ de Bruyn R (ed): *Pediatric Ultrasound: How, Why and When*, 2nd edition (e-book). Philadelphia, Churchill Livingstone/Elsevier, 2010, pp 331–334.
▶ Rumack CM, Levine D (eds): *Diagnostic Ultrasound*, 5th edition. Philadelphia, Elsevier, 2018, pp 1930–1931.
▶ Siegel MJ (ed): *Pediatric Sonography*, 4th edition. Philadelphia, Lippincott Williams & Wilkins, 2011, pp 624–625.

465. **D. Iliopsoas.**

The iliopsoas *muscle lies directly anterior and superficial to the hip joint capsule. It is formed by the blending of the* iliacus *and the* psoas major *muscles. The iliopsoas inserts on the lesser trochanter of the femur, crossing over the hip joint. The psoas major arises from the lumbar vertebrae and the iliacus arises from the ilium of the pelvis. The muscles of the iliopsoas work together for hip flexion and rotation. The* rectus femoris *muscle is one of the four quadriceps muscles of the thigh and lies anterior to the iliopsoas.*

▶ de Bruyn R (ed): *Pediatric Ultrasound: How, Why and When*, 2nd edition (e-book). Philadelphia, Churchill Livingstone/Elsevier, 2010, p 333.

- Lazo DL: *Fundamentals of Sectional Anatomy: An Imaging Approach*, 2nd edition. Stamford, CT, Cengage Learning, 2015, p 222.
- Rumack CM, Levine D (eds): *Diagnostic Ultrasound*, 5th edition. Philadelphia, Elsevier, 2018, p 1930.
- Siegel MJ (ed): *Pediatric Sonography*, 4th edition. Philadelphia, Lippincott Williams & Wilkins, 2011, pp 499, 626, 635.

466. **D. 12 MHz.**

The way to optimize the resolution of musculoskeletal sonography is with the use of a linear or curvilinear array, high-frequency transducer. High-frequency transducers ranging from 12.0 to 18.0 MHz provide the best resolution in the near field. Dual or split-screen formats are used to show side-by-side comparison views or images with and without color Doppler. A large area or wider field of view can be obtained with panoramic or extended-field-of-view software. Due to the extended reconstruction time, 3D sonography is not a practical routine method.

- de Bruyn R (ed): *Pediatric Ultrasound: How, Why and When*, 2nd edition (e-book). Philadelphia, Churchill Livingstone/Elsevier, 2010, pp 319–320, 322.
- Rumack CM, Levine D (eds): *Diagnostic Ultrasound*, 5th edition. Philadelphia, Elsevier, 2018, p 1922.
- Siegel MJ (ed): *Pediatric Sonography*, 4th edition. Philadelphia, Lippincott Williams & Wilkins, 2011, p 602.

467. **C. Avascular necrosis (AVN).**

Avascular necrosis (AVN) is a condition in which the circulation to the femoral head is partially or completely blocked, causing death to the bone. The blood vessels can also be damaged or the circulation interrupted during a forceful repositioning of the hip. On ultrasound, diminished flow may be seen within the femoral epiphysis. The temporary blood loss can damage the growth plate of the proximal femur. Ischemic necrosis is a severe complication, leading to likely premature arthritis and eventual hip replacement. The incidence of AVN is low (1%), but the risk increases if overvigorous attempts at reduction with severe abduction stress the blood supply to the femoral head.

- de Bruyn R (ed): *Pediatric Ultrasound: How, Why and When*, 2nd edition (e-book). Philadelphia, Churchill Livingstone/Elsevier, 2010, pp 326, 334.
- Rumack CM, Levine D (eds): *Diagnostic Ultrasound*, 5th edition. Philadelphia, Elsevier, 2018, p 1930.
- Siegel MJ (ed): *Pediatric Sonography*, 4th edition. Philadelphia, Lippincott Williams & Wilkins, 2011, p 613.

468. B. Labrum.

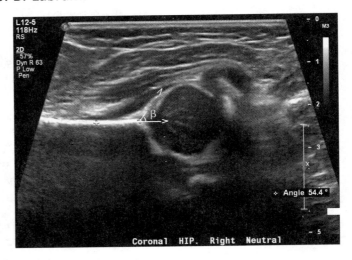

See also the answers to questions 447, 455, and 472.

The beta angle (β) is the angle between the ilium (baseline) and the labrum (fibrocartilaginous roof line); it is also known as the cartilaginous roof angle. In the normal hip the beta angle measures less than 55 degrees. Beta angles increase with the lateral and superior luxation of the femoral head, which pushes the cartilaginous acetabular roof and labrum with it. Although the beta angle is not universally used, a smaller alpha angle (α) accompanied by a larger beta angle is more likely representative of hip dysplasia. Beta angles are important for distinguishing among the more dysplastic hip types.

▶ de Bruyn R (ed): *Pediatric Ultrasound: How, Why and When*, 2nd edition (e-book). Philadelphia, Churchill Livingstone/Elsevier, 2010, p 324.
▶ Rumack CM, Levine D (eds): *Diagnostic Ultrasound*, 5th edition. Philadelphia, Elsevier, 2018, p 1924.
▶ Siegel MJ (ed): *Pediatric Sonography*, 4th edition. Philadelphia, Lippincott Williams & Wilkins, 2011, p 611.

469. B. Type II.

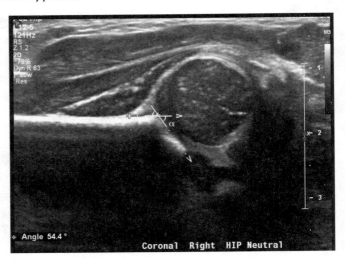

See also the answers to questions 447, 455, and 472.

The alpha angle (α) is formed by the straight edge of the iliac bone and a line drawn on the bony acetabular roof. Alpha angles detect the depth of the acetabulum and indicate the presence and severity of hip dysplasia according to the Graf classification. The normal alpha angle is equal to or greater than 60 degrees (type I). Alpha angles of 43–59 degrees (type II) are considered shallow and stable enough not to require treatment, only follow-up sonography; the notation at the bottom left of the image indicates that the angle in this case is 54.4 degrees and hence it is type II. If the alpha angle is less than 43 degrees, the acetabulum is underdeveloped enough to allow for dislocation (type III). In type IV, the femoral head is dislocated.

▶ de Bruyn R (ed): *Pediatric Ultrasound: How, Why and When*, 2nd edition (e-book). Philadelphia, Churchill Livingstone/Elsevier, 2010, pp 322–326.

▶ Knipe H, Gaillard F, et al: Ultrasound classification of developmental dysplasia of the hip. Radiopaedia. Available from Radiopaedia at http://radiopaedia.org/articles/ultrasound-classification-of-developmental-dysplasia-of-the-hip-1.

▶ Rumack CM, Levine D (eds): *Diagnostic Ultrasound*, 5th edition. Philadelphia, Elsevier, 2018, p 1924.

▶ Siegel MJ (ed): *Pediatric Sonography*, 4th edition. Philadelphia, Lippincott Williams & Wilkins, 2011, pp 611–612.

470. B. Triradiate cartilage.

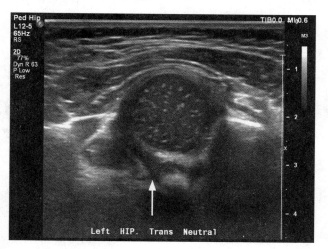

A transverse view of the hip is similar to an axial CT rotated 90 degrees. On a transverse view of the infant hip joint, the acetabulum is V-shaped and composed of the ischium posteriorly, the pubic bone anteriorly, and the triradiate cartilage centrally (arrow). The triradiate cartilage lies central to the femoral head and forms a Y configuration medial to the femoral head in the transverse view. The cartilage appears *hypoechoic to bone and allows sound transmission. The ilium and labrum appear more echogenic. The iliopsoas muscle lies anterior to the femoral head and does not lie within the acetabulum.*

▶ de Bruyn R (ed): *Pediatric Ultrasound: How, Why and When*, 2nd edition (e-book). Philadelphia, Churchill Livingstone/Elsevier, 2010, pp 326–329.
▶ Rumack CM, Levine D (eds): *Diagnostic Ultrasound*, 5th edition. Philadelphia, Elsevier, 2018, p 1923.
▶ Siegel MJ (ed): *Pediatric Sonography*, 4th edition. Philadelphia, Lippincott Williams & Wilkins, 2011, pp 609–610.

471. **C. Supine.**

The success of hip sonography to rule out developmental dysplasia of the hip (DDH) is dependent on the ability to visualize the femoral and acetabular landmarks. Exams are performed with the infant primarily supine, but with a slight upward tilt of the hip being examined. This allows the transducer to be positioned over the posterolateral aspect of the hip.

▶ de Bruyn R (ed): *Pediatric Ultrasound: How, Why and When*, 2nd edition (e-book). Philadelphia, Churchill Livingstone/Elsevier, 2010, pp 322, 326, 327.
▶ Rumack CM, Levine D (eds): *Diagnostic Ultrasound*, 5th edition. Philadelphia, Elsevier, 2018, p 1922.
▶ Siegel MJ (ed): *Pediatric Sonography*, 4th edition. Philadelphia, Lippincott Williams & Wilkins, 2011, pp 607–608.

472. **B. Acetabulum.**

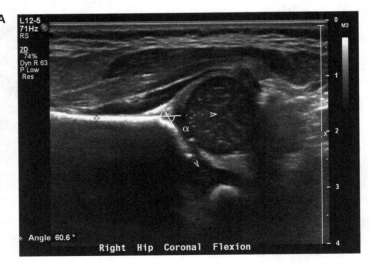

(figure continues . . .)

See also the answers to questions 447, 451, and 469.

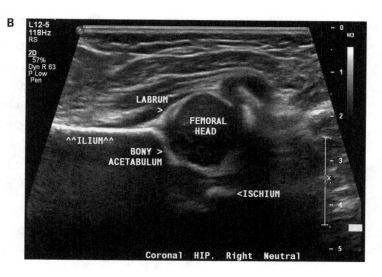

The alpha angle or α (image **A**) is the angle between the ilium and the acetabulum and is also known as the "bony roof" angle. The labrum and the ilium (see image **B**) form the beta angle. The labrum extends laterally to cover the femoral head. The ischium is the lower of the three bones (ilium, ischium, pubis) that form the pelvis. The femoral head should be present and seated in the center of the acetabulum.

▶ de Bruyn R (ed): *Pediatric Ultrasound: How, Why and When*, 2nd edition (e-book). Philadelphia, Churchill Livingstone/Elsevier, 2010, p 324.

▶ Siegel MJ (ed): *Pediatric Sonography*, 4th edition. Philadelphia, Lippincott Williams & Wilkins, 2011, pp 605, 608, 611.

473. **C. Better visualizes the ossified femoral head.**

In neonates and early infants, sonography is the favored method for examining the hip because the majority of the joint components are made up of cartilage and soft tissues that will not be visible on conventional x-rays. Once the femoral head ossifies (usually by 6 months of age), the acetabulum becomes difficult to visualize on ultrasound and an x-ray may be a better imaging method. For patients wearing a harness, diagnostic ultrasound imaging can usually still be obtained. The hip stability, cooperation of the patient, and presence of a harness are all factors that sonographers can work around for successful imaging.

▶ de Bruyn R (ed): *Pediatric Ultrasound: How, Why and When*, 2nd edition (e-book). Philadelphia, Churchill Livingstone/Elsevier, 2010, pp 320, 322.

▶ Rumack CM, Levine D (eds): *Diagnostic Ultrasound*, 5th edition. Philadelphia, Elsevier, 2018, p 1921.

▶ Siegel MJ (ed): *Pediatric Sonography*, 4th edition. Philadelphia, Lippincott Williams & Wilkins, 2011, p 607.

474. A. Acetabulum and femur.

See also the answers to questions 447, 455, and 472.

The position and stability of the femoral head along with the development of the acetabulum are what distinguish a normal from a dysplastic hip. The relationship and articulation of the femoral head and acetabulum are important for normal development. The ilium and ischium are part of the large pelvic bone. The ilium is the upper crest of the hip. The ischium is the "sit bone" and provides stability for the hip. The ilium, ischium, and pubis all join to form the acetabulum.

▸ de Bruyn R (ed): *Pediatric Ultrasound: How, Why and When*, 2nd edition (e-book). Philadelphia, Churchill Livingstone/Elsevier, 2010, p 320.
▸ Siegel MJ (ed): *Pediatric Sonography*, 4th edition. Philadelphia, Lippincott Williams & Wilkins, 2011, p 607.

475. C. Labrum.

See also the answers to questions 447 and 472.

The acetabulum is made up of the ilium, ischium, and pubis. The labrum is the cartilage that lines the cup of the acetabulum to hold the femoral head.

▸ de Bruyn R (ed): *Pediatric Ultrasound: How, Why and When*, 2nd edition (e-book). Philadelphia, Churchill Livingstone/Elsevier, 2010, p 320.
▸ Rumack CM, Levine D (eds): *Diagnostic Ultrasound*, 5th edition. Philadelphia, Elsevier, 2018, p 1923.
▸ Siegel MJ (ed): *Pediatric Sonography*, 4th edition. Philadelphia, Lippincott Williams & Wilkins, 2011, p 608.

476. D. Ilium.

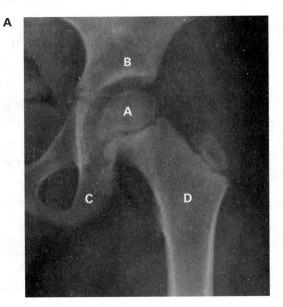

(figure continues . . .)

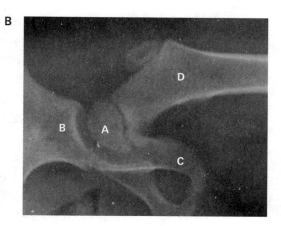

A Rotate this anteroposterior radiograph 90 degrees counterclockwise in your mind, and *B* it will be oriented similarly to a coronal ultrasound image of the hip. The ilium (labeled B) serves as the baseline when calculating the alpha angle. The baseline is drawn along the iliac bone and the second line traces along the bony acetabular roof. In this radiograph, the ischium is labeled C. The acetabulum is formed by the ilium, ischium, and pubis. The femur is labeled D and the femoral head is labeled A.

▶ de Bruyn R (ed): *Pediatric Ultrasound: How, Why and When*, 2nd edition (e-book). Philadelphia, Churchill Livingstone/Elsevier, 2010, p 324.
▶ Rumack CM, Levine D (eds): *Diagnostic Ultrasound*, 5th edition. Philadelphia, Elsevier, 2018, pp 1925–1926.
▶ Siegel MJ (ed): *Pediatric Sonography*, 4th edition. Philadelphia, Lippincott Williams & Wilkins, 2011, p 610.

477. D. Normal.

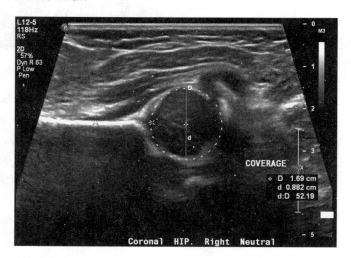

Femoral head coverage by the acetabulum is figured by the acetabular depth in relation to the diameter of the femoral head. Normal coverage should be at least 50%, indicating that 50% of the femoral head is resting within the hip socket.

Coverage less than 50% indicates that the femoral head is not sitting properly within the hip socket and is termed laxity, subluxation, or dislocation. Femoral head coverage measurements are done in a coronal plane. A horizontal line is first drawn across the ilium. A circumference circle (D) is then applied around the femoral head perimeter. Hip tools within the ultrasound system's calculation package automatically assign a femoral head diameter (d). What is important is the percentage of the femoral head diameter (D) that is covered by the osseous acetabular roof (d). The ultrasound system's onboard tool then calculates this percentage. Here that percentage is 52.19% (d:D)—i.e., greater than 50%.

▶ de Bruyn R (ed): *Pediatric Ultrasound: How, Why and When*, 2nd edition (e-book). Philadelphia, Churchill Livingstone/Elsevier, 2010, pp 327–329.

▶ Rumack CM, Levine D (eds): *Diagnostic Ultrasound*, 5th edition. Philadelphia, Elsevier, 2018, p 1924.

478. **C. Proximal focal femoral deficiency (PFFD).**

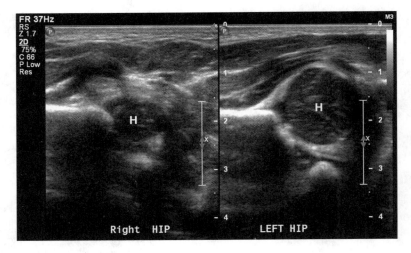

Proximal femoral focal deficiency *(PFFD)* is most often unilateral and presents as a shortened lower extremity. The severity of PFFD varies and is divided into four types, ranging from the absence or underdevelopment of the neck and femoral head (H)—as seen on the right hip in this coronal image, showing an underdeveloped femoral head compared to a normal left femoral head—to a shortened femur. There is no known cause, but PFFD is thought to occur from a vascular accident in utero. This abnormality has been associated with caudal regression syndrome and infants of diabetic mothers. Typically, hip dislocation or developmental dysplasia of the hip (DDH) would not include a shortened femur. Avascular necrosis is a rare complication of DDH treatment and would not be characterized by a shortened femur. The differential diagnosis for PFFD is skeletal dysplasia, although in most cases skeletal dysplasia involves more than one extremity.

▶ Rumack CM, Levine D (eds): *Diagnostic Ultrasound*, 5th edition. Philadelphia, Elsevier, 2018, p 1400.

▶ Siegel MJ (ed): *Pediatric Sonography*, 4th edition. Philadelphia, Lippincott Williams & Wilkins, 2011, pp 613–615.

PART 13

Female Pelvis

479. C. Cervix.

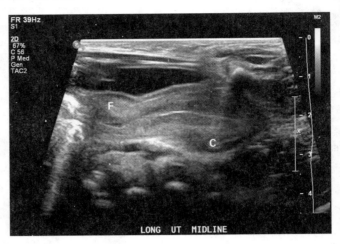

In the neonatal and infant period, the anteroposterior (AP) diameter of the cervix (C) is typically equal to or greater than the diameter of the fundus (F). In this image of an infant uterus, the cervix has a greater AP diameter than the fundus. The endometrium typically appears as a thin echogenic line leading to the vagina. In early infancy the uterus is somewhat larger than it is in a child due to continued stimulation by circulating maternal hormones. During neonatal life the uterus has a prominent cervix and a narrower fundus. Once maternal hormones decline, the uterus regresses in size but still maintains a tubular shape. Up until about age 8, the uterine size remains stable. The uterine body usually begins to grow after age 8. During childhood the anteroposterior dimensions of the cervix and fundus are similar, but the endometrial stripe is not easily seen. After puberty, the fundus will become larger than the cervix, resulting in a pear-shaped structure. The uterus also descends deeper in the pelvis after puberty. Post menarche, the endometrium will change in appearance throughout the menstrual cycle.

▶ Cohen HL, Sivit CJ: *Fetal and Pediatric Ultrasound: A Casebook Approach.* New York, McGraw-Hill, 2001, pp 469–474.

▶ de Bruyn R (ed): *Pediatric Ultrasound: How, Why and When*, 2nd edition (e-book). Philadelphia, Churchill Livingstone/Elsevier, 2010, pp 213–214.

▶ Rumack CM, Levine D (eds): *Diagnostic Ultrasound*, 5th edition. Philadelphia, Elsevier, 2018, pp 1872–1873.

▶ Siegel MJ (ed): *Pediatric Sonography*, 4th edition. Philadelphia, Lippincott Williams & Wilkins, 2011, pp 533–535.

480. **B. Luteinizing hormone (LH).**

Luteinizing hormone *(LH)* is one of the gonadotropins *(gonad-stimulating hormones)*. LH is made by the pituitary gland. In females, it assists in regulating the menstrual cycle. A sudden elevation in LH will trigger ovulation and the development of the corpus luteum. Follicle-stimulating hormone *(FSH)*, another gonadotropin, is also produced in the pituitary gland. FSH helps female eggs to grow. Estrogen *production within the follicle is dependent on FSH. The increase in estrogen tells the pituitary to stop making FSH and make more LH. This spike in LH is what triggers ovulation.* Progesterone *is produced in the ovaries and adrenals and also helps to regulate the menstrual cycle. The corpus luteum releases progesterone to help prepare the body to maintain a pregnancy. In males, LH stimulates Leydig cell production and the release of testosterone. FSH in males assists in sperm production.*

▶ Keough J: *Nursing Laboratory and Diagnostic Tests Demystified*, 2nd edition. New York, McGraw-Hill, 2017, pp 224–226, 228–230, 262–264.

481. **D. 3D ultrasound.**

See Color Plate 29 on page xlv.

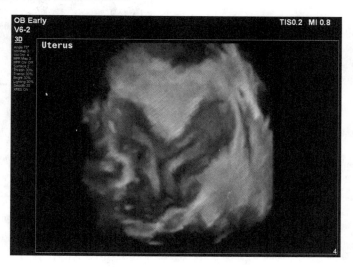

See the diagram "Congenital Anomalies of the Uterus" in answer 500.

A three-dimensional or 3D ultrasound is the modality of choice for evaluating pediatric uterine fusion anomalies. It is a noninvasive technique that can detect and classify congenital anomalies. This image is a coronal 3D ultrasound volume rendering of a uterus didelphys. Uterus didelphys is defined as two complete uteri and cervices that do not communicate with each other. The vagina may or may not be duplicated. If the acoustic window is limited, then magnetic resonance imaging (MRI) would be another modality of choice. A computed tomography *(CT)* scan involves radiation and would not be advised if the diagnosis can be made without it. However, CT and MRI are both helpful in staging malignancies or diagnosing teratomas. Contrast-enhanced ultrasound *(CEUS)* is not needed to image a structural uterine anomaly. Sonohysterography *is used primarily for evaluation of the endometrium and/or polyps, not routinely for uterine anomalies. In the case of a sexually active teen, endovaginal sonography would be appropriate if consent is obtained.*

▶ de Bruyn R (ed): *Pediatric Ultrasound: How, Why and When*, 2nd edition (e-book). Philadelphia, Churchill Livingstone/Elsevier, 2010, p 214.
▶ Rumack CM, Levine D (eds): *Diagnostic Ultrasound*, 5th edition. Philadelphia, Elsevier, 2018, p 1881.
▶ Siegel MJ (ed): *Pediatric Sonography*, 4th edition. Philadelphia, Lippincott Williams & Wilkins, 2011, pp 510, 536.

482. B. Secretory.

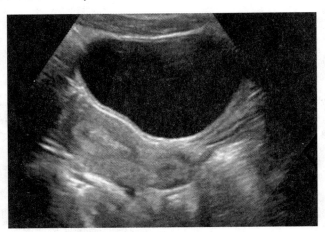

The menstrual phase *is the first phase of the endometrial cycle, days 1–5, when the endometrium is the thinnest, appearing as an echogenic stripe within the uterine fundus. The* proliferative *or* follicular phase *occurs on days 6–14. Leading up to ovulation, the inner layer of the endometrium becomes thicker. During the proliferative phase, the endometrium measures 4–8 mm. Ovulation ideally takes place on day 14 of a 28-day cycle. The* secretory *or* luteinizing phase *of the endometrial cycle occurs after ovulation, usually days 15–28. During this phase, the endometrium reaches its ultimate thickness and is the most echogenic. The endometrium can measure up to 12–15 mm during the secretory phase and is thickened, as seen in this image. The*

luteal phase *is part of the ovarian cycle, taking place during the second half of the menstrual cycle. The corpus luteum forms after ovulation and remains until the ovum is fertilized, or it degenerates after menstruation (becoming the corpus albicans).*

▶ Siegel MJ (ed): *Pediatric Sonography*, 4th edition. Philadelphia, Lippincott Williams & Wilkins, 2011, pp 511–513, 534–535.

483. **A. Broad ligament.**

The broad ligament *is a large and wide peritoneal fold extending from the sides of the uterus to the sides and floor of the pelvis. The ovaries, fallopian tubes, and uterus are all attached to the broad ligament. The uterine and ovarian vessels are also found within the broad ligament. The* round ligament *courses from the uterine horns within the abdominopelvic cavity, through the inguinal canal, and terminates at the labia majora. The* cardinal ligaments *arise from the lateral portions of the cervix and vaginal fornix. The* inguinal ligament *forms the floor of the inguinal canal.*

▶ Rumack CM, Levine D (eds): *Diagnostic Ultrasound*, 5th edition. Philadelphia, Elsevier, 2018, pp 1873–1875.

▶ Siegel MJ (ed): *Pediatric Sonography*, 4th edition. Philadelphia, Lippincott Williams & Wilkins, 2011, pp 510–511.

484. **C. Peritoneal inclusion cyst.**

Peritoneal inclusion cysts *are typically found in patients with pelvic adhesions secondary to pelvic inflammatory disease (PID) or surgery. The majority of peritoneal fluid in young women is produced by the ovaries. This fluid moves through the peritoneal cavity and is absorbed by the mesentery. When this fluid becomes trapped within pelvic adhesions, it cannot be absorbed by the mesentery as it normally would. Instead, a cystic structure is formed. Clinical symptoms are pain and possibly a palpable pelvic mass. On ultrasound, a cystic mass with septations or loculated ascites may be present. The ovary can be located inside or outside of the fluid collection.* Physiologic cysts (follicles) *are typically less than 3 cm in diameter and located within the ovary.* Functional cysts *are follicles that grow larger than 3–5 cm but can become as large as 20 cm. A* functional cyst *can be formed in two different circumstances—either when ovulation fails and the mature*

(Graafian) follicle continues to grow, or when a corpus luteum does not involute after ovulation. Corpus luteal cysts occur at the site where ovulation took place. They may appear complex and can range from 5 cm to 11 cm in diameter.

▸ Rumack CM, Levine D (eds): *Diagnostic Ultrasound*, 5th edition. Philadelphia, Elsevier, 2018, pp 573, 1873, 1875–1876.

▸ Siegel MJ (ed): *Pediatric Sonography*, 4th edition. Philadelphia, Lippincott Williams & Wilkins, 2011, pp 514–519.

485. A. Germ cell tumors.

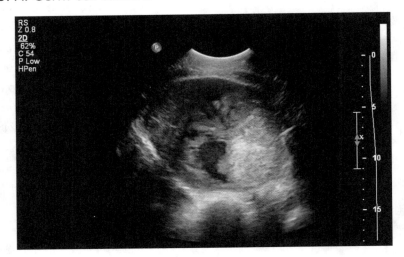

Pediatric ovarian malignancies are very rare, comprising only about 1%–2% of all malignancies in children under the age of 17, but when they do occur, germ cell tumors are the most common type. Germ cell ovarian malignancies may spread to lymph nodes and the liver. When present, they are found in postmenarcheal patients, who commonly present with an abdominal mass. Ovarian malignancies are typically asymptomatic and can grow to be large tumors before they are discovered. Malignant teratomas (dermoids), dysgerminomas, and endodermal sinus tumors (yolk sac tumors) are all germ cell tumors. Only 10% of dermoids will be malignant, with more than 50% of the tumor being composed of soft tissue. They will appear complex or solid and echogenic. Contents may consist of wall nodules, septations, and/or calcifications. Dysgerminomas and endodermal sinus tumors can be homogeneous and echogenic or can appear complex, with areas of hemorrhage or necrosis. An elevated alpha-fetoprotein (AFP) level will be found with endodermal sinus tumors. Sex cord–stromal tumors, such as granulosa cell tumors and Sertoli-Leydig tumors, make up about 13% of pediatric ovarian malignancies. Epithelial carcinomas

comprise only 10% of pediatric ovarian malignancies. Cystadenocarcinomas are extremely rare in childhood and more common in adults.

▶ de Bruyn R (ed): *Pediatric Ultrasound: How, Why and When*, 2nd edition (e-book). Philadelphia, Churchill Livingstone/Elsevier, 2010, pp 228–232.
▶ Rumack CM, Levine D (eds): *Diagnostic Ultrasound*, 5th edition. Philadelphia, Elsevier, 2018, pp 1879–1880.
▶ Siegel MJ (ed): *Pediatric Sonography*, 4th edition. Philadelphia, Lippincott Williams & Wilkins, 2011, pp 522–527.

486. **B. Estrogen.**

Estrogen is produced primarily within the ovary, but it is also produced in the adrenal glands, adipose tissue, testes, and placenta. It is the primary female sex hormone and assists in the development of the reproductive system and secondary sex characteristics, such as breasts and body hair. Estrogen helps regulate the menstrual cycle by controlling the thickness of the endometrial lining. Estrogen levels decrease to encourage menstruation. Lower levels of estrogen are found in polycystic ovary syndrome (PCOS) and Turner syndrome. Estrogen in the form of oral contraceptives is used to prevent and treat ovarian cysts. Luteinizing hormone *(LH) and* follicle-stimulating hormone *(FSH) are produced within the pituitary gland.* Alpha-fetoprotein *(AFP) is a glycoprotein tumor marker found in the blood when produced by specific malignant neoplasms. Increased levels of AFP found in pregnant women are associated with an increased risk for neural tube defects in the fetus.*

▶ Keough J: *Nursing Laboratory and Diagnostic Tests Demystified*, 2nd edition. New York, McGraw-Hill, 2017, pp 224–226, 228–230, 258–264.

487. **D. Gartner duct cyst.**

A Gartner duct cyst *is formed by a remnant of the wolffian duct and most often is located on the anterior upper wall of the vagina. These cysts may protrude out of the vagina. Sonographically, they are anechoic or hypoechoic. For best visualization, a high-frequency transducer should be used. An* inclusion cyst *is typically located in the posterior wall of the lower vagina. Vaginal cysts do not usually occur in the pediatric population.* Nabothian cysts *are located within the cervix.* Cystadenomas *are benign lesions of the ovary.*

▶ Rumack CM, Levine D (eds): *Diagnostic Ultrasound*, 5th edition. Philadelphia, Elsevier, 2018, pp 1883–1884.
▶ Siegel MJ (ed): *Pediatric Sonography*, 4th edition. Philadelphia, Lippincott Williams & Wilkins, 2011, pp 522–523, 525.

488. **A. Fallopian tubes.**

The fallopian tubes *are also known as the* oviducts. *They extend laterally from each uterine cornua and are approximately 10 cm long. Each oviduct is composed of the isthmus, ampulla, and infundibulum. The* isthmus *is the short, thick-walled part of the tube closest to the uterus. The* ampulla *is the wider and longer part of the tube closest to the ovary. The* infundibulum *is the fimbriated end of the fallopian tube. The role of the fallopian tubes is to secrete mucus and, by peristalsis and ciliary movement, transport sperm cells to the egg and then a fertilized egg back to the uterus. Fertilization usually occurs within the ampulla of the tube. Ovaries and testes are gonads. A* follicle *is the fluid-filled sac in an ovary that contains an oocyte (immature egg).*

▶ Rumack CM, Levine D (eds): *Diagnostic Ultrasound*, 5th edition. Philadelphia, Elsevier, 2018, p 565.

489. **C. Assessing the presence of follicles.**

Precocious puberty is the early development of secondary sex characteristics (breast tissue, body hair, menses). The purpose of sonography is to evaluate the uterine size and shape, calculate ovarian volumes, and evaluate the adrenal glands for tumors that might be causing an overproduction of hormones. A large fundus, causing a pear-shaped uterus, is usually not seen until after puberty. Follicles less than 9 mm are present in 50% of all girls and would not be a concern or factor when diagnosing precocious puberty.

There are four classifications of precocious puberty:

- *Central/true isosexual precocity is the early development of the characteristics with menses. This type is usually caused by pituitary lesions or activation of the hypothalamic-pituitary-gonadal axis.*

- *Peripheral/pseudosexual precocity is all of the characteristics without menses and can be caused by ovarian cysts or neoplasms.*

- *Premature adrenarche exhibits isolated pubic hair and elevated androgens, such as testosterone.*

- *Premature thelarche is demonstrated by isolated breast development and normal prepubertal hormones.*

▶ de Bruyn R (ed): *Pediatric Ultrasound: How, Why and When*, 2nd edition (e-book). Philadelphia, Churchill Livingstone/Elsevier, 2010, pp 223–226.

▸ Rumack CM, Levine D (eds): *Diagnostic Ultrasound*, 5th edition. Philadelphia, Elsevier, 2018, pp 1887–1888.

▸ Siegel MJ (ed): *Pediatric Sonography*, 4th edition. Philadelphia, Lippincott Williams & Wilkins, 2011, pp 545–547.

490. **A. Stays intact throughout the menstrual cycle.**

The basalis layer *of the endometrium is also called the* stratum basalis *or basal zone. It is the segment of the endometrium lying closest to the uterine myometrium and contains the vessels that supply the endometrium with blood. It is not shed and stays intact throughout the menstrual cycle. The basalis layer gives rise to the* functionalis layer, *also known as the* stratum functionalis *or functional zone. The functionalis layer lies closest to the uterine cavity. It contains most of the endometrial glands. The functionalis layer is the layer that changes throughout the menstrual cycle and is shed.*

▸ Rumack CM, Levine D (eds): *Diagnostic Ultrasound*, 5th edition. Philadelphia, Elsevier, 2018, pp 1872–1873.

▸ Siegel MJ (ed): *Pediatric Sonography*, 4th edition. Philadelphia, Lippincott Williams & Wilkins, 2011, pp 534–536.

491. **D. Hematometrocolpos.**

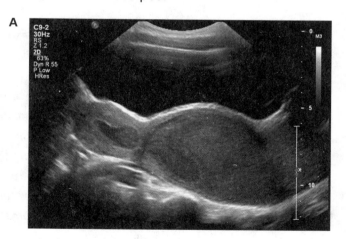

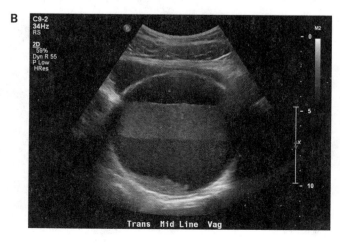

*Hematometrocolpos is the condition that occurs when the uterine cavity, cervix, and vaginal cavity are distended by blood (as demonstrated in image **A**). Hematometrocolpos can be seen in patients with vaginal agenesis, atresia, or obstruction. Vaginal obstruction from imperforate membranes (hymen) or a transverse vaginal septum is more common and surgery is required. Hematocolpos is blood within the cervix and vagina. Hydrocolpos is fluid within the cervix and vagina. Hydrometrocolpos is fluid within the uterine cavity, cervix, and vagina. Blood will appear more echogenic and heterogeneous than the more cystic vaginal secretions. Fluid-debris levels may be present (as demonstrated in image **B**). If the fluid collection is large enough, the fallopian tubes can fill and empty fluid into the peritoneal cavity. A complication of the distention of the uterine cavity would be compression of the ureters, causing hydronephrosis.*

▶ de Bruyn R (ed): *Pediatric Ultrasound: How, Why and When*, 2nd edition (e-book). Philadelphia, Churchill Livingstone/Elsevier, 2010, p 216.

▶ Rumack CM, Levine D (eds): *Diagnostic Ultrasound*, 5th edition. Philadelphia, Elsevier, 2018, p 1882.

▶ Siegel MJ (ed): *Pediatric Sonography*, 4th edition. Philadelphia, Lippincott Williams & Wilkins, 2011, pp 540–541.

492. B. Renal anomalies.

During the embryonic stage of human development, a single uterine cavity is formed by 20 weeks' gestation. Congenital uterine anomalies or septal defects are caused by the partial or absolute failure of the fusion of the two müllerian (paramesonephric) ducts or septal regression. Because the development of the müllerian ducts is dependent on the formation of the wolffian (mesonephric) duct, renal anomalies are associated with uterine anomalies. Precocious puberty, cardiac anomalies, and biliary atresia do not have an association with uterine fusion defects.

▶ de Bruyn R (ed): *Pediatric Ultrasound: How, Why and When*, 2nd edition (e-book). Philadelphia, Churchill Livingstone/Elsevier, 2010, pp 214–215.

▶ Rumack CM, Levine D (eds): *Diagnostic Ultrasound*, 5th edition. Philadelphia, Elsevier, 2018, p 1881.

▶ Siegel MJ (ed): *Pediatric Sonography*, 4th edition. Philadelphia, Lippincott Williams & Wilkins, 2011, p 536.

493. **B. Endodermal sinus tumor.**

An endodermal sinus tumor *is also known as a* yolk sac tumor *and can cause elevated alpha-fetoprotein (AFP) levels in the blood.* Granulosa cell tumors *show elevated estrogen levels.* Sertoli-Leydig tumors *show elevated testosterone levels. Other malignant ovarian neoplasms, such as embryonal carcinoma, can cause elevated levels of human chorionic gonadotropin (hCG).* Teratomas *do not have an association with elevated AFP levels.*

▶ Rumack CM, Levine D (eds): *Diagnostic Ultrasound*, 5th edition. Philadelphia, Elsevier, 2018, pp 1879–1880.

▶ Siegel MJ (ed): *Pediatric Sonography*, 4th edition. Philadelphia, Lippincott Williams & Wilkins, 2011, pp 522–527.

494. **C. Displaces the bowel out of the pelvis.**

During transabdominal pelvic sonography on a pediatric patient, a well-distended bladder is helpful. It not only acts as an acoustic window but also displaces gas-filled bowel out of the pelvis for better visualization of the pelvic organs. Filling the bladder does not change the position of the ovaries, since they are suspended within the broad ligament. Patients are scanned in the supine position with the most adequate highest-frequency transducer available. Vaginal sonography is not performed unless a complete exam cannot be obtained and there are abnormalities or pathology that requires additional imaging or a closer look.

▶ de Bruyn R (ed): *Pediatric Ultrasound: How, Why and When*, 2nd edition (e-book). Philadelphia, Churchill Livingstone/Elsevier, 2010, pp 210–211.

▶ Rumack CM, Levine D (eds): *Diagnostic Ultrasound*, 5th edition. Philadelphia, Elsevier, 2018, pp 1870–1872.

▶ Siegel MJ (ed): *Pediatric Sonography*, 4th edition. Philadelphia, Lippincott Williams & Wilkins, 2011, pp 509–510.

495. **A. Graafian.**

A Graafian follicle *is the dominant follicle within an ovary. The* corpus luteum *forms at the site of ovulation. A functional cyst forms from a Graafian follicle when it fails to ovulate. Functional cysts typically measure 3–5 cm. Physiologic cysts are follicles smaller than 3 cm.*

▶ de Bruyn R (ed): *Pediatric Ultrasound: How, Why and When*, 2nd edition (e-book). Philadelphia, Churchill Livingstone/Elsevier, 2010, p 212.

▶ Rumack CM, Levine D (eds): *Diagnostic Ultrasound*, 5th edition. Philadelphia, Elsevier, 2018, pp 1873, 1875–1876.

▶ Siegel MJ (ed): *Pediatric Sonography*, 4th edition. Philadelphia, Lippincott Williams & Wilkins, 2011, p 514.

496. **C. Peritoneal inclusion.**

Peritoneal inclusion cysts *are usually secondary to adhesions caused by pelvic inflammatory disease (PID) or surgery. Peritoneal fluid released from the ovaries becomes trapped within the adhesions, forming a cyst-like structure containing septations. Symptoms include pain, and a palpable mass may be felt. The ovary can be seen alongside the fluid collection or within in it.* Cystadenomas *(mucinous or serous) are large cysts and are rare under the age of 20.* Cystic teratomas *are composed of germ layers and occur within the ovary. Sonographically, they can range from cystic to solid in appearance, but the majority are complex.* Para-ovarian cysts *arise from the mesothelium of the broad ligament or fallopian tube and typically occur in middle-aged women but can occur at any age. The ovary can be visualized separately or alongside the cyst. On ultrasound, para-ovarian cysts are round or oval, anechoic or hypoechoic. They have thin walls and posterior enhancement. Para-ovarian cysts can become hemorrhagic.*

▶ Rumack CM, Levine D (eds): *Diagnostic Ultrasound*, 5th edition. Philadelphia, Elsevier, 2018, pp 573, 1885–1887.

▶ Siegel MJ (ed): *Pediatric Sonography*, 4th edition. Philadelphia, Lippincott Williams & Wilkins, 2011, pp 517–522.

497. **A. Stein-Leventhal syndrome.**

Stein-Leventhal syndrome *is also known as* polycystic ovary syndrome (PCOS). *The classic clinical signs are amenorrhea, hirsutism, and obesity. Amenorrhea is consistent in all patients, with a combination of one or more of the other clinical signs appearing late in puberty. A decreased level of follicle-stimulating hormone (FSH) and increased luteinizing hormone (LH) cause a relative increase in testosterone (androgen) production and anovulation. Patients with PCOS have an increased risk for endometrial cancer. Most patients have bilaterally enlarged ovaries with a large number of immature or degenerated follicles. Sonographically, they appear more round than oval in shape. A normal ovary can have approximately three follicles present measuring less than 8 mm in size. An ovary with PCOS will have more than five follicles measuring 5–8 mm and located lining the periphery of the ovary, resulting in a "string of pearls"* appearance on ultrasound. *In the center stroma of the ovary, the echogenicity is increased. Turner and Noonan syndromes are genetic syndromes.* Turner syndrome *is associated with gonadal dysgenesis, where the ovaries are either absent or replaced with connective tissue streaks. Dysplastic ovaries may be seen in* Noonan syndrome. Mayer-Rokitansky-Küster-Hauser syndrome *results in an underdeveloped or absent uterus and vagina, although external genitalia will appear normal.*

▶ de Bruyn R (ed): *Pediatric Ultrasound: How, Why and When*, 2nd edition (e-book). Philadelphia, Churchill Livingstone/Elsevier, 2010, pp 228–229.

▶ Rumack CM, Levine D (eds): *Diagnostic Ultrasound*, 5th edition. Philadelphia, Elsevier, 2018, p 1877.

▶ Siegel MJ (ed): *Pediatric Sonography*, 4th edition. Philadelphia, Lippincott Williams & Wilkins, 2011, pp 541, 548–549.

498. **D. Functional cyst.**

The functional cyst *is the most common benign mass of the ovary, whether the origin is follicular, corpus luteal, or theca-lutein in nature. Functional cysts include* follicular cysts, *which do not rupture to release an egg but continue to grow, and* corpus luteum cysts, *which occur when the corpus luteum doesn't involute but continues to grow. When the cysts are larger than 3 cm in diameter, they are considered functional cysts. Follicular and corpus luteal cysts are typically solitary and unilateral.* Theca-lutein cysts *are multiple, bilateral, and the result of human chorionic gonadotropin (hCG).* Cystic teratomas, *also known as* dermoids, *are the most common benign neoplasm (an abnormal growth of tissue) of the ovary. Most cysts resolve on their own over time, but some continue to grow. The most common complication of ovarian cysts is torsion, but bowel obstruction and urinary tract obstruction are also possible.* Cystadenomas *are rarely seen in females younger than 20 years old.* Para-ovarian cysts *are not ovarian in nature; rather, they usually arise from the fallopian tube or broad ligament. A* dysgerminoma *is a malignant, not benign, ovarian tumor.*

▶ Rumack CM, Levine D (eds): *Diagnostic Ultrasound*, 5th edition. Philadelphia, Elsevier, 2018, pp 573, 1873, 1875–1876, 1880.

▶ Siegel MJ (ed): *Pediatric Sonography*, 4th edition. Philadelphia, Lippincott Williams & Wilkins, 2011, pp 511–514, 517–521.

499. B. Ovarian torsion.

See Color Plate 5 on page xxxv.

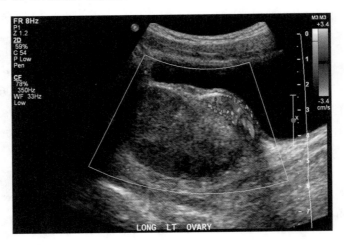

Ovarian torsion can occur in neonates and children with existing masses or cysts but occurs more often in adolescents and younger women. Torsion is almost always unilateral and can involve the ovary (ovarian torsion) or the ovary and fallopian tube (adnexal torsion). The vascular pedicle (composed of the tube, broad ligament, and blood vessels) becomes twisted and restricts the flow of blood and lymph to the ovary. The loss of blood flow can result in infarction or tissue death. The presence of an ovarian mass increases the risk of torsion. If supporting ligaments of the ovary are loose or lax, there is an increased risk that a normal ovary will undergo torsion. Clinical symptoms are the acute onset of pelvic or lower abdominal pain, nausea, vomiting, and leukocytosis. On ultrasound, acute ovarian torsion demonstrates an enlarged edematous ovary with increased posterior enhancement due to vascular congestion. The torsed ovary can become up to six times larger than the unaffected ovary. In the majority of cases multiple peripheral small follicles are present along the perimeter of the ovary. Free fluid within the cul-de-sac may be noted. Venous flow on color Doppler may be extremely diminished or completely absent. In this image, there is an edematous ovary with no flow seen within the ovary. The twisted vascular pedicle is seen outside of the ovary with color flow present. Occasionally, there may be a small amount of arterial flow seen within the ovary or adnexa, but that is not as common. Machine settings (scale, sensitivity, and wall filter) should be adjusted to pick up low frequency shifts for slower blood flow. Precocious puberty and polycystic ovaries do not have the same clinical symptoms

as torsion, but polycystic ovaries can appear enlarged with peripheral follicles. A dermoid can cause pain and an enlarged ovary, but a mass will be visualized.

▶ Rumack CM, Levine D (eds): *Diagnostic Ultrasound*, 5th edition. Philadelphia, Elsevier, 2018, pp 1875–1877, 1880, 1887–1888.

▶ Siegel MJ (ed): *Pediatric Sonography*, 4th edition. Philadelphia, Lippincott Williams & Wilkins, 2011, pp 519–521, 530–531, 545–549.

500. C. Septate uterus.

Congenital Anomalies of the Uterus

Normal uterus

Formation Defects	Fusion Defects	Resorption Defects
Unicornuate with Rudimentary Horn	Partial Bicornuate (Unicollis)	Arcuate
Unicornuate	Complete Bicornuate (Bicollis)	Partial Septate
Complete Uterine Agenesis	Uterus Didelphys	Complete Septate

The most common müllerian fusion anomaly is the septate uterus. A single uterus, cervix, and vagina are present with a midline septum causing a division and separating the uterus into two endometrial compartments. The septation will appear hypoechoic when compared to the myometrium. The contour of the fundal endometrium in the transverse plane can appear flat or convex, showing a concavity of up to 1 cm in depth. With a septate uterus, there is an increased risk of spontaneous abortion. Treatment is hysteroscopic resection of the abnormal septum. A bicornuate uterus demonstrates a concave cleft of greater than 1 cm in the central fundus, causing two symmetric uterine horns. These horns merge caudally to form one cervix. A bicornuate uterus is asymptomatic and does not require surgical repair, but there is an increased risk of spontaneous abortion. In uterus didelphys, there are two complete uteri and cervices that do not communicate with each other. The vagina may or may not be duplicated. Surgery is not performed unless there is an obstructing vaginal septum. An arcuate uterus is the mildest anomaly and considered a normal variant. It is asymptomatic and demonstrates no uterine abnormality of contour or any separation defects. 3D sonography is commonly used to diagnose uterine anomalies.

▶ de Bruyn R (ed): *Pediatric Ultrasound: How, Why and When*, 2nd edition (e-book). Philadelphia, Churchill Livingstone/Elsevier, 2010, pp 214–216.
▶ Rumack CM, Levine D (eds): *Diagnostic Ultrasound*, 5th edition. Philadelphia, Elsevier, 2018, p 1881.
▶ Siegel MJ (ed): *Pediatric Sonography*, 4th edition. Philadelphia, Lippincott Williams & Wilkins, 2011, pp 536–541.

501. **A. Posterior and lateral to the uterus.**

    In a postmenarcheal patient, the ovaries increase in size and descend deeper into the pelvis in a posterior and lateral position relative to the uterus. Ovaries are typically suspended within the superior portion of the broad ligament. The outer layer (cortex) will contain follicles. The central inner layer (medulla) is composed of fibrous tissue and does not contain follicles.

    ▶ Rumack CM, Levine D (eds): *Diagnostic Ultrasound*, 5th edition. Philadelphia, Elsevier, 2018, pp 1873–1875.
    ▶ Siegel MJ (ed): *Pediatric Sonography*, 4th edition. Philadelphia, Lippincott Williams & Wilkins, 2011, p 511.

502. **B. Adenomyosis.**

    Adenomyosis *consists of abnormal endometrial glands found within the myometrium of the uterus. It is more common for adenomyosis to be diffuse than it is for it to be focal (i.e., as an* adenomyoma *or adenomyotic cyst). On ultrasound, diffuse adenomyosis presents as an enlarged uterus with thickened walls. In certain cases, only the posterior aspect of the uterus is affected. An adenomyoma will appear as a hypoechoic or anechoic nodular mass within the myometrium. Clinical symptoms are pelvic pain, dysmenorrhea, and menorrhagia.* Leiomyomas *(fibroids) are composed of connective tissue* and smooth muscle. Endometritis *is the inflammation of the endometrial lining and can be seen with pelvic inflammatory disease (PID).* Endometriomas (chocolate cysts) *are ovarian cysts made up of endometrial tissue and are commonly seen in patients with endometriosis.*

▸ Rumack CM, Levine D (eds): *Diagnostic Ultrasound*, 5th edition. Philadelphia, Elsevier, 2018, pp 575, 1885–1887.

▸ Siegel MJ (ed): *Pediatric Sonography*, 4th edition. Philadelphia, Lippincott Williams & Wilkins, 2011, pp 528, 541–542.

503. D. Vaginal obstruction.

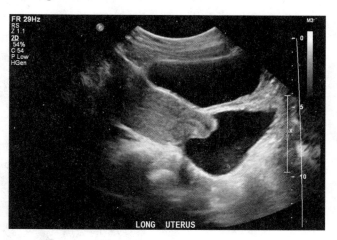

In an adolescent patient, the presence of a fluid-filled, dilated or distended vagina seen when scanning midline and posterior to the bladder is commonly the result of vaginal obstruction due to imperforate membranes. In this image, the external orifice of the cervix is clearly delineated by the surrounding fluid. The thin vaginal walls can be seen surrounding the fluid and a small portion of the distal vagina is seen. Hydrocolpos or hematocolpos *is typically diagnosed by transabdominal sonography, although in some cases transperineal sonography with a high-frequency transducer may be helpful in evaluating the level or extent of obstruction. An* ovarian cyst *would not abut the cervical os.* Rhabdomyosarcoma, *the most common malignancy of the pediatric bladder, would appear as a solid mass distorting the vaginal or uterine contour. A* Gartner duct cyst *would be located on the upper anterior lateral wall of the vagina and most often appears as a solitary oval cystic structure with vaginal tissue surrounding it.*

▸ Rumack CM, Levine D (eds): *Diagnostic Ultrasound*, 5th edition. Philadelphia, Elsevier, 2018, pp 1882–1884.

▸ Siegel MJ (ed): *Pediatric Sonography*, 4th edition. Philadelphia, Lippincott Williams & Wilkins, 2011, pp 540–541, 544–545.

504. A. Submucosal.

Submucosal leiomyomas *(also known as* submucosal fibroids*) involve the endometrium by projecting into the endometrial canal.* Subserosal fibroids *are located beneath the serosal layer of the uterus.* Intramural fibroids *are located within the myometrium.* Pedunculated fibroids *have a stalk that attaches them to the uterine wall, but they develop outside of the uterus. Leiomyomas are round solid masses composed of connective tissue and smooth muscle. They commonly cause dysmenorrhea and menorrhagia. On ultrasound, fibroids tend to appear hypoechoic to the myometrium, but they can be isoechoic or even have a heterogeneous appearance. Adult fibroids can have calcifications or areas of necrosis. If they are large enough, distortion of the uterine contour can occur.*

▸ Siegel MJ (ed): *Pediatric Sonography*, 4th edition. Philadelphia, Lippincott Williams & Wilkins, 2011, pp 542–544.

505. C. Lymphadenopathy.

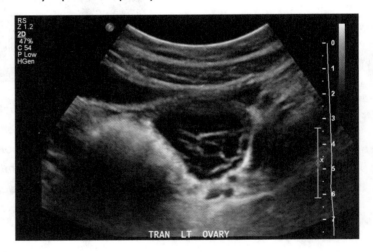

Hemorrhagic cysts *are avascular masses that occur after bleeding takes place within an ovarian cyst or corpus luteum. A hemorrhagic cyst appears complex on ultrasound, with low-level echoes, fluid-debris levels, or a cobweb appearance of fibrin strands (as seen in this image). Included in the differential diagnoses for complex cystic masses of the pelvis are appendiceal abscess, cystic teratoma, tubo-ovarian abscess, and ectopic pregnancy. Ectopic pregnancy and pelvic abscesses can usually be ruled out based on clinical and laboratory signs. Serial sonography can be used to differentiate between a hemorrhagic cyst and a teratoma,*

since hemorrhagic cysts tend to decrease in size and change in echogenicity over time. Lymphadenopathy would appear as multiple hypoechoic areas but demonstrates a vascular center or hilum, whereas hemorrhagic cysts are avascular.

▶ Cohen HL, Sivit CJ: *Fetal and Pediatric Ultrasound: A Casebook Approach*. New York, McGraw-Hill, 2001, pp 499–502.

▶ de Bruyn R (ed): *Pediatric Ultrasound: How, Why and When*, 2nd edition (e-book). Philadelphia, Churchill Livingstone/Elsevier, 2010, p 220.

▶ Rumack CM, Levine D (eds): *Diagnostic Ultrasound*, 5th edition. Philadelphia, Elsevier, 2018, pp 1873, 1875–1878.

▶ Siegel MJ (ed): *Pediatric Sonography*, 4th edition. Philadelphia, Lippincott Williams & Wilkins, 2011, pp 516–518, 621.

506. **B. Rhabdomyosarcoma.**

The most common malignancy of the pediatric uterus or vagina is rhabdomyosarcoma. *These bulky tumors are of mesenchymal origin, originating from the anterior wall of the vagina. They arise adjacent to the cervix and can protrude out of the vagina or extend up into the uterine cavity. The more common embryonal rhabdomyosarcoma occurs primarily in infants and younger children. Metastasis occurs within the liver, lymph nodes, bone, and/or lungs. Clinical symptoms are vaginal bleeding and a protruding mass. On ultrasound, rhabdomyosarcomas appear as solid masses that distort the vaginal and uterine contours. They are homogeneous but may contain cystic areas of necrosis. Extension into the bladder is more common than into the rectum.* Adenocarcinoma *is a common endometrial cancer found in adult females.* Granulosa cell *and* Sertoli-Leydig *tumors are sex cord ovarian tumors of lower incidence and malignancy. Granulosa cell tumors increase estrogen levels and cause precocious puberty. Sertoli-Leydig tumors cause increased androgen production resulting in virilization of patients.*

▶ Rumack CM, Levine D (eds): *Diagnostic Ultrasound*, 5th edition. Philadelphia, Elsevier, 2018, pp 1879–1880, 1883.

▶ Siegel MJ (ed): *Pediatric Sonography*, 4th edition. Philadelphia, Lippincott Williams & Wilkins, 2011, pp 526–527, 544.

507. **C. Arcuate uterus.**

Primary amenorrhea *is the absence of menstruation by age 16. The many causes of primary amenorrhea include pituitary or hypothalamic lesions, polycystic ovary syndrome (PCOS), cytotoxic drugs, radiation therapy, androgen-producing* adrenal tumors, obstructive vaginal or uterine anomalies, and gonadal dysgenesis. Arcuate uterus is the mildest fusion anomaly of the uterus and is not associated with amenorrhea. An arcuate uterus is a mildly variant shape of the uterus that can be considered as a normal variant.

▶ de Bruyn R (ed): *Pediatric Ultrasound: How, Why and When*, 2nd edition (e-book). Philadelphia, Churchill Livingstone/Elsevier, 2010, pp 227–228.

▶ Rumack CM, Levine D (eds): *Diagnostic Ultrasound*, 5th edition. Philadelphia, Elsevier, 2018, pp 1881, 1887.

▶ Siegel MJ (ed): *Pediatric Sonography*, 4th edition. Philadelphia, Lippincott Williams & Wilkins, 2011, pp 547–548.

508. **A. Left renal vein.**

Multiple veins within the ovarian hilum form a pampiniform plexus within the broad ligament. These small veins merge to form one ovarian vein on each side (left and right) in the abdominal cavity. In females, the left ovarian vein drains directly into the left renal vein. In males, the left gonadal vein drains into the left renal vein. The right ovarian and gonadal veins drain into the inferior vena cava (IVC), inferior to the right renal vein. The arterial blood supply of the ovaries comes from the main ovarian arteries, from the aorta and the adnexal branches of the uterine artery.

▶ Rumack CM, Levine D (eds): *Diagnostic Ultrasound*, 5th edition. Philadelphia, Elsevier, 2018, pp 1873–1875.

▶ Siegel MJ (ed): *Pediatric Sonography*, 4th edition. Philadelphia, Lippincott Williams & Wilkins, 2011, pp 513–514.

509. **D. Uterus.**

Intersex disorders are those that are identified by ambiguous external genitalia and gonads, such as hypospadias, cryptorchidism, labial fusion, and clitoromegaly. Ultrasound plays an important role in identifying the presence or absence of a uterus. Uterine presence helps in assigning a gender and distinguishing causes of hermaphroditism. There are four classifications of intersex disorders: female pseudohermaphrodite, male pseudohermaphrodite, true hermaphrodite, *and* mixed gonadal dysgenesis.

▶ de Bruyn R (ed): *Pediatric Ultrasound: How, Why and When*, 2nd edition (e-book). Philadelphia, Churchill Livingstone/Elsevier, 2010, pp 219, 221, 222.

▶ Siegel MJ (ed): *Pediatric Sonography*, 4th edition. Philadelphia, Lippincott Williams & Wilkins, 2011, pp 549–550.

510. **B. Follicle-stimulating hormone (FSH).**

Follicle-stimulating hormone *(FSH) is produced by the anterior pituitary gland and released into blood and urine. It assists in pubertal development and ovarian or testicular function. In females, FSH stimulates follicles to grow and mature. It also helps the Sertoli cells in males to make sperm.* Luteinizing hormone *(LH) is also produced by the pituitary. The sudden rise of LH is what triggers ovulation. FSH and LH are gonadotropins.* Estrogen *and* progesterone *are not pituitary hormones; they are produced by the ovaries and adrenal glands.*

▶ Keough J: *Nursing Laboratory and Diagnostic Tests Demystified*, 2nd edition. New York, McGraw-Hill, 2017, pp 224–226, 228–230, 262–264.

511. **A. Cystic teratoma.**

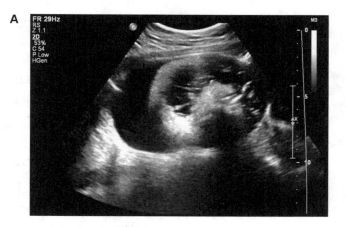

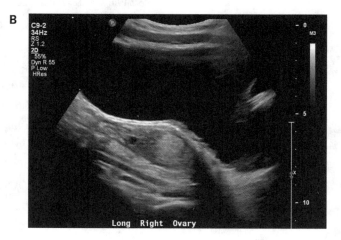

A cystic teratoma *is also known as a* dermoid *cyst or* dermoid. *Teratomas are the most common benign neoplasm in pediatrics, with only 10% of those becoming malignant. Teratomas are germ cell masses composed of ectoderm, mesoderm, and endoderm. Clinical symptoms are usually an*

*asymptomatic palpable pelvic or lower abdominal mass. If hemorrhage, necrosis, or torsion occurs, pelvic pain may be present. Teratomas are usually unilateral, and most measure between 5 and 10 cm. Because of the different germ layers, they can contain serous fluid, oil-like sebum, calcium, hair, and/or fat. This mixture of tissue types is what makes the majority of teratomas look complex on ultrasound (as seen in image **A**). The remainder of teratomas appear as either hypoechoic areas or hyperechoic solid masses (as seen in image **B**). Teratomas may have nodules located centrally or along the wall. A "tip of the iceberg" sign occurs when posterior shadowing from a solid element obscures the back wall of the mass. Teratomas typically have a well-defined border. Uncommon in adolescents, a* fibroid *could be a midline mass but would appear more solid and homogeneous, and the uterus would be identifiable around or adjacent to it. Para-ovarian cysts are most commonly found in women between the ages of 30 and 40 years, and they tend to be anechoic and not complex unless hemorrhagic. A palpable mass is not a clinical symptom of a* pyosalpinx, *which would appear tubular in shape.*

▶ de Bruyn R (ed): *Pediatric Ultrasound: How, Why and When*, 2nd edition (e-book). Philadelphia, Churchill Livingstone/Elsevier, 2010, pp 229–231.

▶ Rumack CM, Levine D (eds): *Diagnostic Ultrasound*, 5th edition. Philadelphia, Elsevier, 2018, p 1880.

▶ Siegel MJ (ed): *Pediatric Sonography*, 4th edition. Philadelphia, Lippincott Williams & Wilkins, 2011, pp 518–521, 528, 542–544.

512. **C. Menstrual.**

The menstrual phase *is the first phase of the endometrial cycle, days 1–5, when the endometrium is the thinnest, appearing as a thin echogenic stripe within the uterine fundus. The* proliferative *or* follicular phase *occurs on days 6–14. Leading up to ovulation, the inner layer of the endometrium becomes thicker. During the proliferative phase, the endometrium measures 4–8 mm. Ovulation ideally takes place on day 14 of a 28-day cycle. The* secretory or luteinizing phase *of the endometrial cycle occurs after ovulation, usually days 15–28. During this phase, the endometrium reaches its ultimate thickness and is the most echogenic. The endometrium can measure 12–15 mm during the secretory phase.*

▶ Siegel MJ (ed): *Pediatric Sonography*, 4th edition. Philadelphia, Lippincott Williams & Wilkins, 2011, pp 533–536.

513. **D. Granulosa cell tumor.**

> Granulosa cell tumors *are sex cord–stromal tumors of low-grade malignancy. They can occur premenarcheally and cause elevated estrogen levels, leading to precocious puberty. Sonographically, granulosa cell tumors appear heterogeneous, with cystic areas containing thick septations as well as solid components. They can appear more cystic than solid and are most often unilateral. Low-resistance peripheral or central flow is present. Metastasis would be uncommon but may occur within the liver or peritoneum. Teratomas, dysgerminomas,* and *endodermal sinus tumors are germ cell tumors that do not cause precocious puberty or virilization.*

▶ Rumack CM, Levine D (eds): *Diagnostic Ultrasound*, 5th edition. Philadelphia, Elsevier, 2018, pp 1879–1880.

▶ Siegel MJ (ed): *Pediatric Sonography*, 4th edition. Philadelphia, Lippincott Williams & Wilkins, 2011, pp 522–524, 526–527.

514. **C. Internal iliac arteries.**

> *The uterus is supplied by the* uterine arteries, *which descend from the anterior division of the* internal iliac arteries. *The anterior division or branch of the internal iliac is also called the* hypogastric artery. *The uterine artery travels through the cardinal ligament and crosses over the ureter anteriorly before reaching the uterus.*

▶ Rumack CM, Levine D (eds): *Diagnostic Ultrasound*, 5th edition. Philadelphia, Elsevier, 2018, pp 1872–1873.

▶ Siegel MJ (ed): *Pediatric Sonography*, 4th edition. Philadelphia, Lippincott Williams & Wilkins, 2011, p 536.

515. **D. The size.**

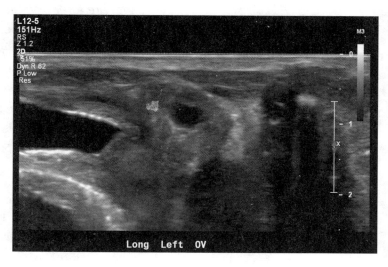

The size of the cyst is usually what differentiates a physiologic from a functional cyst. Physiologic cysts, *also known as* follicular cysts, *are typically less than 3 cm in size, while* functional cysts *are greater than 3 cm in size and can grow to be quite large. Cysts may also be characterized as simple or complex.* Simple cysts *are anechoic and thin-walled, demonstrating posterior enhancement. Simple cysts (as seen in this image) are uncomplicated by hemorrhage or torsion and usually resolve on their own within a few months. Cysts complicated by hemorrhage are called* complex cysts. Hemorrhagic cysts *occur when bleeding takes place within an ovarian cyst or corpus luteum. A hemorrhagic cyst appears complex on ultrasound, with low-level echoes and fluid-debris levels, or can demonstrate a cobweb appearance of fibrin strands. In cases of* torsion, *a twisted vascular pedicle may be identified with color Doppler. Both physiologic and functional cysts contain serous fluid and are lined by granulosa and theca cells. The age of the patient is irrelevant.*

▶ Rumack CM, Levine D (eds): *Diagnostic Ultrasound*, 5th edition. Philadelphia, Elsevier, 2018, pp 1873, 1875–1876.

▶ Siegel MJ (ed): *Pediatric Sonography*, 4th edition. Philadelphia, Lippincott Williams & Wilkins, 2011, pp 514–517.

516. **D. Progesterone.**

Progesterone *is produced primarily within the ovaries but also by the adrenal glands and the placenta. Its purpose is to help the body regulate the menstrual cycle and prepare for a pregnancy. Progesterone levels are elevated after ovulation as the corpus luteum continues to produce and release more progesterone. The progesterone signals the endometrium to prepare for implantation. If estrogen and progesterone levels drop, the endometrium will break down, triggering a menstrual cycle.* Estrogen *is the primary female hormone that assists in the development of secondary sex characteristics and the reproductive system and helps regulate the menstrual cycle.* Follicle-stimulating hormone *(FSH) promotes the maturation of the follicle to release the egg.* Human chorionic gonadotropin *(hCG) is found in a pregnant female's blood or urine.*

▶ Keough J: *Nursing Laboratory and Diagnostic Tests Demystified*, 2nd edition. New York, McGraw-Hill, 2017, pp 224–226, 262–264.

517. B. Pelvic inflammatory disease (PID).

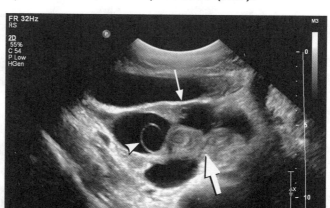

Pelvic inflammatory disease (PID) is an infection ascending from the genital tract, usually caused by a sexually transmitted disease (STD) such as gonorrhea or chlamydia. PID causes endometritis and inflammation of the fallopian tubes. If infected peritoneal fluid or pus spills out from the tubes into the peritoneal cavity, adhesions can form. A rare complication would be spread of the infected fluid into the perihepatic or perisplenic space. Clinical symptoms are pain and tenderness, fever, and vaginal discharge. PID is typically found in females of reproductive age. Sonographic findings of the uterus include poor definition of the uterine borders with endometrial fluid or thickening. There can be a hydrosalpinx (fluid-filled tube) that typically appears anechoic or a pyosalpinx (pus-filled tube) usually demonstrating low-level echoes and a thickened wall seen adjacent to the ovary. These are typically tubular-shaped unless they become large, and then they may appear round. If a tubo-ovarian abscess forms, a rounded complex intraovarian mass can demonstrate internal debris, septations, and even mobile hyperechoic foci that shadow, representing gas within the abscess. In this image, a tubo-ovarian complex depicts an ovary (thin arrow) located amongst a complex, irregular adnexal mass (thick arrow) adjacent to a fluid-filled tube (arrowhead). Appendicitis, dermoid cysts, and hemorrhagic cysts do not have an association with sexually transmitted diseases.

▶ Rumack CM, Levine D (eds): *Diagnostic Ultrasound*, 5th edition. Philadelphia, Elsevier, 2018, pp 1885–1887.

▶ Siegel MJ (ed): *Pediatric Sonography*, 4th edition. Philadelphia, Lippincott Williams & Wilkins, 2011, pp 366–371, 516–517, 528.

518. A. Uterus didelphys.

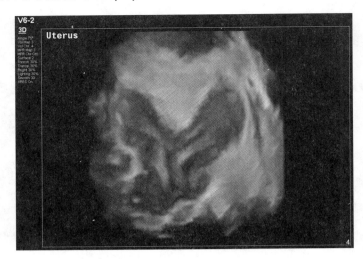

See Color Plate 29 on page xlv.

See also the diagram "Congenital Anomalies of the Uterus" in answer 500.

Uterine fusion anomalies include agenesis, hypoplasia, duplications, and septal defects. These abnormalities are congenital and the result of poor or improper müllerian duct fusion during organogenesis. Uterus didelphys *is defined as two complete uteri and cervices that do not communicate with each other. There can be two vaginas or, in some cases, a single vagina. A deep cleft is seen between the upper and mid uterine bodies.* A bicornuate uterus *has two uterine horns that are symmetric in size but fuse and communicate caudally.* A unicornuate uterus *occurs when there is only one uterine horn that communicates with the vagina. A contralateral smaller rudimentary horn may be present, but in most cases the uterus is curved and banana-shaped. An* arcuate uterus *is the mildest anomaly, usually with a small indentation (depth varies) into the fundal portion of the endometrial cavity, without any separation of the uterine horns or abnormal contour of the uterus.*

▶ de Bruyn R (ed): *Pediatric Ultrasound: How, Why and When*, 2nd edition (e-book). Philadelphia, Churchill Livingstone/Elsevier, 2010, pp 214–215.
▶ Rumack CM, Levine D (eds): *Diagnostic Ultrasound*, 5th edition. Philadelphia, Elsevier, 2018, p 1881.
▶ Siegel MJ (ed): *Pediatric Sonography*, 4th edition. Philadelphia, Lippincott Williams & Wilkins, 2011, pp 536–541.

519. D. Cystadenoma.

Cystadenomas *are a very uncommon finding in females younger than 20 years old. Cystadenomas are typically large masses that can reach 20 cm in size. There are two types.* Serous cystadenomas *are unilocular and composed of thin, watery fluid surrounded by thin walls.* Mucinous cystadenomas *are composed of a thicker, mucinous fluid and are multilocular* masses with septations. Both types may demonstrate wall nodules. Hemorrhagic *and* functional cysts *are commonly found in pediatric sonography.* Cystic teratomas (dermoids) *make up almost 70% of pediatric ovarian masses and are usually found after age 10.*

▶ Rumack CM, Levine D (eds): *Diagnostic Ultrasound*, 5th edition. Philadelphia, Elsevier, 2018, pp 1873, 1875–1876, 1880.

▶ Siegel MJ (ed): *Pediatric Sonography*, 4th edition. Philadelphia, Lippincott Williams & Wilkins, 2011, pp 511–514, 519–523.

520. **D. Daughter cyst.**

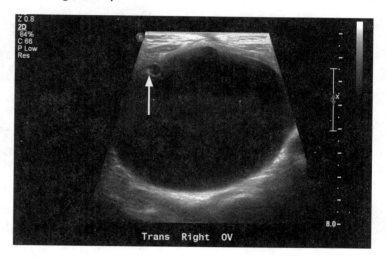

Daughter cyst *(arrow) is the term used for the presence of a follicle within an ovarian cyst. An* oocyte *is an immature egg that develops within a follicle. A* Graafian follicle *is the mature follicle that ruptures during ovulation to release an egg.* Theca-lutein cysts *occur bilaterally in patients with gestational trophoblastic disease or those with hyperstimulated ovaries.*

▶ Rumack CM, Levine D (eds): *Diagnostic Ultrasound*, 5th edition. Philadelphia, Elsevier, 2018, pp 1873, 1875–1876.

▶ Siegel MJ (ed): *Pediatric Sonography*, 4th edition. Philadelphia, Lippincott Williams & Wilkins, 2011, pp 516–518.

521. **C. Round ligament.**

The vascular pedicle of the ovary *is composed of the fallopian tube, broad ligament, and ovarian arteries and veins. Twisting of the vascular pedicle is a sonographic feature seen in cases of adnexal torsion. The* round ligament *originates from the uterine horns and exits the pelvis through the inguinal canal.*

▶ Rumack CM, Levine D (eds): *Diagnostic Ultrasound*, 5th edition. Philadelphia, Elsevier, 2018, pp 1872–1875.

▶ Siegel MJ (ed): *Pediatric Sonography*, 4th edition. Philadelphia, Lippincott Williams & Wilkins, 2011, p 532.

522. B. Bicornuate uterus.

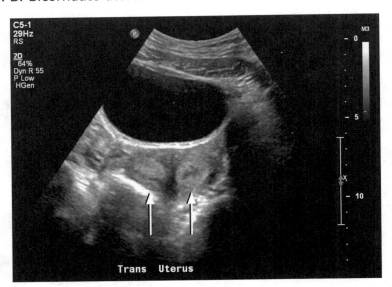

See the diagram "Congenital Anomalies of the Uterus" in answer 500.

A bicornuate uterus *consists of two symmetric uterine horns that communicate with each other caudally. There are two types.* Uterus duplex bicollis *is two uteri, two cervices, and one vagina.* Uterus duplex unicollis *is two uteri, one cervix, and one vagina.* Uterus didelphys *is the term for two uteri, two cervices, and two vaginas that do not communicate.* Septate uterus *is a single uterus whose endometrial cavity is divided by a septum of at least 1 cm.* Uterine agenesis *is the absence of a uterus.*

▸ de Bruyn R (ed): *Pediatric Ultrasound: How, Why and When*, 2nd edition (e-book). Philadelphia, Churchill Livingstone/Elsevier, 2010, p 215.

▸ Rumack CM, Levine D (eds): *Diagnostic Ultrasound*, 5th edition. Philadelphia, Elsevier, 2018, p 1881.

▸ Siegel MJ (ed): *Pediatric Sonography*, 4th edition. Philadelphia, Lippincott Williams & Wilkins, 2011, pp 536–541.

PART 14

Male Pelvis, Scrotum, and Testes

523. **C. Left renal vein.**

See Color Plate 13, "The Abdominal Vasculature," on page xxxviii.

The left testicular vein drains into the left renal vein and then the left renal vein into the inferior vena cava. For this reason, when a left varicocele is seen, evaluation of the left kidney should be performed. The left adrenal vein, as well as the left testicular vein, drains into the left renal vein. The right testicular vein drains directly into the inferior vena cava at a level inferior to the renal veins. The internal and external iliac veins drain into the common iliac vein bilaterally, and the right and left common iliac veins merge to form the inferior vena cava.

▶ de Bruyn R (ed): *Pediatric Ultrasound: How, Why and When*, 2nd edition (e-book). Philadelphia, Churchill Livingstone/Elsevier, 2010, pp 239–240.

▶ Siegel MJ (ed): *Pediatric Sonography*, 4th edition. Philadelphia, Lippincott Williams & Wilkins, 2011, p 556.

524. **A. Hypoechoic.**

Testicular torsion can have a different appearance based on the length of time that the testis has been twisted. Usually, when the testis is scanned within the first four hours from the time of the initial symptoms, the testicular echogenicity appears normal, but with decreased or absent color flow. Between 4 and 6 hours of torsion, the testis usually appears hypoechoic and enlarged. At this stage, if surgery for detorsion is performed, the salvage rate is 100%. A testis that has been torsed over 24 hours will appear heterogeneous and is usually not salvageable.

▶ de Bruyn R (ed): *Pediatric Ultrasound: How, Why and When*, 2nd edition (e-book). Philadelphia, Churchill Livingstone/Elsevier, 2010, pp 243–245.

▶ Rumack CM, Levine D (eds): *Diagnostic Ultrasound*, 5th edition. Philadelphia, Elsevier, 2018, p 1894.

▶ Siegel MJ (ed): *Pediatric Sonography*, 4th edition. Philadelphia, Lippincott Williams & Wilkins, 2011, p 573.

525. C. Decrease pulse repetition frequency.

See Color Plate 6 on page xxxv.

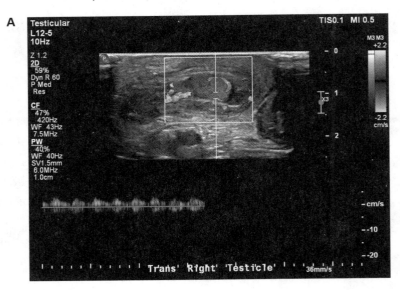

See Color Plate 30 on page xlvi.

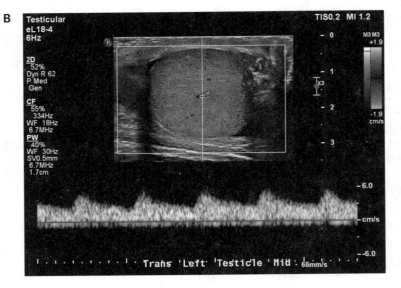

*When you are performing spectral Doppler evaluation of the testis, optimization of the scale is very important for an accurate diagnosis. Decreasing the pulse repetition frequency (PRF) will help with recognition of the low signals that may be missed when a higher PRF is used. Image **A** is an example of spectral Doppler of the testis with a suboptimal PRF. The original 2D image could have been improved by zooming in on the testis prior to applying any color or spectral Doppler. Decreasing the size of the gate or sample volume, decreasing the scale/PRF (seen as 2.2 cm/sec), and making the color box smaller around the testis would also enhance the Doppler results. Image **B** was optimized by decreasing the PRF or scale to 1.9 cm/sec. This 2D image is more focused on the*

testis itself, the color box is fitted more tightly around the testis, and the gate is smaller. Decreasing the gain and increasing the wall filter will eliminate lower signals and will not improve the quality of image **A**.

▶ Rumack CM, Levine D (eds): *Diagnostic Ultrasound*, 5th edition. Philadelphia, Elsevier, 2018, p 1890.

▶ Siegel MJ (ed): *Pediatric Sonography*, 4th edition. Philadelphia, Lippincott Williams & Wilkins, 2011, pp 557–558.

526. **D. Dartos.**

See Color Plate 31 on page xlvi.

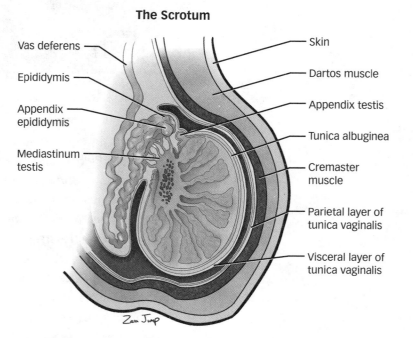

The cremaster and the dartos are two muscles in the scrotum that control its involuntary contraction and relaxation. The dartos muscle is more superficially located under the skin, and the cremaster muscle is more internally located between the two spermatic fascial layers (internal and external). The dartos and cremaster muscles allow the scrotum to contract or move upward when it is cold and relax or move downward when it is hot. This helps control the temperature of the testes so that the sperm can remain in ideal conditions. The internal oblique muscle is located in the abdominal wall and does not help with the movement of the scrotal sac. The raphe is a layer or ridge of fibrous tissue (not a muscle) located in the middle of the scrotum and dividing it into two sacs.

▶ Marcin J, Jewell T: Scrotum overview. Available at https://www.healthline.com/human-body-maps/scrotum.

▶ Siegel MJ (ed): *Pediatric Sonography*, 4th edition. Philadelphia, Lippincott Williams & Wilkins, 2011, pp 554–555.

527. B. Testicular appendage.

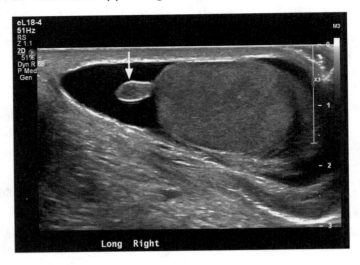

In this longitudinal image of the scrotum, the arrow points to a testicular appendage. A testicular appendage or appendix testis is an embryologic remnant of the müllerian duct that is located in the superior portion of the testis. The appendix testis is a pedunculated structure prone to torsion. Testicular appendages are usually easier to identify when they appear within a hydrocele, as in this image. Sonographically, an appendix testis is seen attached to the testis between the head of the epididymis and the upper pole of the testis. The appendix testis may demonstrate vascularity on color Doppler. The epididymal head *appears as a separate triangular structure superior to the upper pole of the testis and is not attached to the testis. A* scrotolith *is a free-floating macrocalcification found within the scrotum. Scrotoliths are hyperechoic and are seen resting in the dependent portion of the scrotum when accompanied by a hydrocele. The* epididymal tail *is usually seen in the posterolateral and inferior aspect of the testis, and it is not a pedunculated structure extending from the testis.*

▶ de Bruyn R (ed): *Pediatric Ultrasound: How, Why and When*, 2nd edition (e-book). Philadelphia, Churchill Livingstone/Elsevier, 2010, p 240.
▶ Rumack CM, Levine D (eds): *Diagnostic Ultrasound*, 5th edition. Philadelphia, Elsevier, 2018, p 1897.
▶ Siegel MJ (ed): *Pediatric Sonography*, 4th edition. Philadelphia, Lippincott Williams & Wilkins, 2011, p 556.

528. A. Orchitis.

Orchitis *is the inflammation of the testis and is most often seen with epididymitis. When the two conditions occur together they are known as* epididymo-orchitis, *which is more common than isolated orchitis. Epididymo-orchitis results from* the spread of the epididymal inflammation to the testis. When orchitis is isolated, it is commonly associated with mumps. The sonographic appearance of orchitis is a hypoechoic enlarged testis with increased color flow when acute and heterogeneous in appearance over time. Intratesticular neoplasms *and* "bell-clapper" deformity *are associated with testicular torsion, not with epididymitis. A resolved* testicular torsion *(detorsion) can have an effect called reactive hyperemia, whereby there is increased color flow within the testis on Doppler interrogation, which can mimic the increased flow of epididymo-orchitis. The clinical findings can help differentiate between these two conditions because with testicular detorsion, the sudden onset of testicular pain resolves; with epididymo-orchitis, the pain is usually gradual and will still be present at the time of the examination.*

▶ de Bruyn R (ed): *Pediatric Ultrasound: How, Why and When*, 2nd edition (e-book). Philadelphia, Churchill Livingstone/Elsevier, 2010, pp 243–244.
▶ Rumack CM, Levine D (eds): *Diagnostic Ultrasound*, 5th edition. Philadelphia, Elsevier, 2018, pp 1896–1897.
▶ Siegel MJ (ed): *Pediatric Sonography*, 4th edition. Philadelphia, Lippincott Williams & Wilkins, 2011, pp 574, 580, 583.

529. B. Cryptorchidism.

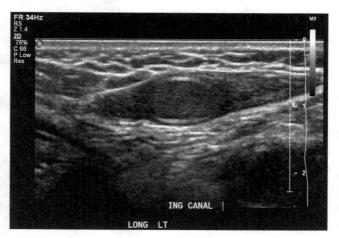

Cryptorchidism *(undescended testes) is a congenital condition in which the testes do not descend into the scrotum. Normally, the testes descend between the 25th and the 32nd weeks of gestation. At birth, the testes may still not be within the scrotum, but the descent can continue up to the first year of age. Patients with testes that have not descended after the first year of life have true cryptorchidism. As seen in this image, an undescended testis is located within the inguinal canal, which is most common. Patients with cryptorchidism have a higher risk of developing testicular malignancy,*

infertility, and torsion. Cryptorchidism has been associated with Prader-Willi syndrome, prune belly syndrome, and abdominal wall defects. Testicular torsion *is demonstrated by the absence of color and spectral Doppler on ultrasound, and this image shows a testis that lies within the inguinal canal.* Crossed testicular ectopia *refers to the abnormal location of a contralateral testis within the same side of the scrotum.* Polyorchidism, *also known as* supernumerary testis, *is a testicular duplication, usually on one side of the scrotum.*

▶ de Bruyn R (ed): *Pediatric Ultrasound: How, Why and When*, 2nd edition (e-book). Philadelphia, Churchill Livingstone/Elsevier, 2010, pp 236–237, 241, 242, 246.

▶ Rumack CM, Levine D (eds): *Diagnostic Ultrasound*, 5th edition. Philadelphia, Elsevier, 2018, p 1890.

▶ Siegel MJ (ed): *Pediatric Sonography*, 4th edition. Philadelphia, Lippincott Williams & Wilkins, 2011, pp 559–562.

530. D. Visceral and parietal layers of the tunica vaginalis.

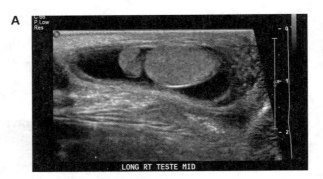

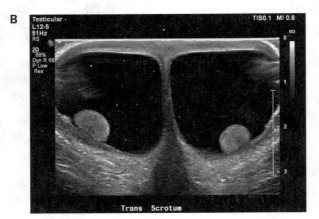

See Color Plate 31, "The Scrotum," on page xlvi.

A hydrocele *is an abnormal fluid accumulation between the visceral and parietal layers of the tunica vaginalis.* Image **A** *represents a longitudinal image of the right hemiscrotum with fluid within it.* Image **B** *demonstrates bilateral hydroceles on a transverse plane. Hydroceles are usually isolated to the scrotum but can sometimes be seen with associated abdominal fluid due to a ventriculo-peritoneal shunt, hemorrhage, or* infection. The fluid from the abdomen can descend to the scrotum via a patent tunica vaginalis. Hydroceles are typically anechoic or composed of serous fluid but can have debris and septations due to hemorrhage and infections. When the fluid collection is composed of blood, they are called **hematoceles**, and when composed of lymph fluid they are known as **lymphoceles**. Lymphoceles are usually due to a leakage of lymph fluid into the scrotum following a renal transplant.

▶ de Bruyn R (ed): *Pediatric Ultrasound: How, Why and When*, 2nd edition (e-book). Philadelphia, Churchill Livingstone/Elsevier, 2010, pp 241–243.
▶ Rumack CM, Levine D (eds): *Diagnostic Ultrasound*, 5th edition. Philadelphia, Elsevier, 2018, pp 1899, 1902.
▶ Siegel MJ (ed): *Pediatric Sonography*, 4th edition. Philadelphia, Lippincott Williams & Wilkins, 2011, pp 587–590.

531. **D. Hernia.**

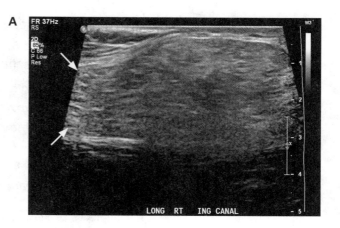

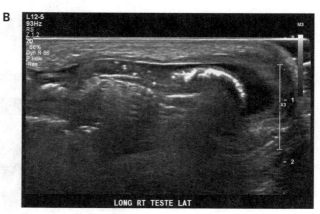

Image **A** demonstrates the presence of omental fat within the scrotal sac, herniated through an inguinal defect (arrows), which is consistent with an inguinal hernia. Inguinal hernias in children are usually associated with a patent processus vaginalis (vaginal process) and are more common on the right side. Inguinal hernias can be easily identified with ultrasound when bowel or omentum is present within the *scrotum, as seen in image* **B**. *The presence of peristalsing bowel loops within the scrotal sac suggests viable bowel, whereas nonperistalsing bowel may represent an incarcerated hernia.* Varicoceles *are dilated veins of the pampiniform plexus and appear as tubular cystic structures in the spermatic cord region.* Epididymitis *is the inflammation of the epididymis, and on ultrasound an enlarged heterogeneous epididymis is usually seen with hyperemia.* Hydroceles *are fluid collections within the two layers of tunica vaginalis and normally appear as simple fluid surrounding the testis.*

▶ de Bruyn R (ed): *Pediatric Ultrasound: How, Why and When*, 2nd edition (e-book). Philadelphia, Churchill Livingstone/Elsevier, 2010, pp 241–243.

▶ Rumack CM, Levine D (eds): *Diagnostic Ultrasound*, 5th edition. Philadelphia, Elsevier, 2018, p 1902.

▶ Siegel MJ (ed): *Pediatric Sonography*, 4th edition. Philadelphia, Lippincott Williams & Wilkins, 2011, pp 590–591.

▶ Zihni I, Duran A, Soysal V: A rare cause of inguinal hernia: scrotal cystocele. Ulus Cerrahi Derg 32:137–139, 2016.

532. **C. Medium-level echoes.**

The normal echogenicity of the testes in patients older than 8 (including adults) would be medium-level echoes. In infancy and early childhood, the testicular echogenicity is more low-level to medium-level echoes and will increase with age. The normal testes have an ovoid shape and should always have a homogeneous appearance.

▶ Rumack CM, Levine D (eds): *Diagnostic Ultrasound*, 5th edition. Philadelphia, Elsevier, 2018, p 1888.

▶ Siegel MJ (ed): *Pediatric Sonography*, 4th edition. Philadelphia, Lippincott Williams & Wilkins, 2011, pp 555–556.

533. **A. Embryonal rhabdomyosarcoma.**

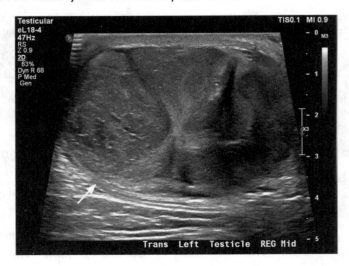

Embryonal rhabdomyosarcomas *are the most common type of paratesticular malignant neoplasms affecting children 5 years old or younger. In general, paratesticular tumors are rare and typically involve the spermatic cord. An embryonal rhabdomyosarcoma clinically presents as a rapidly growing but painless scrotal mass. Sonographically, paratesticular embryonal rhabdomyosarcomas vary and can be homogeneous, heterogeneous, hypoechoic, hyperechoic, or isoechoic to the testis. This image of an embryonal rhabdomyosarcoma demonstrates a heterogeneous appearing mass. Embryonal rhabdomyosarcomas appear as well-circumscribed, solid masses, often displaying hyperemic color flow.* Adenomatoid tumors *and* neurofibromas *are benign masses and are uncommon.* Seminomas *are a type of intratesticular neoplasm occurring more commonly in adults. Paratesticular masses are difficult to differentiate based only on their ultrasound appearance and require more testing for final diagnosis.*

▶ de Bruyn R (ed): *Pediatric Ultrasound: How, Why and When*, 2nd edition (e-book). Philadelphia, Churchill Livingstone/Elsevier, 2010, pp 247–248.

▶ Rumack CM, Levine D (eds): *Diagnostic Ultrasound*, 5th edition. Philadelphia, Elsevier, 2018, pp 1903–1904.

▶ Siegel MJ (ed): *Pediatric Sonography*, 4th edition. Philadelphia, Lippincott Williams & Wilkins, 2011, pp 563, 568–569.

534. D. Nutcracker syndrome.

The "nutcracker" syndrome is a condition in which the left renal vein is compressed as it courses between the superior mesenteric artery (SMA) and the aorta. Because the left testicular vein drains into the left renal vein, this compression can cause increased backflow pressure into the testicular pampiniform plexus of veins, predisposing the patient to the formation of scrotal varices. Patients with nutcracker syndrome are at risk of recurrence of varicoceles even after treatment. With epididymo-orchitis, *hyperemia within the testes and adjacent tissues can be seen, but not varicoceles.* Hydrocele *is an accumulation of fluid within the scrotum and does not cause a varicocele. A* bell-clapper deformity *increases the risk of testicular torsion, not varicoceles.*

▶ Kurklinsky AK, Rooke TW: Nutcracker phenomenon and nutcracker syndrome. Mayo Clin Proc 85:552–559, 2010.

▶ Siegel MJ (ed): *Pediatric Sonography*, 4th edition. Philadelphia, Lippincott Williams & Wilkins, 2011, p 590.

535. B. Epididymitis.

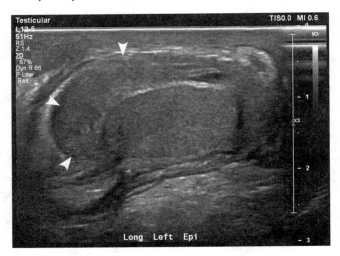

Acute epididymitis *is the inflammation of the epididymis and is a common cause of acute scrotal pain in adolescents. Epididymitis is more common in pubertal than in prepubertal patients, and in older patients it is often associated with sexually transmitted organisms. When epididymitis is present in children, it may be associated with genitourinary infections or abnormalities. Patients with epididymitis may also present with scrotal edema and pyuria. Sonographically, the epididymis (most commonly the head) may appear enlarged and heterogeneous (arrowheads). With color Doppler, the affected side appears hyperemic in comparison to the contralateral side.* Orchitis *is the inflammation of the testis; symptoms and sonographic findings similar to epididymitis are seen, but affecting the testis instead.* Testicular torsion *and* testicular appendage torsion *typically present with a sudden onset of testicular pain, and on ultrasound diminished or absent color flow within these structures is seen.*

▶ de Bruyn R (ed): *Pediatric Ultrasound: How, Why and When*, 2nd edition (e-book). Philadelphia, Churchill Livingstone/Elsevier, 2010, pp 245–246.
▶ Rumack CM, Levine D (eds): *Diagnostic Ultrasound*, 5th edition. Philadelphia, Elsevier, 2018, pp 1895–1897.
▶ Siegel MJ (ed): *Pediatric Sonography*, 4th edition. Philadelphia, Lippincott Williams & Wilkins, 2011, pp 578, 580.

536. D. Androgen.

The embryologic process in which the testes descend from the abdomen to the scrotum is controlled by androgens. The fetal testes develop within the abdomen and start migrating downward between conceptual weeks 8 and 16. At this stage, this process is controlled mainly by the insulin-like factor 3 (Insl3) and testosterone, hormones regulated by Leydig cells.

As the testes continue traveling caudally into the inguinal canal opening, the second phase of testicular descent starts and is controlled by androgens. At this stage the testes move through the inguinal canal into the scrotal sac. The testicular descent is normally completed by week 32. During fetal development, conditions associated with lower gonadotropin levels, such as Prader-Willi syndrome, can be accompanied by cryptorchidism. During embryonic development testosterone plays an important role in development of external genitalia but not in testicular descent. Follicle-stimulating hormone (FSH) is important for fertility. Human chorionic gonadotropin (hCG) is the hormone produced by the placenta during early pregnancy; its main function is to promote progesterone production. FSH and hCG do not contribute to the testicular descent into the scrotum.

▶ Bay K, Main KM, Toppari J, et al: Testicular descent: INSL3, testosterone, genes and the intrauterine milieu. Nat Rev Urol 8:187–196, 2011.
▶ de Bruyn R (ed): *Pediatric Ultrasound: How, Why and When*, 2nd edition (e-book). Philadelphia, Churchill Livingstone/Elsevier, 2010, p 236.
▶ Patni P, Mohanty SK, Singh R: Embryonic development of the testis. In Singh R, Singh K (eds): *Male Infertility: Understanding, Causes and Treatment*. Singapore, Springer, 2017, pp 13–24.
▶ Siegel MJ (ed): *Pediatric Sonography*, 4th edition. Philadelphia, Lippincott Williams & Wilkins, 2011, p 561.

537. **A. Epididymis.**

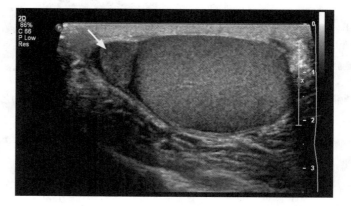

The epididymis is a bowed, tubular structure composed of ductules. It lies posterolateral to the testis. The epididymis appears as an isoechoic structure when compared to the testicular echogenicity on ultrasound. The epididymal head (arrow) can be seen lying superior to the testis as a triangular-shaped structure that is continuous with the epididymal body, which lies along the posterolateral margin of the testis. The tail of the epididymis is located in the inferior aspect of the testis. The epididymal body and tail may be difficult to *delineate, especially if there is no fluid around them or if the patient is young and the scrotum is small. The* mediastinum *is an echogenic linear structure located posteriorly within the testis and merges with the tunica albuginea. The* spermatic cord *is a cord-like structure that extends from the testis to the inguinal canal. The spermatic cord contains the testicular arteries, the pampiniform plexus of veins, lymphatics, and the vas deferens.*

▶ de Bruyn R (ed): *Pediatric Ultrasound: How, Why and When*, 2nd edition (e-book). Philadelphia, Churchill Livingstone/Elsevier, 2010, pp 235, 236, 238–240.

▶ Healthline: Epididymis. Available at https://www.healthline.com/human-body-maps/epididymis#1.

▶ Rumack CM, Levine D (eds): *Diagnostic Ultrasound*, 5th edition. Philadelphia, Elsevier, 2018, p 1890.

▶ Siegel MJ (ed): *Pediatric Sonography*, 4th edition. Philadelphia, Lippincott Williams & Wilkins, 2011, pp 555, 557.

538. A. Epididymal cyst.

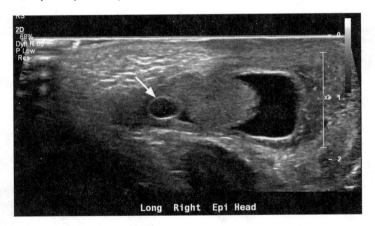

Epididymal cysts *are simple cystic structures (arrow) that can be found anywhere in the epididymis and are usually seen as an incidental finding. Epididymal cysts are dilated efferent tubules that contain clear serous fluid. These cystic structures appear as simple anechoic structures with thin, well-defined walls.* Spermatoceles *can have an appearance similar to that of an epididymal cyst, but they occur only in pubertal patients and are located in the head of the epididymis.* Epididymal cystadenomas *and* lymphangiomas *are more complex cystic masses.*

▶ Rumack CM, Levine D (eds): *Diagnostic Ultrasound*, 5th edition. Philadelphia, Elsevier, 2018, pp 1902–1903.

▶ Siegel MJ (ed): *Pediatric Sonography*, 4th edition. Philadelphia, Lippincott Williams & Wilkins, 2011, pp 569–570.

539. B. Intravaginal testicular torsion.

An intravaginal testicular torsion *is a testicular torsion inside the tunica vaginalis. An* extravaginal testicular torsion *occurs when the torsion is outside of the tunica vaginalis. The "bell-clapper" deformity is an abnormality associated with insertion of the tunica vaginalis higher than normal on the spermatic cord instead of the lower pole. The tunica then surrounds the entire testis and the testis hangs within it like a clapper in a bell. This is the most common cause of intravaginal testicular torsion because the surrounding tunica prevents fixation of the testis to the scrotum and allows free testicular rotation. Extravaginal testicular torsion (spermatic cord level) most commonly occurs in utero and in neonates when there is poor fixation of the spermatic cord to the inguinal canal.*

▶ de Bruyn R (ed): *Pediatric Ultrasound: How, Why and When*, 2nd edition (e-book). Philadelphia, Churchill Livingstone/Elsevier, 2010, pp 243–246.

▶ Rumack CM, Levine D (eds): *Diagnostic Ultrasound*, 5th edition. Philadelphia, Elsevier, 2018, p 1893.

▶ Siegel MJ (ed): *Pediatric Sonography*, 4th edition. Philadelphia, Lippincott Williams & Wilkins, 2011, pp 572–576.

540. C. Compression.

See Color Plate 7 on page xxxvi.

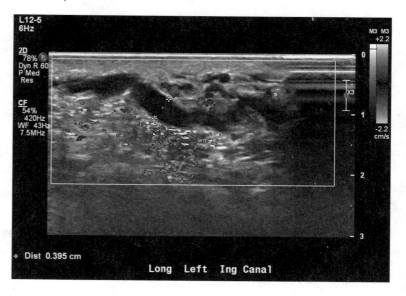

Varicocele *is the enlargement of the veins in the pampiniform plexus of the testis. Maneuvers that increase the visibility of blood flow on Doppler and help with the diagnosis of varicocele are the Valsalva maneuver and placing the patient in a standing or reverse Trendelenburg position. Varicocele is more common on the left side, and it affects primarily adolescents and young adults. Sonographically varicoceles*

appear as tortuous tubular structures (as seen in this image) adjacent to the testis that usually measure more than 2 mm in diameter. Compression does not help with the diagnosis of varicocele because there is no increased blood flow to the spermatic cord. Compression may cause decreased visibility of the varicocele.

▶ de Bruyn R (ed): *Pediatric Ultrasound: How, Why and When*, 2nd edition (e-book). Philadelphia, Churchill Livingstone/Elsevier, 2010, p 243.
▶ Rumack CM, Levine D (eds): *Diagnostic Ultrasound*, 5th edition. Philadelphia, Elsevier, 2018, p 1902.
▶ Siegel MJ (ed): *Pediatric Sonography*, 4th edition. Philadelphia, Lippincott Williams & Wilkins, 2011, p 590.

541. **B. True hermaphroditism.**

An *ovotestis is a gonad that contains ovarian and testicular tissue at the same time. Ovotestes are seen with* true hermaphroditism, *an intersex disorder. Patients with true hermaphroditism usually have ambiguous genitalia and can also have separate testicular and ovarian gonads (not just an ovotestis).* Hypospadias, cryptorchidism, *and* monorchidism *are not associated with ovotestes.*

▶ Rumack CM, Levine D (eds): *Diagnostic Ultrasound*, 5th edition. Philadelphia, Elsevier, 2018, p 1891.
▶ ScienceDirect: True hermaphroditism. Available at https://www.sciencedirect.com/topics/medicine-and-dentistry/true-hermaphroditism.

542. **C. Aorta.**

The testicular arteries *arise directly from the aorta and travel down in the abdomen, passing through the inguinal ring. Within the spermatic cord, the testicular artery courses posterior to the testis, entering the mediastinum testis. The testicular artery supplies the majority of the oxygenated blood to the testis. The* cremasteric artery *and the* deferential artery *are also within the spermatic cord; the cremasteric artery arises from the inferior epigastric artery and the deferential artery arises from the vesicular artery. These supply the epididymis, vas deferens, and paratesticular tissue. All three arteries—testicular, cremasteric, and deferential—anastomose. The inferior epigastric artery and the vesicular artery arise from the external iliac artery and internal iliac artery respectively.*

▶ de Bruyn R (ed): *Pediatric Ultrasound: How, Why and When*, 2nd edition (e-book). Philadelphia, Churchill Livingstone/Elsevier, 2010, p 238.
▶ Siegel MJ (ed): *Pediatric Sonography*, 4th edition. Philadelphia, Lippincott Williams & Wilkins, 2011, pp 555–556.

543. D. Teratoma.

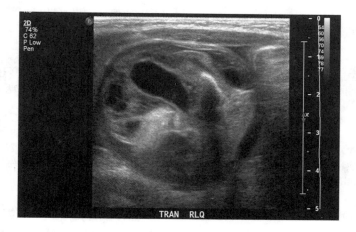

Teratomas *are the most common benign germ cell tumor of the testis.* Germ cell tumors *account for the majority of the primary testicular neoplasms in children.* Teratomas *typically demonstrate good differentiation of the three embryonal cell layers (epithelium, bone/cartilage, and muscle). They appear as well-defined heterogeneous masses with hypoechoic areas, cystic areas, and calcifications, as seen in this image. An endodermal sinus tumor (also known as a yolk sac tumor) can have the same sonographic appearance as a teratoma but (unlike most teratomas) is a malignant neoplasm. Seminomas are also malignant and are rare in the pediatric population. Seminomas commonly appear hypoechoic and homogeneous on ultrasound. While* epidermoid cysts *may also resemble teratomas or have a hypoechoic appearance with an echogenic rim, they are extremely rare masses in children.*

▶ de Bruyn R (ed): P*ediatric Ultrasound: How, Why and When*, 2nd edition (e-book). Philadelphia, Churchill Livingstone/Elsevier, 2010, p 238.

▶ Rumack CM, Levine D (eds): *Diagnostic Ultrasound*, 5th edition. Philadelphia, Elsevier, 2018, pp 1899, 1901.

▶ Siegel MJ (ed): *Pediatric Sonography*, 4th edition. Philadelphia, Lippincott Williams & Wilkins, 2011, pp 562–563, 566.

544. A. Penis.

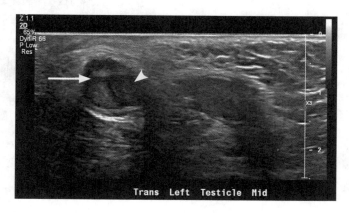

This image of the scrotum demonstrates the left testis in the left side of the transverse image, with the penis indicated by the arrow. In pediatric patients, the penis is commonly imaged incidentally during a scan of the scrotum; thus, recognition of its anatomy is important. The penis appears as a tubular structure that contains the two corpora cavernosa (seen on either side of the arrow), one corpus spongiosum (arrowhead), and the urethra. In a transverse cross-section image, most of these structures can be appreciated. Testicular tissue is homogeneous, so if you are imaging the left testis and see a heterogeneous structure medially, penile tissue should be considered. The epididymis and testicular appendages are normally seen within the scrotum adjacent to the testis, not separated and medial to it.

▶ Abdominal Key: Penile ultrasound. Available at https://abdominalkey.com/penile-ultrasound/.

545. B. 2.5 cm.

The prepubertal testis normally measures between 2.0 and 3.0 cm in length and about 1.2 cm in width. The testis maintains about the same size from age 3 months to puberty. The normal testicular length in a neonate is considered to be about 0.7–1.5 cm, with a width of 1.0 cm. In older postpubertal children the mean testicular length is about 3–5 cm and the mean width is about 2–3 cm. A normal testicular volume for an infant is approximately 1.0 cm³ and for a postpubertal child and adolescent up to 30 cm³.

▶ Rumack CM, Levine D (eds): *Diagnostic Ultrasound*, 5th edition. Philadelphia, Elsevier, 2018, p 1888.

▶ Siegel MJ (ed): *Pediatric Sonography*, 4th edition. Philadelphia, Lippincott Williams & Wilkins, 2011, p 556.

546. A. Klinefelter syndrome.

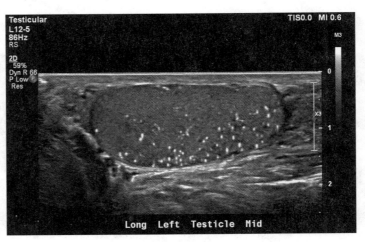

Testicular microlithiasis *is a condition characterized by multiple echogenic foci throughout the testis, as seen in this image. Usually bilateral, microlithiasis may be unilateral or isolated to a focal area within a testis. Microlithiasis may be an isolated condition or associated with Down syndrome, Klinefelter syndrome, cystic fibrosis, or cryptorchidism. Microlithiasis in the testis appears on ultrasound as tiny calcifications within the seminiferous tubules that measure between 1 and 3 mm. These small calcifications may, but more often do not, present posterior shadowing. They are commonly seen scattered throughout the testis. Microlithiasis has been associated with an increased risk of testicular malignancy.* Eagle-Barrett syndrome, Prader-Willi syndrome, *and* Noonan syndrome *are associated with cryptorchidism and not with microlithiasis.*

▶ de Bruyn R (ed): *Pediatric Ultrasound: How, Why and When*, 2nd edition (e-book). Philadelphia, Churchill Livingstone/Elsevier, 2010, p 246.

▶ Rumack CM, Levine D (eds): *Diagnostic Ultrasound*, 5th edition. Philadelphia, Elsevier, 2018, pp 1904, 1906.

▶ Siegel MJ (ed): *Pediatric Sonography*, 4th edition. Philadelphia, Lippincott Williams & Wilkins, 2011, pp 593–594.

547. **D. Tunica albuginea.**

Testicular rupture *occurs when the tunica albuginea is disrupted. Testicular rupture is a surgical emergency that is often the result of a sports injury. Sonographically, the echogenic* tunica albuginea *that surrounds the testis will appear interrupted, and the testis may appear heterogeneous with irregular borders. The difference between testicular fracture and testicular rupture is that with a testicular fracture, the tunica albuginea is not affected or disrupted. The external spermatic fascia, cremasteric fascia, and tunica vaginalis are more external layers and do not determine whether there is testicular rupture or not.*

▶ Rumack CM, Levine D (eds): *Diagnostic Ultrasound*, 5th edition. Philadelphia, Elsevier, 2018, pp 1897–1898.

▶ Siegel MJ (ed): *Pediatric Sonography*, 4th edition. Philadelphia, Lippincott Williams & Wilkins, 2011, pp 585–587.

548. **D. Tunica albuginea.**

See Color Plate 31, "The Scrotum," on page xlvi.

The mediastinum testis *is a portion of fibrous tissue located in the posterior aspect of the testis. The tunica albuginea is the most internal layer that covers the testis. The mediastinum testis is formed when the tunica albuginea wraps around the testis from an anterior to posterior aspect and invaginates* into the testis in that posterior area. The mediastinum testis is the site where the vessels and ducts enter and exit the testis. On ultrasound, the mediastinum testis appears as an echogenic line along the posteromedial aspect of the testis. The cremasteric fascia and cremasteric muscle form a layer of the scrotum and spermatic cord located between the internal and external spermatic fascia. The cremasteric muscle and fascia give support to the scrotum and testes and allow contraction of the scrotal sac for protection and temperature regulation. The internal spermatic fascia is located between the tunica vaginalis (internal) and the cremaster muscle and fascia (superficial) in the scrotum, and in the spermatic cord this layer is the most internal and covers the spermatic cord directly. The tunica vaginalis has two layers, and they surround the testis except for the mediastinum area (posterior). Between the two layers of the tunica vaginalis—the visceral and parietal layers—hydroceles can form.

▶ de Bruyn R (ed): *Pediatric Ultrasound: How, Why and When*, 2nd edition (e-book). Philadelphia, Churchill Livingstone/Elsevier, 2010, p 238.
▶ Rumack CM, Levine D (eds): *Diagnostic Ultrasound*, 5th edition. Philadelphia, Elsevier, 2018, p 1888.
▶ Siegel MJ (ed): *Pediatric Sonography*, 4th edition. Philadelphia, Lippincott Williams & Wilkins, 2011, pp 554–555.

549. **C. Testosterone.**

Testosterone *is a hormone produced by the testes which initiates development of, and maintains, secondary male sexual characteristics. These characteristics include body and facial hair, boosted musculature, deep voice, and enlargement of the genitals.* Estrogen *is the hormone in charge of the female secondary sexual characteristics. Estrogen is also present in men, in whom it helps control spermatogenesis in the testes. Although* luteinizing hormone *is often thought of as a female hormone, in men it helps the testes to form testosterone.* Inhibin *is the hormone responsible for the maturation and health of the sperm.*

▶ Bellman G: Male hormones and their functions. Available at https://www.maleantiaginginstitute.com/blog/Male-Hormones—Their-Functions.html.

550. **B. Anorchidism.**

Bilateral agenesis of the testes is also known as anorchidism (or anorchism). *This is a congenital anomaly and is associated with abnormal external genitalia. Anorchidism occurs in 1:20,000 newborn males.* Monorchidism *refers to the absence of one testis.* Cryptorchidism *occurs when the testes have not descended into the scrotum.* Triorchidism *refers to an additional accessory testis in addition to the normal two.*

▶ Rumack CM, Levine D (eds): *Diagnostic Ultrasound*, 5th edition. Philadelphia, Elsevier, 2018, pp 1890–1891.

▶ Siegel MJ (ed): *Pediatric Sonography*, 4th edition. Philadelphia, Lippincott Williams & Wilkins, 2011, pp 559, 561.

551. A. Seminoma.

Seminomas *are the most common testicular tumor in adults but are rare in the pediatric population. Seminomas are associated with undescended testes.* Teratomas *are the most common benign tumor of the testis in children.* Embryonal carcinomas *usually occur in adolescence and are not associated with cryptorchidism.* Endodermal sinus tumors *are common in the prepubertal age group and again are not associated with undescended testes.*

▶ de Bruyn R (ed): *Pediatric Ultrasound: How, Why and When*, 2nd edition (e-book). Philadelphia, Churchill Livingstone/Elsevier, 2010, p 241.

▶ Rumack CM, Levine D (eds): *Diagnostic Ultrasound*, 5th edition. Philadelphia, Elsevier, 2018, p 1899.

552. B. Testicular torsion.

See Color Plate 8 on page xxxvi.

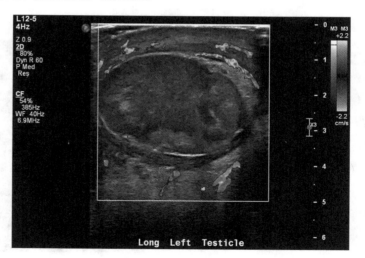

Absence of color Doppler flow in an acutely painful testis is consistent with the diagnosis of testicular torsion. Testicular torsion is a common cause of acute testicular pain and swelling in children and adolescents (most commonly in adolescents and young adults). Patients with testicular torsion will present with an acute onset of testicular pain, often accompanied by vomiting. Clinically, a transverse and higher lie of the twisted testis can be seen due to shortening of the

vascular pedicle. Sonography is the imaging modality of choice when the diagnosis cannot be done clinically. Comparison of both testes with color Doppler should be performed in all patients with possible torsion, because this will show the asymmetry in flow between the normal and affected testes. Also, with partial torsion of the spermatic cord (360 degrees or less), arterial flow may be seen, but it will appear diminished when compared to the unaffected testis. Orchitis *is an inflammatory process in which the testis appears hyperemic on ultrasound. With a* testicular hematoma, *focal areas of absent color Doppler may be seen, but this will not affect the entire testicular tissue and vascularity.* Appendiceal torsion *presents with symptoms similar to those of testicular torsion but on ultrasound demonstrates normal perfusion of the testis with an avascular appendage.*

▸ Cohen HL, Sivit CJ: *Fetal and Pediatric Ultrasound: A Casebook Approach.* New York, McGraw-Hill, 2001, pp 533–537.

▸ de Bruyn R (ed): *Pediatric Ultrasound: How, Why and When,* 2nd edition (e-book). Philadelphia, Churchill Livingstone/Elsevier, 2010, pp 243–245.

▸ Rumack CM, Levine D (eds): *Diagnostic Ultrasound,* 5th edition. Philadelphia, Elsevier, 2018, pp 1895–1898.

▸ Siegel MJ (ed): *Pediatric Sonography,* 4th edition. Philadelphia, Lippincott Williams & Wilkins, 2011, pp 571–578, 580.

553. C. Cryptorchidism.

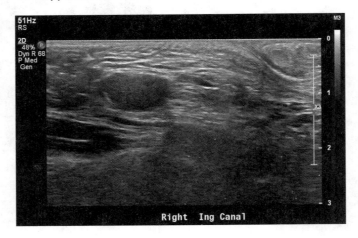

In this image, the testis can be visualized within the inguinal canal, supporting the diagnosis of cryptorchidism, *also known as* undescended testes. *Undescended testes are common in premature infants weighing less than 2500 grams at birth. With undescended testes, the scrotal sac is empty (unilaterally or bilaterally) and one or both testes are found within the inguinal canal, up in the abdomen, or in the pelvis near the bladder. For the diagnosis of* herniated bowel *or* omentum, *these structures are seen within the scrotum adjacent to*

the normal scrotal contents. Peristalsing bowel within the scrotum is diagnostic of an inguinal herniation. Hydrocele is an accumulation of fluid within the scrotum between the two layers of the tunica vaginalis.

▶ de Bruyn R (ed): *Pediatric Ultrasound: How, Why and When*, 2nd edition (e-book). Philadelphia, Churchill Livingstone/Elsevier, 2010, pp 237–238, 241.

▶ Rumack CM, Levine D (eds): *Diagnostic Ultrasound*, 5th edition. Philadelphia, Elsevier, 2018, p 1890.

▶ Siegel MJ (ed): *Pediatric Sonography*, 4th edition. Philadelphia, Lippincott Williams & Wilkins, 2011, p 561.

554. **D. Monorchidism.**

Monorchidism is a congenital anomaly in which there is unilateral agenesis of a testis. Monorchidism is associated with a blind-ending spermatic cord and vessels. This is thought to be caused by the development and subsequent disappearance of the testis. It may be due to an in utero testicular torsion or a vascular accident. Anorchidism *is bilateral testicular agenesis.* Polyorchidism *is a supernumerary testis.* Cryptorchidism *is the failure of the testes to descend into the scrotal sac. Anorchidism, polyorchidism, and cryptorchidism are not associated with a blind-ending spermatic cord.*

▶ Rumack CM, Levine D (eds): *Diagnostic Ultrasound*, 5th edition. Philadelphia, Elsevier, 2018, pp 1890–1891.

▶ Siegel MJ (ed): *Pediatric Sonography*, 4th edition. Philadelphia, Lippincott Williams & Wilkins, 2011, pp 559, 561.

555. **B. Spermatocele.**

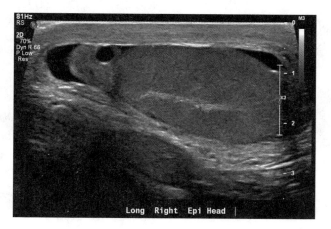

Spermatoceles are cystic structures found in the head of the epididymis in postpubertal patients. Patients with spermatoceles may present with a painless palpable mass in the superior portion of the testis, although these masses are most commonly found incidentally. Spermatoceles are dilated

efferent tubules that contain spermatozoa. Sonographically, spermatoceles appear as thin-walled anechoic or hypoechoic structures with posterior enhancement, located in the head of the epididymis (as seen in this image). Epididymal cystadenomas *are complex cystic masses, not simple.* Testicular cysts *are located within the testes (not epididymis) and are rare in the pediatric population.* Lymphangiomas *are paratesticular cystic structures that usually contain septations.*

▸ Rumack CM, Levine D (eds): *Diagnostic Ultrasound*, 5th edition. Philadelphia, Elsevier, 2018, pp 1902–1903.

▸ Siegel MJ (ed): *Pediatric Sonography*, 4th edition. Philadelphia, Lippincott Williams & Wilkins, 2011, pp 569–570.

556. **A. Testicular appendage torsion.**

The "blue dot sign" refers to a bluish discoloration of a small, firm testicular nodule (often in the upper pole of the testis/scrotum) that is visible through the skin. This is a classic clinical finding of testicular appendage torsion. Patients with a torsed appendage will present with symptoms similar to those of testicular torsion. On ultrasound, torsion of the appendix testis appears as an avascular ovoid mass near the superior aspect of the testis with surrounding hypervascularity. Testicular torsion, infarction, and trauma *are not clinically associated with the blue dot sign.*

▸ Cohen HL, Sivit CJ: *Fetal and Pediatric Ultrasound: A Casebook Approach.* New York, McGraw-Hill, 2001, p 553.

▸ de Bruyn R (ed): *Pediatric Ultrasound: How, Why and When*, 2nd edition (e-book). Philadelphia, Churchill Livingstone/Elsevier, 2010, p 246.

▸ Rumack CM, Levine D (eds): *Diagnostic Ultrasound*, 5th edition. Philadelphia, Elsevier, 2018, p 1897.

▸ Siegel MJ (ed): *Pediatric Sonography*, 4th edition. Philadelphia, Lippincott Williams & Wilkins, 2011, pp 577–578.

557. **C. Gonadoblastoma.**

Gonadoblastomas *are rare tumors commonly associated with undescended testes, phenotypic females with streak testes, and an abnormal male karyotype. Gonadoblastomas have malignant potential but are usually benign and typically are found during surgery for removal of dysplastic abdominal gonads.* Teratomas, juvenile granulosa cell tumors, *and* Sertoli cell tumors *are not associated with the male karyotype.*

▸ Rumack CM, Levine D (eds): *Diagnostic Ultrasound*, 5th edition. Philadelphia, Elsevier, 2018, p 1900.

▸ Siegel MJ (ed): *Pediatric Sonography*, 4th edition. Philadelphia, Lippincott Williams & Wilkins, 2011, p 569.

PART 15

Soft Tissue

558. D. Pilonidal cyst.

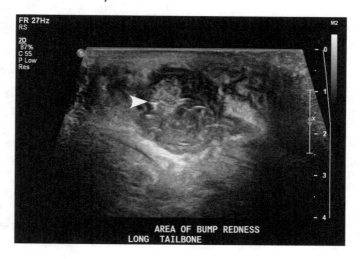

A pilonidal cyst *(arrowhead)* is a cystic structure located in the sacrococcygeal (tailbone) region that contains hair, as seen in this image. Pilonidal (meaning "nest of hair") cysts are also known as pilonidal sinuses. Patients with pilonidal cysts may present with swelling and tenderness in the tailbone area. The cysts can become infected and form a pilonidal abscess. Sacrococcygeal teratomas *are germ cell tumors that arise from the coccyx and are typically found prenatally. Most sacrococcygeal tumors have an external component and would be found at birth, not in the teenage years.* Synovial cysts *can be found anywhere in the body but most often are located in the spine.* A meniscal cyst *occurs in the knee adjacent to a meniscal tear.*

▸ Conley S: Sonographic evaluation of a pilonidal cyst: a case study. J Diagn Med Sonogr 32:279–282, 2016. Available at http://journals.sagepub.com/doi/pdf/10.1177/8756479316662648.

▸ Rumack CM, Levine D (eds): *Diagnostic Ultrasound*, 5th edition. Philadelphia, Elsevier, 2018, pp 869–870.

▸ Siegel MJ (ed): *Pediatric Sonography*, 4th edition. Philadelphia, Lippincott Williams & Wilkins, 2011, pp 622–623, 662.

559. **A. Gastrocnemius and calcaneus.**

The Achilles tendon *is the largest tendon in the body and connects the* gastrocnemius *and* soleus muscles *(calf muscles) to the* calcaneus *(heel bone). The Achilles tendon is prone to tendinosis (degeneration of the tendon), making it more vulnerable to tearing. The* rotator cuff *is a group of muscles (including the subscapularis) and tendons that are connected to the humerus. The* quadriceps muscle *and the* patella *are attached by the quadriceps tendon anteriorly in the lower end of the upper leg. The two* peroneal tendons *connect the* peroneal muscles *to the first and fifth* metatarsals *and run along the lateral aspect of the ankle posterior to the fibula.*

▶ Anatomy Medicine: The patella. Available at https://anatomy-medicine.com/musculoskeletal-system/79-the-patella.html.
▶ Rumack CM, Levine D (eds): *Diagnostic Ultrasound*, 5th edition. Philadelphia, Elsevier, 2018, pp 859–861.
▶ Siegel MJ (ed): *Pediatric Sonography*, 4th edition. Philadelphia, Lippincott Williams & Wilkins, 2011, p 606.

560. **A. Umbilical hernia.**

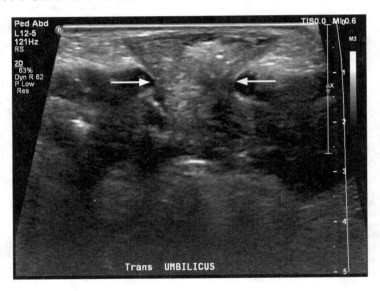

Umbilical hernias *(arrows) result from a defect in the umbilical ring. In infants and young children, umbilical hernias usually regress spontaneously. If the hernia has not regressed by age 4, surgical repair may be needed. With large defects, intraperitoneal contents may be herniated and evaluation of the bowel may be needed to assess for incarceration.* Spigelian hernias *occur in the Spigelian facia at the level of the arcuate line (not the umbilical region). A* linea alba hernia arises in the linea alba (midline abdomen) and can occur superior to the umbilicus (epigastric hernia) or inferior to the umbilicus (hypogastric hernia). An inguinal hernia occurs in the groin area.

▶ Rumack CM, Levine D (eds): *Diagnostic Ultrasound*, 5th edition. Philadelphia, Elsevier, 2018, pp 483, 488, 491.

561. **B. Hypervascularity.**

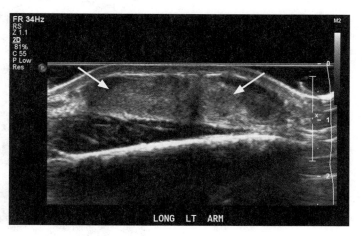

Lipomas *are tumors of fatty tissue and in children are most commonly found in the subcutaneous soft tissues. Their sonographic appearance is of an isoechoic or slightly hyperechoic mass (arrows) compared to the adjacent fat. Lipomas are homogeneous, well defined, compressible, mobile, painless, and avascular. A liposarcoma may be suspected when a lipoma has a complex and hyperemic appearance.*

▶ de Bruyn R (ed): *Pediatric Ultrasound: How, Why and When*, 2nd edition (e-book). Philadelphia, Churchill Livingstone/Elsevier, 2010, pp 337, 338.
▶ Rumack CM, Levine D (eds): *Diagnostic Ultrasound*, 5th edition. Philadelphia, Elsevier, 2018, p 870.
▶ Siegel MJ (ed): *Pediatric Sonography*, 4th edition. Philadelphia, Lippincott Williams & Wilkins, 2011, p 622.

562. **C. Hemangioma.**

During infancy, hemangiomas *are the most common vascular tumor and appear as a purplish or reddish mass within the skin. Hemangiomas can be present at birth or appear during the first week of life; usually they appear within the first decade of life. Sonographically, hemangiomas are hypervascular masses with monophasic venous flow (no arteriovenous fistulas). Hemangiomas have two phases,* proliferative *and* involutive.

The growth (proliferative) phase usually starts shortly after birth and might last up to 9 months. The regression (involutive) phase, can last up to 10 years. Hematomas *are not vascular tumors.* Aneurysms *and* arteriovenous malformations *(AVMs) are less common than hemangiomas.*

▸ de Bruyn R (ed): *Pediatric Ultrasound: How, Why and When*, 2nd edition (e-book). Philadelphia, Churchill Livingstone/Elsevier, 2010, pp 288–289, 337–338.

▸ Rumack CM, Levine D (eds): *Diagnostic Ultrasound*, 5th edition. Philadelphia, Elsevier, 2018, pp 1742–1743.

▸ Siegel MJ (ed): *Pediatric Sonography*, 4th edition. Philadelphia, Lippincott Williams & Wilkins, 2011, pp 618–619.

563. C. Ganglion cyst.

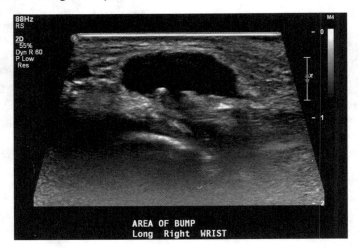

Ganglion cysts *are mucin-filled cysts most commonly located at the dorsal aspect of the hand and wrist. On ultrasound, ganglion cysts appear as cystic structures with well-defined borders and posterior enhancement. Ganglion cysts may have low-level echoes or internal septations. A* Baker's cyst, *also known as a popliteal cyst, is a fluid collection located posterior to the knee joint. Popliteal cysts are avascular and may appear on ultrasound as anechoic or hypoechoic with a distinctive narrow neck. Doppler should always be used to rule out vascularity. A* meniscal cyst *occurs adjacent to a meniscal tear (in the knee) and appears as an anechoic, well-defined structure.* Sebaceous cysts *originate from sebaceous glands and contain yellow sebum. They commonly occur in the trunk, neck, or face.*

▸ Rumack CM, Levine D (eds): *Diagnostic Ultrasound*, 5th edition. Philadelphia, Elsevier, 2018, pp 869–870.

▸ Siegel MJ (ed): *Pediatric Sonography*, 4th edition. Philadelphia, Lippincott Williams & Wilkins, 2011, pp 622–623.

564. D. Standoff pad.

The use of a standoff pad *is helpful when structures are located in the near field just below the skin. Highly reflective near-field structures can cause reverberation artifact, thus minimizing the ability to visualize this area. Standoff pads increase the distance between the transducer and the area of interest, making it easier to evaluate. Compression with the transducer is a technique used to evaluate the collapsibility. A panoramic or* extended-field-of-view image *expands the field of view instead of optimizing the near field.* Harmonic imaging *helps improve lateral resolution and reduces artifacts.*

▶ Rumack CM, Levine D (eds): *Diagnostic Ultrasound*, 5th edition. Philadelphia, Elsevier, 2018, p 767.

565. A. Cellulitis.

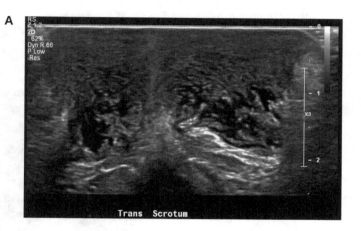

See Color Plate 32 on page xlvii.

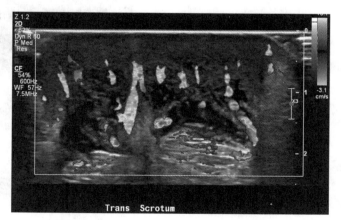

Cellulitis *is an infection of the subcutaneous tissue that is most commonly caused by* Staphylococcus aureus, *but in neonates* Streptococcus (group B) *is most common. In most cases, cellulitis is diagnosed based on the clinical symptoms.* Phlebitis *is inflammation involving the veins. Ultrasound is helpful*

in the evaluation of abscess formation. **A** Sonographically, cellulitis appears as thickened subcutaneous tissue with an increase in echogenicity and **B** may demonstrate increased color Doppler flow. Within the inflamed tissue, small fluid collections can be seen, appearing irregular, round, or oval-shaped. Like cellulitis, an abscess *is caused by an infection but can be distinguished from cellulitis on ultrasound by its characteristic focal collection of complex-appearing material (pus).* Dermatitis *is the inflammation of the skin (not the subcutaneous soft tissues).* Pyomyositis *is a bacterial infection within the muscle causing a pus-filled sac.*

▶ Rumack CM, Levine D (eds): *Diagnostic Ultrasound*, 5th edition. Philadelphia, Elsevier, 2018, pp 872–874.

▶ Siegel MJ (ed): *Pediatric Sonography*, 4th edition. Philadelphia, Lippincott Williams & Wilkins, 2011, pp 626–628.

▶ Stephenson SR, Dahiya N: *Musculoskeletal Sonography Review: A Q&A Review for the ARDMS Musculoskeletal Sonographer Exam*. Pasadena, CA, Davies Publishing, 2019, pp 301, 306, 317–319.

566. B. 2.

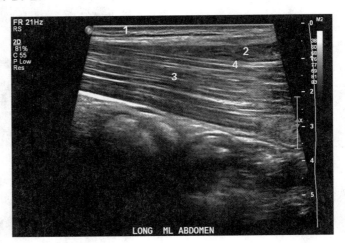

The hypodermis, *also known as the* subcutaneous tissue, *is a superficial facia that lies beneath the dermis and is represented with the number 2 in this image.* The subcutaneous tissue is composed of connective tissue and fat. The fatty component of the hypodermis appears hypoechoic, whereas the fibrous connective tissue appears as echogenic septae that can be seen scattered throughout the subcutaneous fat. The number 1, marking the most superficial echogenic layer, represents the skin, which is composed of the epidermis and dermis. These two layers of the skin cannot be differentiated with ultrasound and instead appear as one echogenic layer. The number 3 in this image represents the muscle. Muscles on *ultrasound appear as hypoechoic structures that have fibrous tissue along the long axis of the muscle. The echogenic sheath that surrounds the muscle is known as the* epimysium, *which is represented by the number 4.*

▶ Rumack CM, Levine D (eds): *Diagnostic Ultrasound*, 5th edition. Philadelphia, Elsevier, 2018, pp 857–858.

▶ Siegel MJ (ed): *Pediatric Sonography*, 4th edition. Philadelphia, Lippincott Williams & Wilkins, 2011, p 603.

567. A. Hematoma.

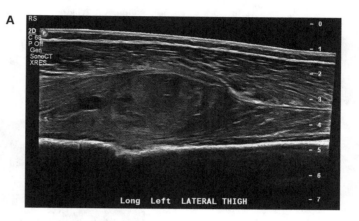

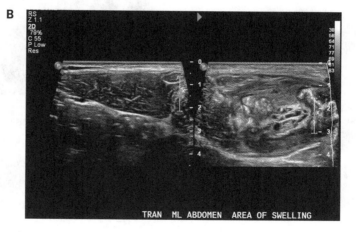

Ultrasound can be used as an imaging method to evaluate muscles, tendons, and ligaments after sports injuries; it can help with the diagnosis of small fractures, strains, tears, and hematomas. **A** *The abnormality represented in this image is a hematoma located within the thigh muscle. Within the first few hours of formation hematomas appear homogeneous and echogenic. After a few days a clot forms and appears complex. After a few weeks the hematoma liquefies and may appear anechoic or with low-level echoes.* **B** *This image compares the appearances of a normal muscle (right) and an injured muscle containing a hematoma (left).*

Seromas *are collections of serous fluid and appear anechoic on ultrasound.* Foreign bodies *appear as linear echogenic structures and may have posterior shadowing. An* abscess *can have a sonographic appearance similar to that of a hematoma (heterogeneous), but given the indication for the exam posed by the question—a sports injury—abscess is less likely to be the diagnosis.*

▸ Rumack CM, Levine D (eds): *Diagnostic Ultrasound*, 5th edition. Philadelphia, Elsevier, 2018, p 858.

▸ Siegel MJ (ed): *Pediatric Sonography*, 4th edition. Philadelphia, Lippincott Williams & Wilkins, 2011, pp 631–632.

▸ Stephenson SR, Dahiya N: *Musculoskeletal Sonography Review: A Q&A Review for the ARDMS Musculoskeletal Sonographer Exam*. Pasadena, CA, Davies Publishing, 2019, pp 315–316.

568. **D. Splinter.**

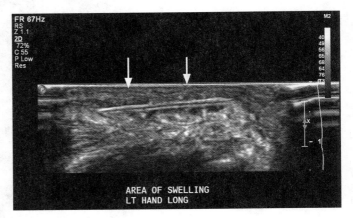

Although radiography is the preferred imaging method for evaluating foreign bodies, ultrasound is also very helpful when the object is radiolucent (invisible on x-ray). In children, some of the more common materials that can become embedded as foreign bodies are glass, metal, and wood. On radiography, glass and metal are usually visible (radiolucent). Wood is not easily seen on radiography, and therefore ultrasound may be needed to identify the object.

Ultrasound can be used both to localize foreign bodies and to assist during the removal procedure. On ultrasound, foreign bodies appear as linear echogenic structures (arrows), sometimes with posterior shadowing and sometimes without, as demonstrated in this image. Wood is initially visualized as a hyperechoic foreign body within tissue. As infection takes hold, a hypoechoic "halo" surrounds the wood, and its echogenicity decreases during decomposition; there is minimal posterior shadowing with wood. Glass demonstrates an echogenic focus with a comet-tail artifact, while a metallic object typically presents as an echogenic structure with a posterior reverberation artifact.

▶ Rumack CM, Levine D (eds): *Diagnostic Ultrasound*, 5th edition. Philadelphia, Elsevier, 2018, p 872.

▶ Shah V, Knipe H: Glass foreign bodies. Radiopaedia.org. Available from Radiopaedia at https://radiopaedia.org/articles/glass-foreign-bodies.

▶ Siegel MJ (ed): *Pediatric Sonography*, 4th edition. Philadelphia, Lippincott Williams & Wilkins, 2011, p 635.

▶ Stephenson SR, Dahiya N: *Musculoskeletal Sonography Review: A Q&A Review for the ARDMS Musculoskeletal Sonographer Exam*. Pasadena, CA, Davies Publishing, 2019, pp 315–316.

569. **C. Hypoechoic.**

In general, on ultrasound a muscle appears as a hypoechoic structure that has internal thin bands along its longitudinal orientation. In a transverse plane, the internal muscle bands are seen as speckled echoes throughout the overall hypoechoic muscle. The external thick, fibrous echogenic sheath of connective tissue that surrounds the muscle is known as the epimysium.

▶ Rumack CM, Levine D (eds): *Diagnostic Ultrasound*, 5th edition. Philadelphia, Elsevier, 2018, pp 857–858.

▶ Siegel MJ (ed): *Pediatric Sonography*, 4th edition. Philadelphia, Lippincott Williams & Wilkins, 2011, p 603.

570. **A. Ligament.**

Ligaments *connect bone to bone.* Tendons *are fibrous bands of connective tissue that connect muscles to bones.* Cartilage *is a smooth type of connective tissue located at the ends of the bones in the joints (serving as a cushion). The* epimysium *is a sheath of connective tissue fascia that surrounds the skeletal muscles and fat.*

▶ MedlinePlus: Cartilage disorders. Available at https://medlineplus.gov/cartilagedisorders.html.

▶ Rumack CM, Levine D (eds): *Diagnostic Ultrasound*, 5th edition. Philadelphia, Elsevier, 2018, pp 859–865.

▶ Siegel MJ (ed): *Pediatric Sonography*, 4th edition. Philadelphia, Lippincott Williams & Wilkins, 2011, pp 603–604.

571. B. Lymphadenopathy.

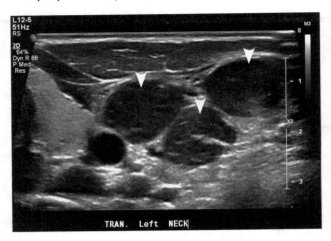

Lymphadenopathy *is one of the most common pediatric inflammatory masses of the neck and sonographically appears as multiple enlarged lymph nodes (arrowheads). Lymphadenopathy is commonly seen in the anterior, lateral, and posterior regions of the neck. Enlarged lymph nodes can be a result of viral and bacterial infections or cancers such as non-Hodgkin lymphoma.* Fibromatosis colli, thyroglossal duct cysts, *and* hemangiomas *are not inflammatory masses of the neck.*

▶ de Bruyn R (ed): *Pediatric Ultrasound: How, Why and When*, 2nd edition (e-book). Philadelphia, Churchill Livingstone/Elsevier, 2010, pp 278, 280, 284–285.

▶ Rumack CM, Levine D (eds): *Diagnostic Ultrasound*, 5th edition. Philadelphia, Elsevier, 2018, pp 1660–1662.

▶ Siegel MJ (ed): *Pediatric Sonography*, 4th edition. Philadelphia, Lippincott Williams & Wilkins, 2011, pp 130–132, 137–138, 141, 143.

572. C. Split-screen.

Split-screen, *or* dual screen, *imaging provides a side-by-side comparison of a normal and an affected extremity on one image.* Panoramic *and* extended-field-of-view *imaging are the same type of imaging technique, allowing for a wider or longer field of view.* 3D imaging *is used to obtain volumetric measurements of structures, resulting in a three-dimensional appearance. 3D, panoramic, and extended-field-of-view imaging methods do not offer a side-by-side function (comparison views) on a single image.*

▶ Rumack CM, Levine D (eds): *Diagnostic Ultrasound*, 5th edition. Philadelphia, Elsevier, 2018, p 769.

▶ Siegel MJ (ed): *Pediatric Sonography*, 4th edition. Philadelphia, Lippincott Williams & Wilkins, 2011, pp 602–603.

573. **D. Color flow in tear region.**

With tendon tears, the sonographic appearance is discontinuity of the tendon, and the area of the tear appears hypoechoic when it fills with blood. In a torn tendon, the free ends may be seen floating within the blood, which is termed the "bell-clapper" sign. A tendon tear will not exhibit color flow.

▶ Rumack CM, Levine D (eds): *Diagnostic Ultrasound*, 5th edition. Philadelphia, Elsevier, 2018, pp 485–486.

▶ Siegel MJ (ed): *Pediatric Sonography*, 4th edition. Philadelphia, Lippincott Williams & Wilkins, 2011, pp 635–636.

574. **D. 2 weeks.**

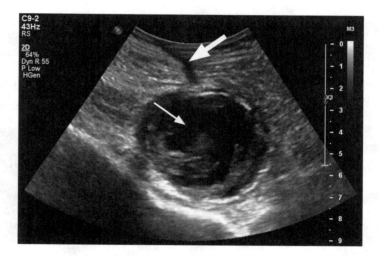

The sonographic appearance of the hematoma distal to the stab wound (thick arrow) evolves after the initial injury. Within the first few hours of formation the hematoma will appear homogeneous and echogenic. After a few days, a clot forms, and it will appear complex. After a few weeks, the hematoma liquefies and may appear anechoic or with low-level echoes. This hematoma exhibits areas of liquefaction centrally (thin arrow).

▶ Rumack CM, Levine D (eds): *Diagnostic Ultrasound*, 5th edition. Philadelphia, Elsevier, 2018, p 858.

▶ Siegel MJ (ed): *Pediatric Sonography*, 4th edition. Philadelphia, Lippincott Williams & Wilkins, 2011, pp 631–632.

575. **B. Abscess.**

An abscess is a focal collection of pus caused by an infection. If the organism causing the infection produces gas, then gas within the fluid collection can be seen. Therefore, the presence of gas within a fluid collection is most indicative of an infectious process (abscess). Abscesses on ultrasound may appear hypoechoic, anechoic, or echogenic with well or poorly defined margins. Hyperemia of the surrounding tissue may be seen. Myositis *refers to a diffuse infection of muscle and is not associated with the presence of abscess. Myositis appears as a thickened muscle with heterogeneous echogenicity. A* hematoma *is a collection of blood that, depending on the stage, can have a variable appearance—from anechoic or hypoechoic to septated and/or complex—depending on the age of the injury and the hematoma's stage of resolution; however, gas formation is not one of the characteristics of hematoma.* Seromas *are collections of serous fluid and on ultrasound usually appear anechoic without internal gas.*

▶ Rumack CM, Levine D (eds): *Diagnostic Ultrasound*, 5th edition. Philadelphia, Elsevier, 2018, pp 874, 1936.

▶ Siegel MJ (ed): *Pediatric Sonography*, 4th edition. Philadelphia, Lippincott Williams & Wilkins, 2011, pp 628, 632.

576. **A. Baker's cyst.**

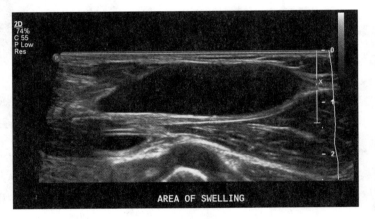

A Baker's cyst, *also known as a* popliteal cyst, *is a common fluid collection located posterior to the knee joint in the gastrocnemius-semimembranosus bursa, as seen in this image. For correct diagnosis, a Baker's cyst must be seen to originate between the medial head of the gastrocnemius muscle and the semimembranosus tendon; color Doppler helps differentiate the Baker's cyst from vessels, as the cyst lacks flow. Baker's cysts may appear anechoic or hypoechoic on ultrasound, with a distinctive narrow neck. Although Baker's cysts usually appear isolated from other conditions, they may be associated with juvenile rheumatoid arthritis. A* meniscal cyst *occurs adjacent to a meniscal tear (in the knee) and appears as an anechoic, well-defined structure.* Ganglion cysts *can be found anywhere in the body but are most often located at the dorsal aspect of the hand and wrist.*

On ultrasound, ganglion cysts appear as cystic structures with well-defined borders and posterior enhancement. Ganglion cysts may have low-level echoes or internal septations. Sebaceous cysts are typically located in the torso, neck, or face and arise from sebaceous glands.

▶ Fan RSP, Ryu RKN: Meniscal lesions: diagnosis and treatment. Available at https://www.medscape.com/viewarticle/408520_8.

▶ Rumack CM, Levine D (eds): *Diagnostic Ultrasound*, 5th edition. Philadelphia, Elsevier, 2018, pp 869–870, 1939.

▶ Siegel MJ (ed): *Pediatric Sonography*, 4th edition. Philadelphia, Lippincott Williams & Wilkins, 2011, pp 622–623.

▶ Stephenson SR, Dahiya N: *Musculoskeletal Sonography Review: A Q&A Review for the ARDMS Musculoskeletal Sonographer Exam*. Pasadena, CA, Davies Publishing, 2019, pp 253, 255, 264–265, 302, 347.

577. A. Tendon.

Tendons are fibrous bands of connective tissue that connect muscles to bones. Ligaments are similar to tendons but connect bone to bone. Cartilage, located at the ends of bones in the joints, is a smooth type of connective tissue that serves as a cushion. Nerves are bundles of fibers that allow communication between the brain and other organs by transmitting signals throughout the body.

▶ MedlinePlus: Cartilage disorders. Available at https://medlineplus.gov/cartilagedisorders.html.

▶ Rumack CM, Levine D (eds): *Diagnostic Ultrasound*, 5th edition. Philadelphia, Elsevier, 2018, pp 859–865.

▶ Siegel MJ (ed): *Pediatric Sonography*, 4th edition. Philadelphia, Lippincott Williams & Wilkins, 2011, pp 603–604.

PART 16

Vasculature of the Extremities

578. **B. Tunica adventitia.**

The tunica adventitia *is the outer layer of the venous and arterial walls, composed of loose connective tissue, smooth muscle fibers, and elastic tissue. The* tunica media *is the middle layer, containing smooth muscle, elastic fibers, and collagen. The inner layer is called the* tunica intima; *it has three layers—endothelial cells that line the lumen, connective tissue, and elastic fibers. The* tunica elastica *is not a layer within the walls of veins and arteries; all of the layers contain elastic tissue or fibers.*

▸ Rice University: Structure and function of blood vessels. Available at https://opentextbc.ca/anatomyandphysiology/chapter/20-1-structure-and-function-of-blood-vessels/.

579. **C. Hepatic vein.**

A peripherally inserted central catheter (PICC) line is used to administer long-term antibiotics, chemotherapy, and total parenteral nutrition (TPN) to patients who are have serious chronic diseases such as cancer. It is an intravenous line that starts in a peripheral vessel and ends in a central vessel near the heart. Blood can also be drawn from a PICC line. A transjugular intrahepatic portosystemic shunt (TIPS) is a catheter that is inserted into the internal jugular vein and runs into the hepatic veins. A stent is then placed in a tract made to connect the portal vein to a hepatic vein. TIPS procedures are used in patients with portal hypertension and esophageal varices as a method of decompressing the portal system.

▸ de Bruyn R (ed): *Pediatric Ultrasound: How, Why and When*, 2nd edition (e-book). Philadelphia, Churchill Livingstone/Elsevier, 2010, pp 354, 355, 356, 360–361.

▸ Infusion Solutions Inc.: What is a PICC line? Available at https://www.infusionsolutionsinc.com/what-is-a-picc-line.

▸ Pal N: Femoral central venous access. Available at https://emedicine.medscape.com/article/80279-overview.

▸ Rumack CM, Levine D (eds): *Diagnostic Ultrasound*, 5th edition. Philadelphia, Elsevier, 2018, pp 993, 1757, 1764, 1955–1957.

▸ Siegel MJ (ed): *Pediatric Sonography*, 4th edition. Philadelphia, Lippincott Williams & Wilkins, 2011, pp 254–255, 694–696.

580. **A. Arteriovenous malformation.**

An arteriovenous malformation *(AVM) is defined as a network of multiple abnormal, thin-walled, tangled channels between feeding arteries and draining veins. The network of abnormal channels is termed a* nidus. *AVMs are high-flow abnormalities that can occur within the brain, spine, or extremities and disrupt normal blood flow. They can be congenital or post-traumatic. Clinically, a bruit or pulsatile mass may be appreciated.* Pseudoaneurysms *and* arteriovenous (AV) fistulas *are typically a result of a penetrating injury or catheterization, not a malformation of vessels. A pseudoaneurysm results from an injury to the vessel wall and demonstrates a localized hematoma that communicates with an artery. An AV fistula is a direct connection between an artery and a vein. AV fistulas shunt blood from a high-pressure artery to a low-pressure vein. AV fistulas can also be congenital. A thrombus is a blood clot that occurs within a vessel and can impede blood flow.*

▶ Rumack CM, Levine D (eds): *Diagnostic Ultrasound*, 5th edition. Philadelphia, Elsevier, 2018, pp 973–974.

▶ Siegel MJ (ed): *Pediatric Sonography*, 4th edition. Philadelphia, Lippincott Williams & Wilkins, 2011, pp 81–83, 619, 642–643.

581. **D. Distal to the stenosis.**

A tardus parvus waveform *can be seen distal to an arterial stenosis. The tardus parvus waveform demonstrates decreased pulsatility, delayed acceleration time, a rounded systolic peak, and low velocity. A stenosis greater than 50% is associated with an increased peak systolic velocity at the site of stenosis. If an occlusion is present, an absence of color flow or spectral signal will be demonstrated. In screening for stenosis or occlusion, ultrasound has a sensitivity and specificity of up to 95%. Higher resistance is visualized proximal to the stenosis, and turbulence is seen within the site of the stenosis.*

▶ Rumack CM, Levine D (eds): *Diagnostic Ultrasound*, 5th edition. Philadelphia, Elsevier, 2018, p 966.

▶ Siegel MJ (ed): *Pediatric Sonography*, 4th edition. Philadelphia, Lippincott Williams & Wilkins, 2011, pp 641–642.

582. **B. Valsalva.**

The Valsalva maneuver is used to evaluate for thrombus within a vein. In a Valsalva maneuver, the patient takes in a deep breath and then bears down (as if having a bowel movement) while holding the breath. During Valsalva, a normal vein will demonstrate a temporary reversal of flow, followed by a quick halting of flow; when the patient releases the breath and stops bearing down, there is a quick increase of forward flow, resulting in augmentation of the venous signal. If reversal of flow or reflux is present following the Valsalva maneuver, grading is performed based on the amount of time reflux is present to determine pathologic versus nonpathologic conditions. The flow augmentation technique (squeezing of the calf) is another method utilized to show patency distal to the interrogation site. When the calf is squeezed, there is normally an increase in flow.

Pumping of the fists helps make the veins of the arms more visible but does not demonstrate patency. Limb elevation will normally decrease the hydrostatic pressure in the leg so that fluid can be moved through the capillaries and absorbed. Applying a blood pressure cuff to the extremity would not allow ultrasound evaluation of the area under the cuff and therefore would not provide any diagnostic information.

▸ Rumack CM, Levine D (eds): *Diagnostic Ultrasound*, 5th edition. Philadelphia, Elsevier, 2018, p 989.

▸ Siegel MJ (ed): *Pediatric Sonography*, 4th edition. Philadelphia, Lippincott Williams & Wilkins, 2011, p 639.

583. **C. Pseudoaneurysm.**

See Color Plate 33 on page xlvii.

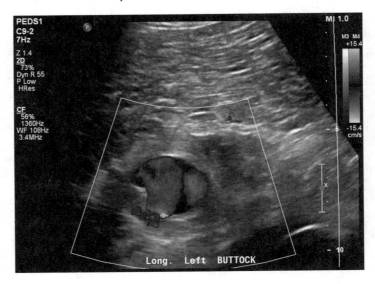

A pseudoaneurysm is a hematoma that communicates with an artery, resulting from injury to a blood vessel wall. Pseudoaneurysms are typically complications of penetrating injuries and femoral artery catheterizations. On ultrasound, a hypoechoic or complex fluid collection appears in the region of the affected artery. Because they communicate with an artery, a swirling blood flow pattern is seen in the shape of the yin-yang sign, demonstrated by the blue and red colors in this image. Blood is flowing both toward and away from the transducer, resulting in two different colors. This pattern is typical for a pseudoaneurysm. Perivascular tissue vibrations, resulting in mixed color pixel signals within the surrounding soft tissues, can also be seen. Deep venous thrombosis *(DVT)* and arteriovenous malformations *(AVMs)* are not associated with penetrating injuries. A nidus is the network of abnormal blood vessels within an AVM.

▸ Kalva S: Venous physiology. Available at http://www.phlebology.org/wp-content/uploads/2015/03/02-Physiology-Function-Normal-Venous-Hemodynamics-Venous-Pumps-Lymphatic-System-Kalva.pdf.

▸ Rumack CM, Levine D (eds): *Diagnostic Ultrasound*, 5th edition. Philadelphia, Elsevier, 2018, pp 972–973.

▸ Siegel MJ (ed): *Pediatric Sonography*, 4th edition. Philadelphia, Lippincott Williams & Wilkins, 2011, pp 81–83, 639, 642–643.

584. B. Brachial.

See Color Plate 34 on page xlviii.

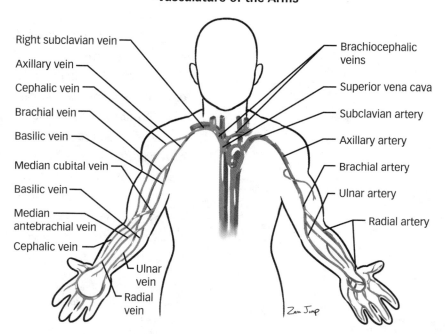

Vasculature of the Arms

The brachial artery *gives rise to the radial and ulnar arteries. The* subclavian artery *gives rise to the* axillary artery, *which gives rise to the brachial artery. The* basilic *is not an artery but a large superficial vein in the upper arm.*

▶ Rumack CM, Levine D (eds): *Diagnostic Ultrasound*, 5th edition. Philadelphia, Elsevier, 2018, pp 975–976, 990–992.

▶ Siegel MJ (ed): *Pediatric Sonography*, 4th edition. Philadelphia, Lippincott Williams & Wilkins, 2011, pp 640–641.

585. C. Popliteal.

See Color Plate 35 on page xlviii.

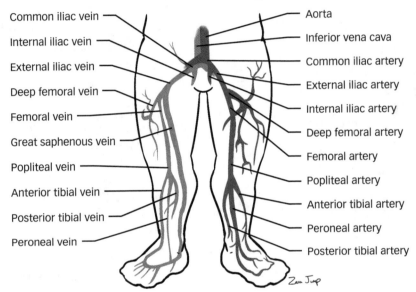

Vasculature of the Legs

The popliteal vein *lies deep to the gastrocnemius (calf) muscle. It is formed by the merging of the anterior and posterior tibial veins posterior and distal to the knee. The* femoral, saphenous, *and* deep profunda *(also known as the deep femoral) veins are located within the upper thigh. All of the paired veins (anterior and posterior tibial and peroneal) form confluences (tibioperoneal trunk) and empty into the popliteal vein. When performing sonography of veins, use light pressure to avoid undesired compression. Longitudinal and transverse images are obtained with and without Doppler imaging. The femoral, saphenous, and deep profunda veins are all located within the thigh, not the calf.*

▶ Rumack CM, Levine D (eds): *Diagnostic Ultrasound*, 5th edition. Philadelphia, Elsevier, 2018, pp 980–982.

▶ Siegel MJ (ed): *Pediatric Sonography*, 4th edition. Philadelphia, Lippincott Williams & Wilkins, 2011, pp 627–638.

586. **D. Deep venous thrombosis (DVT).**

Deep venous thrombosis (DVT) is associated with immobilization and central venous catheterization. DVT is uncommon in pediatrics. Clinical symptoms are pain, erythema, and swelling. The D-dimer test evaluates the level of protein produced when a blood clot is breaking down. A negative D-dimer test rules out DVT, but a positive D-dimer test is nonspecific. While a positive D-dimer test can occur with a DVT, extravascular bleeding (bruising) can also cause a positive test. Pulmonary embolisms are the most life-threatening complication of DVT. Ultrasound has up to a 95% sensitivity and specificity for diagnosing DVT. To interrogate for DVT with ultrasound, the sonographer uses a high-frequency transducer; an enlarged vein is present with an echogenic thrombus. The vein will be noncompressible, which is best demonstrated in the transverse plane. Since compression is operator-dependent, it is important for the sonographer to apply proper and adequate compression to avoid false positives. If complete occlusion is present, no color flow will be demonstrated. Arteriovenous malformations (AVMs), arteriovenous fistulas, and pseudoaneurysms are not associated with immobilization.

▶ Lab Tests Online: D-dimer. Available at https://labtestsonline.org/tests/d-dimer.

▶ Rumack CM, Levine D (eds): *Diagnostic Ultrasound*, 5th edition. Philadelphia, Elsevier, 2018, pp 983–984.

▶ Siegel MJ (ed): *Pediatric Sonography*, 4th edition. Philadelphia, Lippincott Williams & Wilkins, 2011, pp 619, 639, 642–643.

587. **A. Arteries.**

Atherosclerosis is a disease in which fatty deposits or plaque affects the inner walls of arteries. This buildup within the arterial walls can obstruct the arterial lumen and hinder blood flow, causing stenosis or occlusion. Veins, capillaries, and lymphatic vessels are not affected by atherosclerosis.

▶ National Heart, Lung, and Blood Institute: Atherosclerosis. Available at https://www.nhlbi.nih.gov/health-topics/atherosclerosis.

▶ Rumack CM, Levine D (eds): *Diagnostic Ultrasound*, 5th edition. Philadelphia, Elsevier, 2018, p 968.

ANSWERS

588. D. L5.

The inferior vena cava (IVC) is formed by the union of the common iliac veins. This typically occurs at the level of the L5 vertebra. The IVC is the largest vein in the body and is located within the retroperitoneum. The superior vena cava (SVC) drains the head, neck, thorax, and upper extremities. The IVC drains the remainder of the body.

▶ Hapugoda S, Jones J, et al: Inferior vena cava. Available from Radiopaedia at https://radiopaedia.org/articles/inferior-vena-cava-1.

▶ Siegel MJ (ed): *Pediatric Sonography*, 4th edition. Philadelphia, Lippincott Williams & Wilkins, 2011, p 495.

589. B. Triphasic and high-resistance.

Normal peripheral arteries will demonstrate triphasic, high-resistance waveforms. Forward antegrade flow is present during systole. During early diastole, a reversal of flow is seen. In late diastole, low antegrade flow is present. Most normal arteries are not usually biphasic.

▶ Rumack CM, Levine D (eds): *Diagnostic Ultrasound*, 5th edition. Philadelphia, Elsevier, 2018, p 966.

▶ Siegel MJ (ed): *Pediatric Sonography*, 4th edition. Philadelphia, Lippincott Williams & Wilkins, 2011, p 641.

590. C. Right subclavian.

See Color Plate 34, "Vasculature of the Arms," on page xlviii.

The right subclavian artery is not a direct branch off the aortic arch. The innominate artery, also known as the brachiocephalic trunk, bifurcates into the right common carotid and right subclavian arteries. The left common carotid and left subclavian arteries both branch directly off the aortic arch.

▶ Keeley JD, Ashurst JV: Anatomy, thorax, aortic arch. StatPearls. Available at https://www.ncbi.nlm.nih.gov/books/NBK499911/.

▶ Rumack CM, Levine D (eds): *Diagnostic Ultrasound*, 5th edition. Philadelphia, Elsevier, 2018, p 1279.

▶ Siegel MJ (ed): *Pediatric Sonography*, 4th edition. Philadelphia, Lippincott Williams & Wilkins, 2011, p 640.

591. D. Common femoral vein.

See Color Plate 35, "Vasculature of the Legs," on page xlviii.

The deep and superficial veins of the leg empty directly into the common femoral vein. The common femoral vein drains into the external iliac vein, which then empties into the common iliac vein. The popliteal vein becomes the femoral vein at the adductor canal.

▶ Rumack CM, Levine D (eds): *Diagnostic Ultrasound*, 5th edition. Philadelphia, Elsevier, 2018, pp 960–961.

▶ Siegel MJ (ed): *Pediatric Sonography*, 4th edition. Philadelphia, Lippincott Williams & Wilkins, 2011, p 637.

592. B. Great saphenous.

See Color Plate 35, "Vasculature of the Legs," on page xlviii.

The great saphenous vein is the most medial vein of the upper leg. It is a superficial vein—coursing superficial to the muscles of the leg through the subcutaneous tissues beneath the skin—and drains into the common femoral vein. The longest vein of the inner leg and thigh, the great saphenous vein is commonly used in coronary bypass surgeries to create a bypass vessel in the heart. The common femoral, superficial femoral, and deep femoral are all considered deep veins of the leg and are all located lateral to the great saphenous vein.

▶ Rumack CM, Levine D (eds): *Diagnostic Ultrasound*, 5th edition. Philadelphia, Elsevier, 2018, pp 960–961.

▶ Siegel MJ (ed): *Pediatric Sonography*, 4th edition. Philadelphia, Lippincott Williams & Wilkins, 2011, p 637.

PART 17

Physics and Instrumentation

593. B. Lipoma.

A refraction artifact occurs when the ultrasound beam encounters an interface with a different tissue type at a non-perpendicular angle. Sound propagates at different speeds in different media, due to their different densities, and it is the difference in propagation speeds between the two media (i.e., different types of human tissue) that causes the refraction artifact to occur. Should the refracted incident sound wave strike a reflector and cause an echo to return to the transducer, this may be displayed at an incorrect location, since the transducer "assumes" that all echoes have traveled along a direct path. Refraction artifacts are more frequently seen when the sound beam moves from a tissue type in which sound propagates at a higher speed to one in which the beam propagates at a slower speed. The liver is soft tissue, a medium in which sound travels at an average speed of 1540 meters per second (m/sec). In the liver, the lesion that most frequently causes a refraction artifact is the lipoma, which is fat, a tissue in which the beam travels at only 1450 m/sec. Furthermore, the sonographer may see refraction artifacts when interrogating a mass because the beam is often traveling through several different types of tissue (media) that are in close proximity—in this case, the liver (soft tissue), a cyst (fluid), a lipoma (fat), and a hematoma (blood)—so the beam will be propagated at speeds that are continuously changing from faster to slower. To correct the artifact, you must move the transducer so that the beam is perpendicular to the interface with the object of the interrogation, in this case the lipoma. The table lists the speeds of the ultrasound beam through different media.

Approximate speeds of ultrasound waves in the human tissues

Medium	Speed
Air	330 m/sec
Fat	1450 m/sec
Water	1480 m/sec
Soft tissue	1540 m/sec
Blood	1570 m/sec
Muscle	1580 m/sec
Bone	4080 m/sec

▶ Knipe H, O'Gorman P, et al: Propagation speed. Available from Radiopaedia at https://radiopaedia.org/articles/propagation-speed.

▶ Rumack CM, Levine D (eds): *Diagnostic Ultrasound*, 5th edition. Philadelphia, Elsevier, 2018, pp 2–3.

▶ Siegel MJ (ed): *Pediatric Sonography*, 4th edition. Philadelphia, Lippincott Williams & Wilkins, 2011, pp 21–25.

594. **D. Harmonics.**

Tissue harmonic imaging *(THI or harmonics) reduces the width of the beam, which improves lateral resolution and minimizes artifacts. Harmonics can be helpful to improve the resolution of organs or lesions when patients are gassy or obese. A high-frequency sound beam or transducer is typically used for objects at shallower depths.* Extended-field-of-view imaging*, also known as* panoramic imaging*, generates a wider view of a structure that may not fit into a typical field of view.* 3D imaging *provides an additional dimension, allowing for multiplanar reconstruction. 3D imaging can be technically limited by a patient who is difficult to scan due to body habitus.*

▶ Rumack CM, Levine D (eds): *Diagnostic Ultrasound*, 5th edition. Philadelphia, Elsevier, 2018, p 1776.

▶ Siegel MJ (ed): *Pediatric Sonography*, 4th edition. Philadelphia, Lippincott Williams & Wilkins, 2011, pp 11–12, 384–385.

595. **A. M-mode.**

M-mode, or motion mode, is an ultrasound technique that evaluates the time and motion of a structure. Diaphragmatic movement, embryonic heartbeat, and fetal heart anatomy can be evaluated with M-mode ultrasound because these structures are in constant movement. B-mode, or brightness mode, refers to the real-time 2D imaging ultrasound technique that allows us to have gray-scale images. In real-time imaging, the moving structures can be observed, but unlike M-mode, B-mode cannot analyze or calculate movement and time. A-mode, or amplitude mode, displays the position and strength of a structure by using a y-axis and an x-axis to represent (respectively) the depth and the amplitude of the same. Thus, A-mode is not useful for the evaluation of the diaphragmatic movement. D-mode is not an ultrasound technique.

▶ Rumack CM, Levine D (eds): *Diagnostic Ultrasound*, 5th edition. Philadelphia, Elsevier, 2018, pp 9–10, 1716.

596. **D. Low pulse repetition frequency (PRF).**

Also known as velocity scale, pulse repetition frequency (PRF) is the number of pulses that occur in 1 second. A low PRF can help in the detection of lower Doppler frequencies, but aliasing can occur. Aliasing occurs when the frequency shift is greater than half the Doppler PRF (known as the Nyquist limit). With aliasing, these higher frequencies (above the Nyquist limit) "wrap around" the scale and are displayed in the color opposite to the mapped color. Increasing the PRF can help eliminate aliasing artifacts but may decrease or eliminate the detection of lower frequency shifts. PRF changes when the depth is adjusted. The deeper the depth, the lower the PRF. A shallow depth results in a higher PRF. Imaging at a shallower depth, using a transducer with a low Doppler frequency, increases the frequency shift, which helps to eliminate aliasing artifacts, not cause them.

▶ Echocardiographer.org: Aliasing. Available at http://www.echocardiographer.org/Echo%20Physics/Aliasing.html.

▶ Rumack CM, Levine D (eds): *Diagnostic Ultrasound*, 5th edition. Philadelphia, Elsevier, 2018, pp 29–30.

▶ Siegel MJ (ed): *Pediatric Sonography*, 4th edition. Philadelphia, Lippincott Williams & Wilkins, 2011, pp 35–36.

597. **C. The ability to display an entire vessel.**

One of the advantages of color Doppler imaging over pulsed Doppler imaging is the ability to display an entire vessel or most of it. With pulsed Doppler (duplex Doppler ultrasound), the area being evaluated is limited to the Doppler sample, so assessment of the entire vessel simultaneously cannot be done. With color Doppler imaging, measuring velocities is not possible, making this an advantage of pulsed Doppler imaging over color Doppler imaging. Both color and pulsed Doppler are angle-dependent, so inappropriate angles of insonation will affect the accuracy of the results displayed. Very slow capillary flow is not detectable with color Doppler imaging.

▶ Rumack CM, Levine D (eds): *Diagnostic Ultrasound*, 5th edition. Philadelphia, Elsevier, 2018, pp 24–25.

▶ Siegel MJ (ed): *Pediatric Sonography*, 4th edition. Philadelphia, Lippincott Williams & Wilkins, 2011, pp 16, 18.

598. **B. Anisotropy.**

Anisotropy is an artifact that occurs mainly when the tendons are imaged. The tendons are made of parallel collagen bundles and appear as hyperechoic, linear structures perpendicular to the sound beam. If the angle of insonation is not perpendicular when you are scanning the tendons, they may appear hypoechoic (anisotropic effect), causing a false appearance of pathologic findings. Anisotropic artifacts can be avoided by changing the angle of insonation to 90 degrees. Posterior shadowing is an artifact that occurs when the sound waves hit a highly reflective structure, causing posterior attenuation. Reverberation occurs when there is a highly reflective structure in the near field, causing echoes to appear as multiple lines equally separated deeper within the image. A side-lobe artifact may cause false echoes within fluid-filled structures inside the central beam. These false echoes are due to lateral echoes from highly reflective structures located outside the central beam.

▶ Rumack CM, Levine D (eds): *Diagnostic Ultrasound*, 5th edition. Philadelphia, Elsevier, 2018, pp 19, 21, 859.

▶ Siegel MJ (ed): *Pediatric Sonography*, 4th edition. Philadelphia, Lippincott Williams & Wilkins, 2011, pp 30–33.

599. A. Mirror-image.

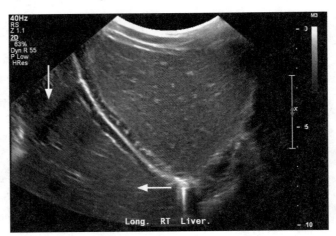

A mirror-image artifact *(arrows)* occurs when the sound beam encounters a highly reflective surface, resulting in a specular reflection. When the specular reflection is trying to return to the transducer but encounters another structure, the sound beam is then redirected and again sent back to the large, smooth interface before being reflected back to the transducer. Because the second reflected pulse takes longer to return to the transducer, it creates a duplicate or a mirror image deeper to the original. Therefore one can falsely assume that the structure is located deeper than it actually is. Mirror-image artifacts are commonly seen during liver scans because the diaphragm is a large, smooth interface. Reverberation artifacts *are multiple repeated reflections that are separated by equal-sized spaces due to a highly reflective interface. Reverberation artifacts are commonly seen in the near field and the bladder.* Refraction artifacts *can cause side duplication of a structure, distortion, or a shadowing artifact. Refraction artifacts occur when the angle between the ultrasound beam and an interface that propagates sound at a different speed is not a 90-degree angle (i.e., the beam and interface are not perpendicular).* A ring-down artifact *occurs when the sound beam encounters fluid located between gas bubbles that cause a vibration, which produces a continuous sound wave to be reflected.*

▸ Bickle I, Goel A, et al: Mirror image artifact. Available from Radiopaedia at https://radiopaedia.org/articles/mirror-image-artifact.

▸ Siegel MJ (ed): *Pediatric Sonography*, 4th edition. Philadelphia, Lippincott Williams & Wilkins, 2011, pp 21–28.

600. D. Enhance blood flow signals.

The purpose of using contrast agents in ultrasound is to enhance blood flow signals within an organ or specific lesion. The use of contrast with ultrasound allows for detection of very small vessels that are not visualized with color or power Doppler ultrasound. Contrast-enhanced ultrasound (CEUS) is especially useful in the evaluation of tumors because it helps identify the vascularity of the lesion when other techniques fail. CEUS involves gas-filled microbubbles that are injected directly into the bloodstream. A big advantage of CEUS over conventional studies is that it does not require the use of radiation, making it an excellent alternative for the pediatric population. Voiding urosonography (VUS) or contrast-enhanced voiding urosonography (ceVUS) is in the early stages of use, and it is anticipated that it will replace the traditional voiding cystourethrogram (VCUG). In the future, this may eliminate the need for fluoroscopy, thereby supporting the ALARA ("as low as reasonably achievable") principle of limiting exposure to ultrasound and radiation beams.

▶ Darge K: Voiding urosonography with ultrasound contrast agents for the diagnosis of vesicoureteric reflux in children. Pediatr Radiol 38:40–53, 2007. Available at https://www.ncbi.nlm.nih.gov/pmc/articles/PMC2292498/.

▶ Duran C, Beltrán VP, González A, et al: Voiding urosonography for vesicoureteral reflux diagnosis in children. RadioGraphics 37:1854–1871, 2017. Available at https://pubs.rsna.org/doi/10.1148/rg.2017170024.

▶ International Contrast Ultrasound Society: What is CEUS? Available at http://www.icus-society.org/about-ceus/what-is-ceus.

▶ Siegel MJ (ed): *Pediatric Sonography*, 4th edition. Philadelphia, Lippincott Williams & Wilkins, 2011, pp 18–19.

601. C. Gallbladder.

Side-lobe artifacts *are usually more visible when displayed within fluid-filled structures. These artifacts occur as result of highly reflective structures located in the lateral aspect of the ultrasound beam (where the least amount of energy is transmitted) but appear within the center of the image. The lateral reflectors are received with strong energy and are displayed as if they belonged to a structure within the center of the beam (where most of the energy is transmitted). This results in echoes misplaced to the center of the image and thus greatest visibility within fluid-filled structures. A very* common side-lobe artifact is seen within the gallbladder and appears as pseudosludge. Side-lobe artifacts cannot be differentiated in soft tissues. As is true for most of the ultrasound artifacts, scanning from a different angle may help clear this artifact. Tendons, air, and the diaphragm are less likely to generate side-lobe artifacts since they are not fluid-filled structures.

▶ Rumack CM, Levine D (eds): *Diagnostic Ultrasound*, 5th edition. Philadelphia, Elsevier, 2018, p 19.
▶ Siegel MJ (ed): *Pediatric Sonography*, 4th edition. Philadelphia, Lippincott Williams & Wilkins, 2011, pp 28–29.

602. **C. Displays the strength of the signal.**

Power Doppler displays the magnitude or strength of flow in color. Power Doppler is not dependent on angle and is sensitive to low flow, but it cannot provide information about flow velocity, direction of flow, or Doppler frequency—as is possible with color Doppler imaging. There is no aliasing with power Doppler, since this mode is not sensitive to the motion of reflectors and thus does not provide information about velocity. Power Doppler is sensitive to noise, however, and therefore it is not ideal for use with children because of the flash artifacts encountered with movement.

▶ Deane C: Doppler ultrasound: principles and practice. Available at https://sonoworld.com/client/Fetus/html/Doppler/capitulos-html/chapter_01.htm.
▶ Morgan MA, Kitamura FC, et al: Power Doppler. Available from Radiopaedia at https://radiopaedia.org/articles/power-doppler-1.
▶ Rumack CM, Levine D (eds): *Diagnostic Ultrasound*, 5th edition. Philadelphia, Elsevier, 2018, pp 25–26.
▶ Siegel MJ (ed): *Pediatric Sonography*, 4th edition. Philadelphia, Lippincott Williams & Wilkins, 2011, pp 17–18.

603. **B. Increase the wall filter.**

The wall filter sets a threshold used to eliminate frequency shifts. Sensitivity to slow flow is decreased when the wall filter is increased. A higher filter will eliminate more of the flow signal, as well as noise. Decreasing, not increasing, the Doppler frequency decreases the sensitivity to slow flow. Pulse repetition frequency (PRF) is the same as the velocity scale. To eliminate low frequency shifts, you would increase the PRF. To evaluate slow flow, a low PRF should be used. Packet size, also known as the dwell time, is the number of sound pulses transmitted per color sector line. To eliminate sensitivity to low flow, you would decrease the packet size or dwell time. An increased packet size will decrease the frame rate and line density, improving the sensitivity to low flow.

▸ Kruskal JB, Newman PA, Sammons LG, et al: Optimizing Doppler and color flow US: application to hepatic sonography. RadioGraphics 24:657–675, 2004. Available at https://pubs.rsna.org/doi/full/10.1148/rg.243035139.

▸ Rumack CM, Levine D (eds): *Diagnostic Ultrasound*, 5th edition. Philadelphia, Elsevier, 2018, pp 29–30.

▸ Siegel MJ (ed): *Pediatric Sonography*, 4th edition. Philadelphia, Lippincott Williams & Wilkins, 2011, p 34.

604. **B. Organ volume.**

Three-dimensional (3D) scanning *(also known as* volume ultrasound *or* volumetric sonography*) allows you to obtain the volumes of tissues or organs. The advantage of the 3D ultrasound over two-dimensional (2D) or B-mode imaging is that 3D acquires multiple planes at the same time, allowing for multiplanar reconstruction. This provides more information than conventional 2D ultrasound and the possibility of obtaining volumetric measurements of lesions. Tissue stiffness may be determined using* elastography. *Blood flow velocities are obtained by using* spectral Doppler *and measuring the desired velocities. To acquire movement and time together in an image (time-motion display),* M-mode *is the technique you would use.*

▸ Rumack CM, Levine D (eds): *Diagnostic Ultrasound*, 5th edition. Philadelphia, Elsevier, 2018, p 15.

▸ Siegel MJ (ed): *Pediatric Sonography*, 4th edition. Philadelphia, Lippincott Williams & Wilkins, 2011, pp 13–15.

605. **A. Cavitation.**

Ultrasound cavitation *is the formation and oscillation of a gas bubble in a liquid. These bubbles can form, move around, expand, and collapse. Pitting of a solid surface can occur during bubble oscillation or collapse. Ultrasound medical devices and their acoustic output are controlled in the United States by the Food and Drug Administration (FDA). The* mechanical index *(MI) on the machine is used to set a threshold and prevent the risk of cavitation. There are no confirmed adverse bioeffects at the diagnostic level. When there is an increase in temperature of more than 1 degree Celsius, thermal effects may include localized heating, which can lead to cell damage or necrosis. Thermal outputs are indicated in the* thermal index *(TI) settings on the machine. With Doppler, there is an increased risk of thermal effects. The terms* infiltration *and* extravasation *describe when blood, medicine, or fluid leaks out of its original and normal vascular pathway and into surrounding tissues.*

▸ Holland CK: Mechanical bioeffects from diagnostic ultrasound: AIUM consensus statements. J Ultrasound Med 19:67–72, 2000. Available at https://www.ncbi.nlm.nih.gov/pmc/articles/PMC1925043?.
▸ Kimmel E: Cavitation bioeffects. Crit Rev Biomed Eng 34:105–161, 2006. Available at https://www.researchgate.net/publication/7032839_Cavitation_Bioeffects.
▸ Rumack CM, Levine D (eds): *Diagnostic Ultrasound*, 5th edition. Philadelphia, Elsevier, 2018, p 35.

606. C. Gas bubbles.

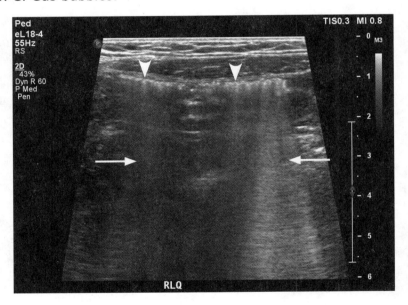

A ring-down artifact *(arrows) is commonly seen when gas (arrowheads) is hit by a sound beam, causing the fluid within a cluster of gas bubbles to vibrate. This vibration produces a continuous sound wave to be reflected. Fluid collections can cause* posterior enhancement *because there is less attenuation of the sound within the fluid, so the sound beam moves quickly through the fluid and hits the tissue deeper to the fluid with a greater intensity. Large, smooth interfaces, such as the diaphragm, are likely to cause* mirror images (see answer 599). Reverberation artifacts *occur when two parallel and highly reflective structures cause the sound beam to bounce back and forth between them. Reverberation commonly occurs in the near field.*

> Bost N, Morgan MA, et al: Ring down artifact. Available from Radiopaedia at https://radiopaedia.org/articles/ring-down-artifact-1.

> Siegel MJ (ed): *Pediatric Sonography*, 4th edition. Philadelphia, Lippincott Williams & Wilkins, 2011, pp 21–28.

607. D. Twinkle artifact.

See Color Plate 9 on page xxxvi.

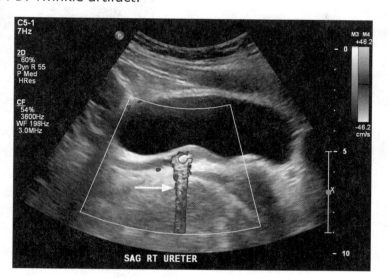

A twinkle artifact *(arrow) is seen posterior to a strong reflective interface when color Doppler is used. Twinkle artifacts appear as a mixture of colors posterior to the strong reflector, mimicking turbulent flow. This artifact is helpful in the detection of urinary tract stones that may not demonstrate posterior shadowing due to size or chemical makeup. Aliasing is an artifact caused when the pulse repetition frequency (PRF), or scale, is set too low. This leaves the received higher frequency shifts out of range, causing them to be displayed in the color opposite to the mapped color.* Doppler noise *can occur as result of pulsations or movement and may give the false appearance of color within adjacent structures. This can occur near the heart, especially in the left lobe of the liver and within cystic structures such as ascites and cysts.* Ring-down *is not a color Doppler artifact and appears as a bright linear echo posterior to a gas.*

> Rumack CM, Levine D (eds): *Diagnostic Ultrasound*, 5th edition. Philadelphia, Elsevier, 2018, pp 29–30.

> Siegel MJ (ed): *Pediatric Sonography*, 4th edition. Philadelphia, Lippincott Williams & Wilkins, 2011, pp 34–35, 37, 39.

608. A. Shadowing

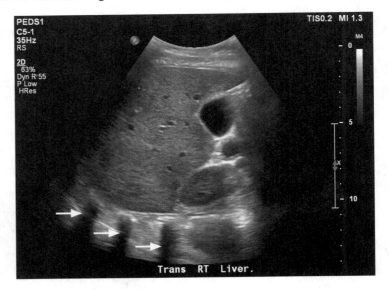

Shadowing *(arrows)* occurs when there is attenuation of the ultrasound beam due to a strong reflector. When the sound beam interacts with a highly reflective structure, the sound is absorbed and penetration of the beam is minimal or impossible. The result is a loss of information from structures deeper to the strong reflector. *Posterior shadowing (as seen here)* is a helpful artifact because it differentiates structures with specific characteristics, such as stones. *Posterior acoustic enhancement is the opposite of shadowing and occurs when the sound travels through a minimally attenuating (fluid-filled) structure, resulting in an intensification of the deeper echoes. Side-lobe artifacts appear as misplaced echoes in the center of the sound beam and are visible within cystic structures as false internal debris. Reverberation artifacts are multiple repeated reflections that are separated by equal spaces due to a highly reflective interface.*

▶ Rumack CM, Levine D (eds): *Diagnostic Ultrasound*, 5th edition. Philadelphia, Elsevier, 2018, pp 19, 21.

▶ Siegel MJ (ed): *Pediatric Sonography*, 4th edition. Philadelphia, Lippincott Williams & Wilkins, 2011, pp 30–31.

609. B. Decreasing the gain.

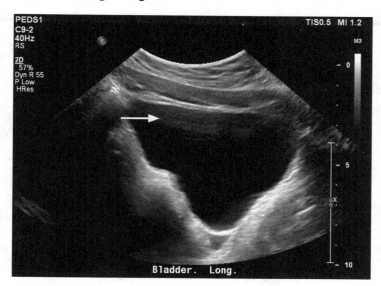

The artifact that is seen in the near field of the bladder is known as reverberation (arrow). Reverberation artifacts occur when the sound beam travels through lower-attenuating structures, such as cystic or soft-tissue structures, and then encounters a highly reflective interface, causing a repetition of the returning echoes. Reverberations are parallel to the sound beam and are always equally spaced because they are a repetition of the first returning signal. Reverberation artifacts are commonly seen in highly reflective near-field structures and also in the near field of the bladder or a cystic area. Decreasing the gain and power output, changing the transducer's position (making the cystic structure deeper), and using a standoff pad are adjustments that can be made to eliminate reverberation artifacts. Dynamic range, or compression, controls the shades of gray within the image. Decreasing the dynamic range will fill in areas of low attenuation with more grays, worsening a reverberation artifact. Increasing the number of focal zones will not help eliminate reverberation artifacts.

▶ Bell DJ, Morgan MA, et al: Reverberation artifact. Available from Radiopaedia at https://radiopaedia.org/articles/reverberation-artifact.

▶ Rumack CM, Levine D (eds): *Diagnostic Ultrasound*, 5th edition. Philadelphia, Elsevier, 2018, pp 9, 19.

▶ Siegel MJ (ed): *Pediatric Sonography*, 4th edition. Philadelphia, Lippincott Williams & Wilkins, 2011, pp 25–27.

610. **D. 60 degrees or less.**

The beam/vessel angle is the angle of insonation. The optimal beam/vessel angle is as close to zero as possible. When you are measuring absolute velocities, the acceptable beam/vessel angle is 60 degrees or less. To measure velocity, you should consider the Doppler frequency shift and angle of insonation in relation to the vessel in the calculation. At an angle of 90 degrees, there is no detectable Doppler frequency shift since there is no flow recognized going to or from the transducer. The more the angle of insonation is aligned with the direction of flow (0 degrees), the more the Doppler frequency increases and the more accurate the velocity measurement will be.

▶ Deane C: Doppler ultrasound: principles and practice. Available at https://sonoworld.com/client/Fetus/html/Doppler/capitulos-html/chapter_01.htm.

▶ Rumack CM, Levine D (eds): *Diagnostic Ultrasound*, 5th edition. Philadelphia, Elsevier, 2018, pp 4–5.

611. **A. Elastography.**

Elastography is an ultrasound technique used to evaluate the stiffness of normal and abnormal tissues. Elastography is helpful in evaluating the liver for fibrosis because the stiffness of the organ is altered with this pathology. With this noninvasive and convenient method, ten separate samples (ultrasound pulses) are obtained from the liver, and the returning information is averaged, recorded, and evaluated by a physician for a suggestive result. Contrast-enhanced ultrasound *(CEUS) is employed to enhance visualization of blood flow in an organ or lesion by using microbubbles.* 3D ultrasound *is used to obtain volumetric measurements of structures.* B-mode ultrasound *is the conventional method that provides 2D images in scales of gray. CEUS, 3D imaging, and B-mode do not provide information about a tissue's stiffness.*

▶ Rumack CM, Levine D (eds): *Diagnostic Ultrasound*, 5th edition. Philadelphia, Elsevier, 2018, pp 15–16.

▶ Siegel MJ (ed): *Pediatric Sonography*, 4th edition. Philadelphia, Lippincott Williams & Wilkins, 2011, pp 13–14, 18–19.

612. **B. Center it within the vessel.**

The gate (or sample volume) determines the Doppler sample, location, and size. When performing spectral Doppler, you should center the gate within the vessel and opened to include the majority of the vessel lumen. A gate that is too large (outside the lumen) can pick up flow from surrounding vessels. Larger sample volumes tend to increase noise and spectral broadening. A gate that is too small will leave out information. Angle correction is always important to utilize for accuracy of targeted velocities.

▶ Deane C: Doppler ultrasound: principles and practice. Available at https://sonoworld.com/client/Fetus/html/Doppler/capitulos-html/chapter_01.htm.

▶ de Bruyn R (ed): *Pediatric Ultrasound: How, Why and When*, 2nd edition (e-book). Philadelphia, Churchill Livingstone/Elsevier, 2010, p 8.

▶ Kruskal JB, Newman PA, Sammons LG, et al: Optimizing Doppler and color flow US: application to hepatic sonography. RadioGraphics 24:657–675, 2004. Available at https://pubs.rsna.org/doi/full/10.1148/rg.243035139.

▶ Siegel MJ (ed): *Pediatric Sonography*, 4th edition. Philadelphia, Lippincott Williams & Wilkins, 2011, pp 15–16.

PART 18

Patient Care and Management

613. C. Bleeding risk.

Coagulation testing *is a standard of care to assess the bleeding risk of a patient prior to surgery or invasive procedures. The body will naturally react to prevent blood loss by forming a thrombus when necessary. Clotting tests such as prothrombin time (PT) and partial thromboplastin time (PTT) are performed to evaluate the appropriate coagulation abilities. If lab values are not ideal, attempts to correct coagulopathy will be made or the procedure may be rescheduled.*

▶ Chee YL, Crawford JC, Watson HG, et al (British Committee for Standards in Haematology): Guidelines on the assessment of bleeding risk prior to surgery or invasive procedures. Brit J Haematol 140:496–504, 2008. Available at http://williams.medicine.wisc.edu/bleeding_risk_assessment_2008.pdf.

▶ Pietrangelo A: Coagulation tests. Available at https://www.healthline.com/health/coagulation-tests.

▶ Siegel MJ (ed): *Pediatric Sonography*, 4th edition. Philadelphia, Lippincott Williams & Wilkins, 2011, p 675.

614. C. Correct method.

The "time out" pre-procedural process is the verification specified by the Universal Protocol to ensure that the correct patient, correct procedure, and correct site have been identified prior to an interventional procedure or operation. A time out should be performed in the operating room or location of the procedure before the procedure is begun. This allows the healthcare team to pause and confirm the patient's identity, the procedure to be performed, and the location, side, or site. The correct method is not *one of the components of the Universal Protocol's time out procedure.*

▶ Chin S: Use "time outs" to re-establish focus and eliminate medical errors. Available at https://stanfordhealthcare.org/health-care-professionals/medical-staff/medstaff-update/2014-february/201402-patient-safety.html.

▶ Joint Commission: The Universal Protocol for preventing wrong site, wrong procedure, and wrong person surgery. Available at https://www.jointcommission.org/assets/1/18/UP_Poster.pdf.

▶ Stahel PF, Mehler PS, Clarke TJ, et al: The 5th anniversary of the "Universal Protocol": pitfalls and pearls revisited. Available at https://pssjournal.biomedcentral.com/articles/10.1186/1754-9493-3-14.

615. **D. Maintaining proper hand hygiene.**

Maintaining proper hand hygiene is the easiest and most effective way to prevent the spread of infectious disease. A large portion of the Standard Precautions addresses this topic, including standards for hand washing and the use of alcohol-based rubbing foam. Hand hygiene should be practiced before and after all patient contact, before entering a patient's room, and after exiting the patient's room. If handling patient equipment or personal belongings, you should also exercise hand hygiene before and after. It is also important to clean your hands following the removal of gloves. Wearing personal protective equipment (PPE) and not recapping needles are other components of the Standard Precautions, but hand hygiene is considered the most effective method of reducing the risk for cross-contamination and the spread of infectious diseases.

▸ Centers for Disease Control and Prevention: Hand hygiene in healthcare settings. Available at https://www.cdc.gov/handhygiene/index.html.

▸ World Health Organization: *WHO Guidelines on Hand Hygiene in Health Care*. Geneva, World Health Organization, 2009. Available at http://apps.who.int/iris/bitstream/handle/10665/44102/9789241597906_eng.pdf;jsessionid=EE15BEEB63FB0EEE158C12AAE9B4240A?sequence=1.

616. **A. Picture archiving and communication system.**

PACS stands for "picture archiving and communication system." PACS is a digital imaging system created for permanent image archiving for hospitals looking to become filmless. Images within the PACS system are permanent and are less likely to be lost, misfiled, or stolen. Reports are linked to the imaging studies. This system allows the images to be retrieved at any time of day from numerous computer terminals.

▸ Nagy P, Farmer J: Demystifying data storage: archiving options for PACS. Available at https://appliedradiology.com/articles/demystifying-data-storage-archiving-options-for-pacs.

▸ Strickland NH: PACS (picture archiving and communication systems): filmless radiology. Arch Dis Child 83:82–86, 2000. Available at https://www.ncbi.nlm.nih.gov/pmc/articles/PMC1718393/pdf/v083p00082.pdf.

617. C. Communicate the findings to the radiologist.

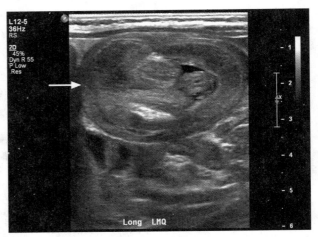

An intussusception (arrow) is a sonographic finding that requires urgent attention, so it is necessary to communicate the findings directly and immediately to the radiologist. Treatment is necessary to resolve the intussusception and avoid further complications. It is not the sonographer's responsibility to communicate results directly to the parents or ordering physician. Leaving the results for the radiologist for the following morning would constitute a delay of patient care and could result in further complications.

▶ del-Pozo G, Albillos JC, Tejedor D, et al: Intussusception in children: current concepts in diagnosis and enema reduction. RadioGraphics 19:299–318, 1999. Available at https://pubs.rsna.org/doi/full/10.1148/radiographics.19.2.g99mr14299.
▶ Shekherdimian S, Lee SL: Management of pediatric intussusception in general hospitals: diagnosis, treatment, and differences based on age. World J Pediatr 7:70–73, 2011. Available at https://www.ncbi.nlm.nih.gov/m/pubmed/21191779/.
▶ Siegel MJ (ed): *Pediatric Sonography*, 4th edition. Philadelphia, Lippincott Williams & Wilkins, 2011, pp 356, 358.

618. B. N95 respirator.

PPE stands for "personal protective equipment," which is worn to reduce the risk of exposure. Tuberculosis falls under airborne precautions, requiring an N95 respirator, a type of respirator that has a tighter-fitting seal than found in a normal mask. N95 respirators protect against infectious respiratory particles that may come from patients who are coughing, sneezing, or talking. Healthcare workers should be fitted yearly for N95 respirators and should know their size. Gloves are important to wear with all patients, but gloves will not protect against airborne particles.

▶ Centers for Disease Control and Prevention: Guidance for the selection and use of personal protective equipment (PPE) in healthcare settings. Available at https://www.cdc.gov/HAI/pdfs/ppe/PPEslides6-29-04.pdf.
▶ Centers for Disease Control and Prevention: Transmission-based precautions. Available at https://www.cdc.gov/infectioncontrol/bsics/transmission-based-precautions.html.
▶ Occupational Safety and Health Administration (OSHA): Personal protective equipment. Available at https://www.osha.gov/SLTC/personalprotectiveequipment/.

619. **A. Umbilical artery catheter (UAC).**

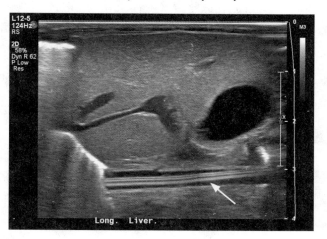

This image demonstrates an umbilical artery catheter or UAC (arrow) within the aorta of this neonate. The purpose of a UAC is to obtain blood gas samples, monitor pressures, administer fluids and drugs, and transfuse blood. Umbilical vein catheters (UVCs) are placed within the inferior vena cava to deliver fluids, blood, medicines, or total parenteral nutrition (TPN). A transjugular intrahepatic portosystemic shunt (TIPS) is utilized in patients with cirrhosis to connect the portal vein to the hepatic vein, bringing blood back to the heart while bypassing the liver. A ventriculoperitoneal shunt (VP shunt) relieves pressure caused by hydrocephalus. The shunt extends from the brain into the peritoneal cavity.

▶ Dagle J: Insertion of umbilical vessel catheters. Available at https://uichildrens.org/health-library/insertion-umbilical-vessel-catheters.
▶ Falck S: Ventriculoperitoneal shunt. Available at https://www.healthline.com/health/ventriculoperitoneal-shunt.

- RadiologyInfo.org: Transjugular intrahepatic portosystemic shunt (TIPS). Available at https://www.radiologyinfo.org/en/pdf/tips.pdf.
- UCSanDiegoHealth: Neonatal umbilical vessel catheterization. Available at https://health.ucsd.edu/medinfo/medical-staff/application/Documents/SP30%20Neonatal%20Umbilical%20Vessel%20Catherization%20(Neonatal).pdf.
- van Schuppen J, Onland W, van Rijn R: Lines and tubes in neonates. Available at http://www.radiologyassistant.nl/en/p526bd2e468b8c/lines-and-tubes-in-neonates.html.

620. **B. Hand washing with soap.**

Clostridium difficile (C. difficile) is a bacterium spread through contact. It can survive for long periods of time on people or objects. Contact precautions should be taken when working with the patient. Following patient care, the correct method of hand hygiene for C. difficile is washing your hands with soap and water. Alcohol-based foams have proven ineffective in killing the C. difficile spores.

- Centers for Disease Control and Prevention: Healthcare-associated infections. Available at https://www.cdc.gov/hai/organisms/cdiff/cdiff_clinicians.html.
- World Health Organization: Clean care is safer care. Available at https://www.who.int/gpsc/tools/faqs/system_change/en/.
- World Health Organization: Guide to appropriate hand hygiene in connection with *Clostridium difficile* spread. In *WHO Guidelines on Hand Hygiene in Health Care*. Geneva, World Health Organization, 2009. Available at https://www.ncbi.nlm.nih.gov/books/NBK144042/.

621. **D. Put the bed rails up in your absence.**

Patients who are at a risk for falls require specific intervention or supervision. Patient safety goals include fall prevention to eliminate additional harm or injury to the patient. Preventing falls reduces fall-related injury reporting in the workplace. Putting up the bed rails before you step away from the patient helps to prevent an accidental fall. Although it is good patient communication and care to tell the patient you will be right back and to leave the exam room door open, these measures will not ensure patient safety and prevent a fall from occurring. Temporarily sitting the patient up while you are away increases the fall risk.

- Agency for Healthcare Research and Quality: Preventing falls in hospitals. Available at https://www.ahrq.gov/professionals/systems/hospital/fallpxtoolkit/fallpxtk3.html.
- Joint Commission: Preventing falls and fall-related injuries in health care facilities. Available at https://www.jointcommission.org/assets/1/18/SEA_55.pdf.
- Stanford Health Care: Fall risk. Available at https://stanfordhealthcare.org/health-care-professionals/nursing/quality-safety/fall-risk.html.

622. C. Discuss your findings with the performing physician.

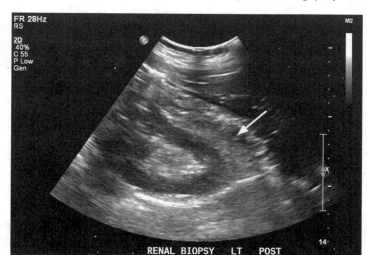

This image demonstrates a post-biopsy subcapsular hematoma (arrow). Acute hematomas are echogenic or hyperechoic. It is the sonographer's responsibility to convey any concerns or findings to the performing physician while in the OR. Although post-biopsy hematomas will usually resolve within a few months, the physician should be made aware of the complication so that patient follow-up or treatment can be performed appropriately. Leaving the finding to be dictated by the radiologist or telling your supervisor is not advised because it places the responsibility on someone else and may delay patient care.

▸ de Bruyn R (ed): *Pediatric Ultrasound: How, Why and When*, 2nd edition (e-book). Philadelphia, Churchill Livingstone/Elsevier, 2010, p 171.

▸ Shamshirgar F, Bagheri SM: Percutaneous ultrasound-guided renal biopsy: a comparison of axial vs. sagittal probe location. Rom J Intern Med 55:96–102, 2017. Available at https://www.degruyter.com/downloadpdf/j/rjim.2017.55.issue-2/rjim-2017-0011/rjim-2017-0011.pdf.

▸ Siegel MJ (ed): *Pediatric Sonography*, 4th edition. Philadelphia, Lippincott Williams & Wilkins, 2011, pp 445, 683.

623. B. Engage with the patient and explain the procedure.

Children under the age of 5 are often unsure or afraid of the process of having a medical exam. Engaging with the patient from the start helps earn the child's trust. Offer a compliment on a cute shirt or sparkly shoes or ask the name of a favorite stuffed animal that the child has brought to the waiting room. Such measures will ease the child's fear and make him or her more comfortable with you. Speaking to children about the exam in simple terms and explaining what you are going to do ahead of time will also help. Show them your "camera," let them touch the surface and see that it won't hurt, and show them the ultrasound gel you are going to use. Warming the gel is more comfortable for the patient. Helping children know what to expect will encourage their cooperation. These efforts go a long way with the parents as well. Seeing that you are trying to comfort their child from the start helps to put some of their own anxiety to rest. Books, TV, and toys can be good distractors. Restraints for children are not suggested; these tend to increase fear, anxiety, and combative behavior. Instead of scolding an uncooperative patient, work with the parent to find a compromise on a patient position or other method of cooperation. On many occasions a child can be scanned while lying beside the parent or being held by the parent. Although there may be times when you have to work to keep focused on the exam of a screaming or unruly child, you should avoid rushing an exam and always try to be as thorough as possible.

▶ de Bruyn R (ed): *Pediatric Ultrasound: How, Why and When*, 2nd edition (e-book). Philadelphia, Churchill Livingstone/Elsevier, 2010, pp 3–5.

▶ Rumack CM, Levine D (eds): *Diagnostic Ultrasound*, 5th edition. Philadelphia, Elsevier, 2018, pp 1628, 1776.

PART 20

Application for CME Credit

Pediatric Sonography Review

Objectives of This Activity
How to Obtain CME Credit
Applicant Information
Evaluation—You Grade Us!
Answer Sheet
CME Quiz

This continuing medical educational (CME) activity is approved for 12 hours of credit by the Society of Diagnostic Medical Sonography. This credit may be applied as follows:

- Sonographers and technologists may apply these Category A hours toward the CME requirements of the ARDMS, APCA, ARRT, and/or CCI, as well as to the CME requirements of most other organizations that may accredit your facility.
- SDMS-approved credit is not applicable toward the AMA Physician's Recognition Award but may be applicable to the CME requirements for physicians associated with accredited ultrasound facilities. Be sure to confirm requirements with the pertinent organizations.
- If you have any questions whatsoever about CME requirements that affect you, please contact the organization that governs your credential directly for current information. CME requirements can and sometimes do change.

Objectives of This Activity

Upon completion of this educational activity, you will be able to:

1. Describe and identify the ultrasound appearance of normal and abnormal pediatric anatomy and physiology.
2. Describe how, why, and when pediatric sonography is used.
3. Differentiate normal from abnormal findings and explain the correlations between these findings and pertinent laboratory and imaging studies.
4. Describe how, when, and why pediatric measurements are made using ultrasound.
5. Explain the role of congenital conditions in the practice of pediatric sonography.
6. Describe the sonographic findings in the presence of specific pediatric diseases, conditions, complications, and associated disorders.
7. Explain how to prepare for, perform, and explain the techniques of pediatric sonography.

How to Obtain CME Credit

To apply for credit, please do all of the following:

1. Read and study the mock exam questions.

2. Be sure to make photocopies of the blank forms below. Then use those photocopies to fill in your information and circle the answers. Keep the original forms in this book blank, and do not share your answers with others. That way you will always have the original set of blank forms in case you wish to make this CME activity available to others for their use.

3. Return the completed "Applicant Information" form, "Evaluation—You Grade Us!" questionnaire, and CME Answer Sheet, together with payment of the administrative processing fee of $39.50 (if you are the book's original purchaser) or $49.50 (for borrowers or purchasers of used books), by one of these methods:

Mail with enclosed paper check or credit card information to:

> Davies Publishing, Inc.
> CME Coordinator
> 32 South Raymond Avenue, Suite 4
> Pasadena, California 91105-1961

Fax the appropriate pages to 626-792-5308 and pay by credit card. Include credit card information on the applicant information form OR call in your credit card after faxing.

Email to cme@daviespublishing.com and pay by credit card. Include credit card information on the applicant information form OR call in your credit card after emailing.

We grade quizzes within 24 business hours of receipt and will email your certificate to the email address you provide in your application form. Questions? Please call us at 626-792-3046 or toll-free (within the continental United States) at 877-792-0005.

Applicant Information

Pediatric Sonography Review

Name _____ Date of birth _____

Your degrees and credentials _____

Address _____

City/State/ZIP _____

Telephone _____ Email (required) _____

ARDMS # _____ ARRT # _____ CCI # _____

SDMS # _____ Sonography Canada # _____

Payment Information

❏ I am the original purchaser of an unused (new) copy of this book (fee is $39.50).

❏ I borrowed the book or purchased it used (fee is $49.50).

Credit card # _____ Exp date _____ 3- or 4-digit code _____

Name and address on credit card (if different from above):

Name _____

Address _____

City/State/ZIP _____

Signature and date certifying your completion of the activity:

_____

NOTE: The original purchaser of this CME activity is entitled to submit this CME application for an administrative fee of $39.50. Please enclose a check payable to Davies Publishing, Inc., or include credit card information with your application. Others may also submit applications for CME credits by completing the activity for an administrative fee of $49.50. The CME administrative fee helps to defray the cost of processing, evaluating, and maintaining a record of your application and the credit you earn. Fees may change without notice. For the current fee, call us at 626-792-3046, email us at **cme@daviespublishing.com**, or write to us at the aforementioned address. We will be happy to help!

Evaluation—You Grade Us!

Please let us know what you think of *Pediatric Sonography Review*. Participating in this quality survey is a requirement for CME applicants, and it benefits future readers by ensuring that current readers are satisfied or, if not, that their comments and opinions are heard and taken into account.

1. Why did you purchase *Pediatric Sonography Review*? (Check your primary reason.)

    ❑ Registry review ❑ Course text

    ❑ Clinical reference ❑ CME activity

2. Have you used *Pediatric Sonography Review* for other reasons, too? (Check all that apply.)

    ❑ Registry review ❑ Course text

    ❑ Clinical reference ❑ CME activity

3. To what extent did *Pediatric Sonography Review* meet its stated objectives and your needs? (Check one.)

    ❑ Greatly ❑ Moderately

    ❑ Minimally ❑ Insignificantly

4. The content of *Pediatric Sonography Review* was (check one):

    ❑ Just right ❑ Too basic

    ❑ Too advanced

5. The quality of the questions, explanations, illustrations, and case examples was mainly (check one):

    ❑ Excellent ❑ Good

    ❑ Fair ❑ Poor

6. The manner in which *Pediatric Sonography Review* presents the material is mainly (check one):

    ❑ Excellent ❑ Good

    ❑ Fair ❑ Poor

7. If you used *Pediatric Sonography Review* to prepare for the registry exam, did you also use other materials or take any exam-preparation courses?

    ❏ No   ❏ Yes

    If yes, please specify what materials and courses:

    _____

    _____

    _____

8. If you used *Pediatric Sonography Review* for a course, please list the course name, the instructor's name, the name of the school or program, and any other textbooks you may have used:

    Course/instructor/school or program:

    _____

    _____

9. What did you like best about *Pediatric Sonography Review*?

    _____

    _____

    _____

    _____

10. What did you like least about *Pediatric Sonography Review*?

    _____

    _____

    _____

    _____

11. If you used *Pediatric Sonography Review* to prepare for your registry exam please answer these questions:

    Which exam did you take?

    ❏ ARDMS's PS exam

    ❏ Other: _____

    Did you pass?

    ❏ Yes   ❏ No   ❏ Haven't yet taken it

12. May we quote any of your comments in our catalogs or promotional material?

    ❏ Yes   ❏ No

    ❏ Further comment:

    _____
    _____
    _____
    _____
    _____
    _____
    _____
    _____
    _____
    _____
    _____

Answer Sheet

Pediatric Sonography Review

Circle the correct answer below and return this sheet to Davies Publishing, Inc. Passing criterion is 70% for attempt 1 and (for those who do not pass on the first attempt) 75% for attempts 2 and 3. Applicant may not have more than 3 attempts to pass.

1. A B C D	31. A B C D	61. A B C D	91. A B C D
2. A B C D	32. A B C D	62. A B C D	92. A B C D
3. A B C D	33. A B C D	63. A B C D	93. A B C D
4. A B C D	34. A B C D	64. A B C D	94. A B C D
5. A B C D	35. A B C D	65. A B C D	95. A B C D
6. A B C D	36. A B C D	66. A B C D	96. A B C D
7. A B C D	37. A B C D	67. A B C D	97. A B C D
8. A B C D	38. A B C D	68. A B C D	98. A B C D
9. A B C D	39. A B C D	69. A B C D	99. A B C D
10. A B C D	40. A B C D	70. A B C D	100. A B C D
11. A B C D	41. A B C D	71. A B C D	101. A B C D
12. A B C D	42. A B C D	72. A B C D	102. A B C D
13. A B C D	43. A B C D	73. A B C D	103. A B C D
14. A B C D	44. A B C D	74. A B C D	104. A B C D
15. A B C D	45. A B C D	75. A B C D	105. A B C D
16. A B C D	46. A B C D	76. A B C D	106. A B C D
17. A B C D	47. A B C D	77. A B C D	107. A B C D
18. A B C D	48. A B C D	78. A B C D	108. A B C D
19. A B C D	49. A B C D	79. A B C D	109. A B C D
20. A B C D	50. A B C D	80. A B C D	110. A B C D
21. A B C D	51. A B C D	81. A B C D	111. A B C D
22. A B C D	52. A B C D	82. A B C D	112. A B C D
23. A B C D	53. A B C D	83. A B C D	113. A B C D
24. A B C D	54. A B C D	84. A B C D	114. A B C D
25. A B C D	55. A B C D	85. A B C D	115. A B C D
26. A B C D	56. A B C D	86. A B C D	116. A B C D
27. A B C D	57. A B C D	87. A B C D	117. A B C D
28. A B C D	58. A B C D	88. A B C D	118. A B C D
29. A B C D	59. A B C D	89. A B C D	119. A B C D
30. A B C D	60. A B C D	90. A B C D	120. A B C D

CME Quiz

Pediatric Sonography Review

Please answer the following questions after you have studied *all* the mock-exam questions in the rest of this book. There is one best answer for each question. Circle it on the answer sheet. The passing criterion is 70% for attempt 1 and (for those who do not pass on the first attempt) 75% for attempts 2 and 3. The applicant can make no more than 3 attempts to pass and earn credit.

1. The largest part of the uterus in neonates and infants is typically the:

    A. Body
    B. Endometrium
    C. Cervix
    D. Fundus

2. In relation to the renal arteries, where are the main renal veins located?

    A. Anterior
    B. Medial
    C. Posterior
    D. Lateral

3. In comparison to adjacent muscle, the thyroid normally appears:

    A. Hypoechoic and heterogeneous
    B. Hypoechoic and homogeneous
    C. Isoechoic and homogeneous
    D. Hyperechoic and homogeneous

4. What is the name of the congenital hernia that occurs in the posterior portion of the diaphragm?

    A. Bochdalek hernia
    B. Morgagni hernia
    C. Spigelian hernia
    D. Hiatal hernia

5. Which bone forms the angle of the jaw?

    A. Vomer
    B. Mandible
    C. Maxilla
    D. Zygoma

6. Liver pathology that appears thick-walled and contains air suggests:

   A. Lymphoma
   B. Pyogenic abscess
   C. Hepatic cyst
   D. Hemangioma

7. The findings in this image (arrow) are from a 2-year-old patient with abdominal pain. What should you do?

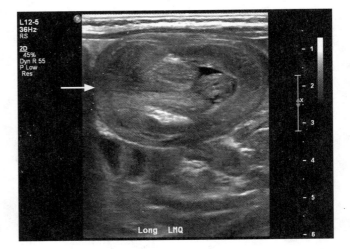

   A. Call the ordering physician with the results.
   B. Leave the results to be read in the morning.
   C. Tell the parent about the findings.
   D. Communicate the findings to the radiologist.

8. In relation to the left kidney, the left adrenal gland lies:

   A. Anteromedial
   B. Posterolateral
   C. Posteromedial
   D. Anterolateral

9. Given the findings in this image, what is the most likely diagnosis?

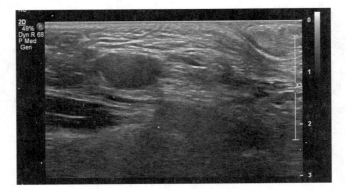

    A. Herniated omentum
    B. Cryptorchidism
    C. Hydrocele
    D. Herniated bowel

10. Ovotestis is associated with:

    A. True hermaphroditism
    B. Monorchidism
    C. Hypospadias
    D. Cryptorchidism

11. The arrows in this image are pointing at which type of artifact?

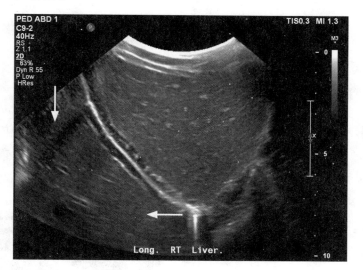

    A. Reverberation
    B. Ring-down
    C. Refraction
    D. Mirror-image

12. Which of the following fontanelles is best for axial imaging of the posterior fossa in the neonatal brain?

    A. Mastoid fontanelle
    B. Posterior fontanelle
    C. Sphenoidal fontanelle
    D. Anterior fontanelle

13. The fascia that covers the kidneys and adrenal glands is:

    A. Gerota's fascia
    B. Scarpa's fascia
    C. Psoas fascia
    D. Extraperitoneal fascia

14. Failure of midline closure of the infraumbilical abdominal wall results in:

    A. Megacystis
    B. Patent urachus
    C. Bladder diverticula
    D. Bladder exstrophy

15. Hepatization of the lungs can be caused by:

    A. Congenital pulmonary airway malformation (CPAM)
    B. Pneumothorax
    C. Empyema
    D. Atelectasis

16. An echogenic triangular focus or line within the renal cortex suggests:

    A. Fetal lobulations
    B. Dromedary hump
    C. Junctional parenchymal defect
    D. Hypertrophied column of Bertin

17. The cystic structure seen in this image is located in the gastrocnemius-semimembranosus bursa. What does it most likely represent?

    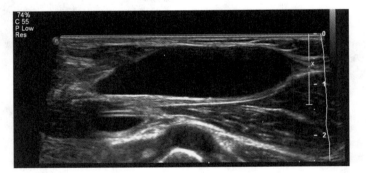

    A. Sebaceous cyst
    B. Meniscal cyst
    C. Ganglion cyst
    D. Baker's cyst

18. Which of the following is a type of subcutaneous soft tissue infection?

    A. Pyomyositis
    B. Phlebitis
    C. Dermatitis
    D. Cellulitis

19. This hypoxic neonate presented with a left abdominal mass and anemia. Given the findings in this postnatal sonogram, what is the most probable diagnosis?

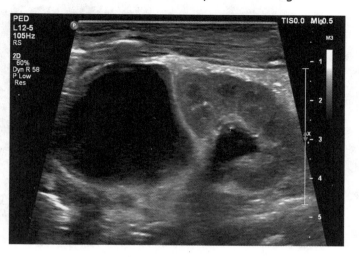

   A. Adrenal hypertrophy
   B. Adrenal hemorrhage
   C. Adrenal cyst
   D. Adrenocortical adenoma

20. Stones within the biliary ducts are known as:

   A. Cholecystitis
   B. Cholangitis
   C. Choledocholithiasis
   D. Cholestasis

21. Which of these sonographic characteristics helps you distinguish between a pancreatoblastoma and an adenocarcinoma?

   A. Presence of metastasis
   B. Presence of ascites
   C. Size
   D. Echogenicity

22. In the presence of liver damage all of the following may be elevated EXCEPT:

   A. Alkaline phosphatase (ALP)
   B. Alanine transaminase (ALT)
   C. Albumin
   D. Aspartate transaminase (AST)

23. What structure is the arrow in this image pointing to?

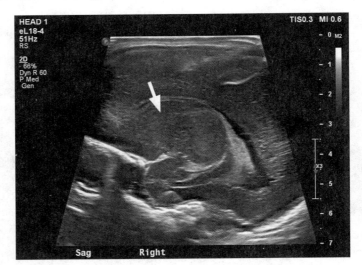

   A. Caudate nucleus
   B. Tentorium
   C. Pons
   D. Putamen

24. The urachus lies midline, superior and anterior to the peritoneum within the:

   A. Space of Retzius
   B. Anterior cul-de-sac
   C. Morison's pouch
   D. Pouch of Douglas

25. The most common malignant tumor of the small intestine in childhood is:

   A. Hodgkin lymphoma
   B. Adenocarcinoma
   C. Non-Hodgkin lymphoma
   D. Leiomyosarcoma

26. A premature infant in the neonatal care unit has an unexpected drop in hematocrit, and you are performing a "stat" head ultrasound. What pathology are you most concerned about?

   A. Hemorrhage
   B. Infection
   C. Hydrocephalus
   D. Malignant tumor

27. A sonographic characteristic that helps distinguish Graves' disease from Hashimoto's thyroiditis is:

    A. Lobulated contours
    B. Nodular formation
    C. Enlarged gland
    D. Hypervascularity

28. The free movement between the visceral and parietal pleura seen on ultrasound during respiration is known as the:

    A. Sliding sign
    B. Visceroparietal pleural sign
    C. Pleural sign
    D. Gliding sign

29. What is the most common malignant liver tumor in children?

    A. Liver metastases
    B. Hepatoblastoma
    C. Embryonal sarcoma
    D. Hepatocellular carcinoma

30. To evaluate for the presence of hip dysplasia in a 9-month-old, what can radiography do better than ultrasound?

    A. Accommodate the presence of a harness
    B. Lower the chances of patient movement during the exam
    C. Demonstrate the ossified femoral head more clearly
    D. Better maintain the infant's hip stability

31. The primary cause of acalculous cholecystitis is:

    A. Trauma
    B. Cholangitis
    C. Cholestasis
    D. Gallstones

32. What is the condition in which abnormal endometrial glands are found within the uterine myometrium?

    A. Endometrioma
    B. Adenomyosis
    C. Endometritis
    D. Leiomyoma

33. In a 10-year-old, the renal artery resistive index (RI) should be equal to or less than:

    A. 0.7
    B. 0.9
    C. 1.0
    D. 0.5

34. Epididymitis is commonly seen with:

    A. Bell-clapper deformity
    B. Intratesticular neoplasm
    C. Orchitis
    D. Testicular torsion

35. Which vessel is the arrow in this image pointing to?

    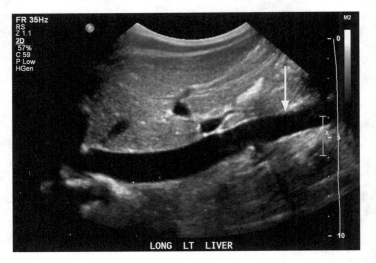

    A. Inferior vena cava (IVC)
    B. Azygos vein
    C. Portal vein
    D. Aorta

36. When you see the blue dot sign, which condition would you suspect?

    A. Testicular torsion
    B. Testicular trauma
    C. Testicular infarction
    D. Testicular appendage torsion

37. A 14-year-old male is undergoing abdominal ultrasound and you see this structure (arrow). This incidental finding is most likely:

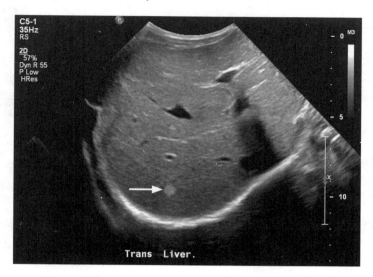

A. Mesenchymal hamartoma
B. Hemangioma
C. Hemangioendothelioma
D. Hepatoblastoma

38. During transabdominal pelvic sonography on a pediatric patient, why is a well-distended bladder important?

A. Eliminates the need for vaginal sonography
B. Displaces the bowel out of the pelvis
C. Displaces the ovaries medially
D. Determines presence of ambiguous genitalia

39. What parasite causes hydatid disease?

A. *Ascaris lumbricoides*
B. Amoeba
C. Schistosoma
D. *Echinococcus granulosus*

40. What type of measurement is possible using three-dimensional (3D) ultrasound?

A. Organ volume
B. Time-motion display
C. Tissue stiffness
D. Blood flow velocity

41. Failure or incomplete cleavage of the prosencephalon into the telencephalon and diencephalon during organogenesis results in:

    A. Lissencephaly
    B. Schizencephaly
    C. Holoprosencephaly
    D. Hydranencephaly

42. The connective tissue that encapsulates the liver is known as:

    A. Mesentery
    B. Glisson's capsule
    C. Peritoneum
    D. Gerota's fascia

43. This image from a 1-year-old patient demonstrates what type of hernia?

    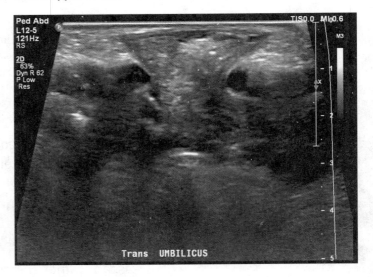

    A. Spigelian hernia
    B. Umbilical hernia
    C. Inguinal hernia
    D. Linea alba hernia

44. On ultrasound the normal newborn adrenal medulla appears thin and:

    A. Hyperechoic
    B. Anechoic
    C. Hypoechoic
    D. Heterogeneous

45. What is the most common cause of splenic vein thrombosis in children?

    A. Portal vein thrombosis
    B. Pancreatitis
    C. Trauma
    D. Infarction

46. Where will you see a tardus parvus waveform in higher-grade arterial stenosis?

    A. At the site of the stenosis
    B. Distal to the stenosis
    C. Nowhere
    D. Proximal to the stenosis

47. You just scanned a patient with *Clostridium difficile*. How should you clean your hands?

    A. Apply Betadine
    B. Wash with soap
    C. Wash with a solution of bleach and water
    D. Apply alcohol foam

48. Which of these abnormalities is NOT associated with prune belly syndrome?

    A. Hypoplastic/absent abdominal wall muscles
    B. Urinary tract anomalies
    C. Cryptorchidism
    D. Bilateral renal agenesis

49. What is the echogenicity of the normal pancreas in relation to that of the liver?

    A. Anechoic to the liver
    B. More than the liver
    C. Less than the liver
    D. Isoechoic to the liver

50. How many parathyroid glands do most people have?

    A. 2
    B. 4
    C. 3
    D. 1

51. What muscle lies immediately anteromedial to the hip capsule?

    A. Psoas major
    B. Iliopsoas
    C. Iliacus
    D. Rectus femoris

52. Where do the uterine arteries originate?

    A. Renal arteries
    B. Aorta
    C. Common iliac arteries
    D. Internal iliac arteries

53. What is the name of the uterine anomaly seen in this image?

    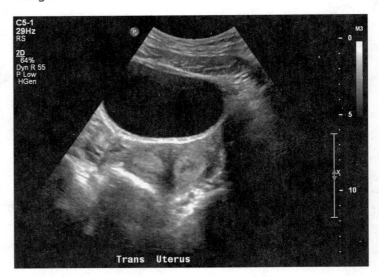

    A. Bicornuate uterus
    B. Septate uterus
    C. Uterine agenesis
    D. Uterus didelphys

54. In a preprandial patient, arteries traveling toward the liver should display:

    A. Hepatopetal low-resistance flow
    B. Hepatofugal low-resistance flow
    C. Hepatopetal high-resistance flow
    D. Hepatofugal high-resistance flow

55. What is the name of the echogenic, string-like extension from the conus medullaris?

   A. Cauda equina
   B. Leptomeninges
   C. Filum terminale
   D. Meninges

56. The arrows in this image are pointing to what type of artifact?

   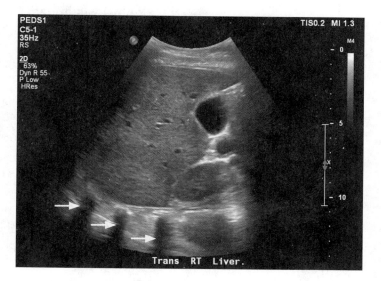

   A. Enhancement
   B. Reverberation
   C. Side-lobe artifact
   D. Shadowing

57. The procedure used to remove ductal stones or place a stent within the bile duct is:

   A. Magnetic resonance cholangiopancreatography (MRCP)
   B. Cholescintography
   C. Endoscopic retrograde cholangiopancreatography (ERCP)
   D. Kasai procedure

58. Which of these liver abnormalities is usually congenital?

   A. Cirrhosis
   B. Focal nodular hyperplasia (FNH)
   C. Arteriovenous malformation (AVM)
   D. Cavernous transformation

59. Increased neonatal head circumference and distention of the lateral and third ventricles with no dilatation of the fourth ventricle suggests:

    A. Cerebrospinal fluid (CSF) malabsorption
    B. Congenital aqueductal stenosis
    C. Chiari malformation
    D. Vein of Galen aneurysm

60. As renal failure progresses and becomes chronic, the kidneys will appear:

    A. Hydronephrotic
    B. Hyperechoic
    C. Hypoechoic
    D. Edematous

61. From which vessel does a vein of Galen malformation develop?

    A. Pericallosal artery
    B. Straight sinus
    C. Primitive prosencephalic vein
    D. Great vein of Galen

62. An ectopic pancreas is most commonly found in the:

    A. Spleen
    B. GI tract
    C. Liver
    D. Umbilicus

63. Biliary atresia is associated with which congenital anomaly?

    A. Gallbladder duplication
    B. Ectopic gallbladder
    C. Septate gallbladder
    D. Gallbladder agenesis

64. You see this echogenic intraluminal structure while scanning a neonate in the NICU. What is the most likely cause of this finding?

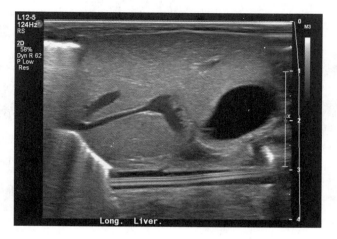

A. Ventriculoperitoneal shunt (VP shunt)
B. Transjugular intrahepatic portosystemic shunt (TIPS)
C. Umbilical artery catheter (UAC)
D. Umbilical vein catheter (UVC)

65. The most common benign ovarian mass in both pediatric and adult females is the:

A. Dysgerminoma
B. Functional cyst
C. Cystadenoma
D. Para-ovarian cyst

66. What structure is identified by the arrow in this longitudinal image of the scrotum?

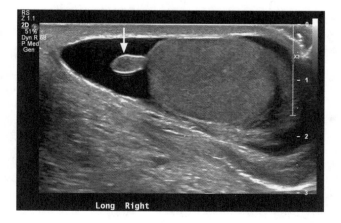

A. Testicular appendage
B. Epididymal tail
C. Scrotolith
D. Epididymal head

67. Which procedure most accurately diagnoses diffuse liver disease?

    A. Percutaneous biopsy
    B. Contrast ultrasound
    C. Abscess drainage
    D. Elastography

68. High-scale color Doppler can be used to demonstrate a twinkling artifact. This is useful in diagnosing which pathology?

    A. Cysts
    B. Abscesses
    C. Hematomas
    D. Stones

69. The calipers in this image indicate:

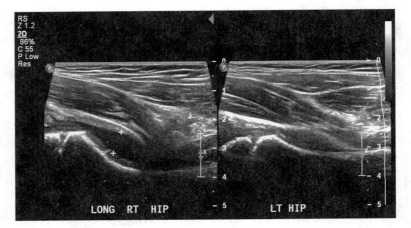

    A. Hip effusion
    B. Popliteal cyst
    C. Cellulitis
    D. Hip dysplasia

70. Gallbladder or liver disease is typically associated with elevated levels of:

    A. Alkaline phosphatase (ALP)
    B. Aldosterone
    C. Amylase
    D. Albumin

71. The typical appearance of a torsed testis after 6 hours is:

    A. Normal
    B. Hyperechoic
    C. Heterogeneous
    D. Hypoechoic

72. What is the name of the fusion anomaly that results in two complete uteri, cervices, and vaginas?

    A. Unicornuate uterus
    B. Bicornuate uterus
    C. Arcuate uterus
    D. Uterus didelphys

73. The brain of a full-term infant with microcephaly appears abnormally smooth on ultrasound. What is the most likely diagnosis?

    A. Lissencephaly
    B. Schizencephaly
    C. Hydranencephaly
    D. Intraparenchymal hemorrhage

74. What normal renal variant is the arrow in this image pointing to?

    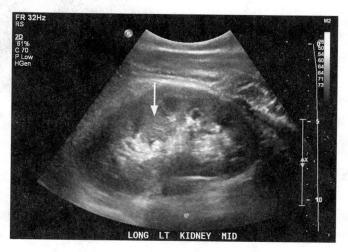

    A. Dromedary hump
    B. Junctional parenchymal defect
    C. Hypertrophied column of Bertin
    D. Fetal lobulation

75. A sonographic sign of air within the gallbladder is:

    A. Clean shadowing
    B. Posterior enhancement
    C. Ring-down artifact without shadowing
    D. Reverberation and ring-down artifact

76. The diameter of the pediatric main pancreatic duct should not exceed:

    A. 1 mm
    B. 2 mm
    C. 3 mm
    D. 4 mm

77. Which Graf classification of hip dysplasia do the findings in this image suggest?

    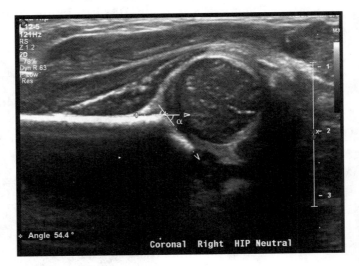

    A. Type I
    B. Type II
    C. Type III
    D. Type IV

78. The most common malignancy of the pediatric uterus or vagina is:

    A. Rhabdomyosarcoma
    B. Granulosa cell tumor
    C. Sertoli-Leydig tumor
    D. Adenocarcinoma

79. Infection within the bile ducts is known as:

    A. Choledocholithiasis
    B. Cholangitis
    C. Cholecystitis
    D. Cholestasis

80. You are performing renal ultrasound on a two-month-old infant. Which of the following is the best frequency for this scan?

    A. 5 MHz
    B. 8 MHz
    C. 9 MHz
    D. 12 MHz

81. This image demonstrates which type of intraventricular hemorrhage (IVH)?

    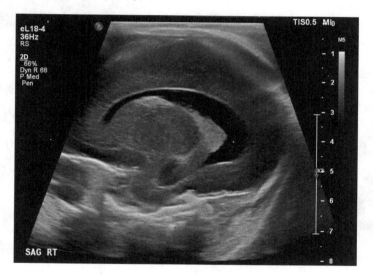

    A. Grade 1
    B. Grade 2
    C. Grade 3
    D. Grade 4

82. What are the characteristics of a normal peripheral arterial waveform?

    A. Biphasic and high-resistance
    B. Triphasic and high-resistance
    C. Triphasic and low-resistance
    D. Biphasic and low-resistance

83. Which renal arteries course between the renal pyramids?

    A. Interlobar
    B. Interlobular
    C. Arcuate
    D. Segmental

84. The duct that drains the gallbladder (arrow) is the:

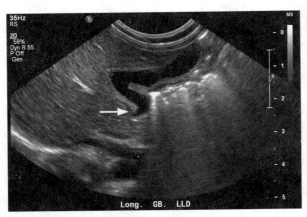

    A. Intrahepatic duct
    B. Common hepatic duct
    C. Common bile duct
    D. Cystic duct

85. By what age should the examination to detect developmental dysplasia of the hip (DDH) be performed?

    A. 4 weeks of age
    B. 6 weeks of age
    C. 8 weeks of age
    D. 12 weeks of age

86. What structure is the arrow in this image pointing to?

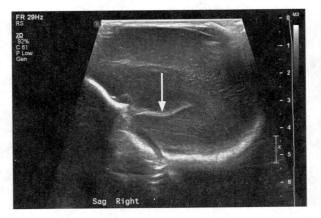

    A. Cingulate gyrus
    B. Sylvian fissure

C. Interhemispheric fissure
D. Cingulate sulcus

87. Which marker, released as a waste product in the blood after muscular exertion, is elevated when kidney function slows?

    A. Glomerular filtration rate (GFR)
    B. Blood urea nitrogen (BUN)
    C. Creatinine (CR)
    D. Alkaline phosphatase (ALP)

88. In this gastrointestinal duplication cyst, what does the echogenic inner layer represent?

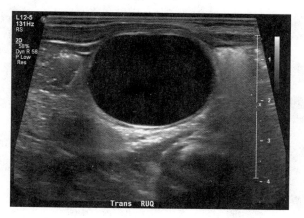

    A. Muscular layer
    B. Mucosal layer
    C. Fibrinous layer
    D. Serosal layer

89. You are scanning a gallbladder and image a polypoid mass. Which sonographic finding increases the risk of malignancy in this scenario?

    A. Hydrops
    B. Wall thickening
    C. Ductal dilatation
    D. Sludge

90. What is the name for abnormal clefts or slits in the brain parenchyma that extend through the entire hemisphere?

    A. Lissencephaly
    B. Schizencephaly
    C. Hydranencephaly
    D. Porencephaly

91. Why is percutaneous nephrostomy drainage performed?

    A. To obtain a biopsy sample
    B. To remove calculi
    C. To catheterize the bladder
    D. To relieve built-up pressure

92. The hormone that induces and maintains male sexual secondary characteristics is:

    A. Inhibin
    B. Luteinizing hormone (LH)
    C. Testosterone
    D. Estrogen

93. How many main sutures are there in the skull?

    A. 2
    B. 3
    C. 5
    D. 8

94. Compared to bone, the infant femoral head is cartilaginous and:

    A. Anechoic
    B. Isoechoic
    C. Hyperechoic
    D. Hypoechoic

95. Multiple abnormal vascular channels located between arteries and veins are known as:

    A. Pseudoaneurysm
    B. Thrombus
    C. Arteriovenous fistula
    D. Arteriovenous malformation

96. During embryonic organogenesis, what structure develops into the cerebrum, thalamus, and hypothalamus?

    A. Prosencephalon
    B. Metencephalon
    C. Rhombencephalon
    D. Mesencephalon

97. The femoral head coverage documented on this image is:

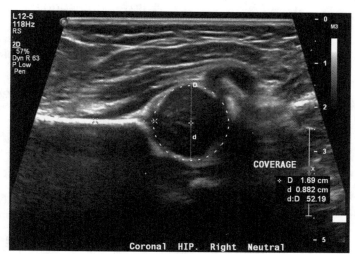

A. Normal
B. Subluxed
C. Dislocated
D. Shallow

98. A neonate presents with torticollis and a palpable mass in the right neck. What is the most likely diagnosis based on this image of the sternocleidomastoid muscle?

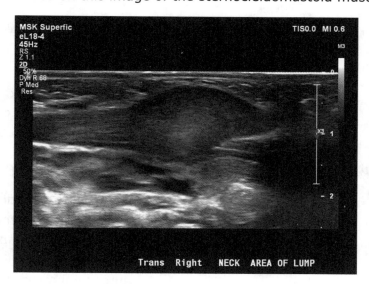

A. Aggressive fibromatosis
B. Nodular fasciitis
C. Inflammatory myofibroblastic tumor
D. Fibromatosis colli

99. A central stellate scar that appears echogenic on ultrasound suggests which benign liver tumor?

    A. Hamartoma
    B. Hemangioendothelioma
    C. Hemangioma
    D. Focal nodular hyperplasia (FNH)

100. An infant with acute reversible respiratory failure does not respond to conventional treatment. What type of technique can be used to treat this patient?

    A. Therapeutic hypothermia and brain cooling
    B. Tracheostomy
    C. Extracorporeal membrane oxygenation (ECMO)
    D. Dialysis

101. Premature infants are at higher than normal risk for which of these diseases?

    A. Pseudomembranous colitis
    B. Imperforate anus
    C. Necrotizing enterocolitis
    D. Intussusception

102. Which of the following is one of the most common pediatric inflammatory masses of the neck?

    A. Hemangioma
    B. Lymphadenopathy
    C. Thyroglossal duct cyst
    D. Fibromatosis colli

103. Which of these conditions is incompatible with life?

    A. Eagle-Barrett syndrome
    B. Bilateral renal agenesis
    C. Autosomal dominant polycystic kidney disease (ADPKD)
    D. Autosomal recessive polycystic kidney disease (ARPKD)

104. An increased risk of neural tube defects is associated an elevated level of:

   A. Inhibin-A
   B. Alpha-fetoprotein (AFP)
   C. Human chorionic gonadotropin (hCG)
   D. Folic acid

105. The best acoustic window for visualizing the pancreas is the:

   A. Right lobe of the liver
   B. Spleen
   C. Stomach
   D. Left lobe of the liver

106. What does this image of a unilateral small kidney with multiple noncommunicating cysts most likely indicate?

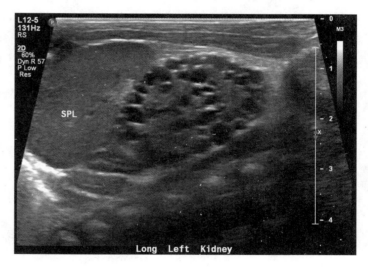

   A. Multicystic dysplastic kidney (MCDK)
   B. Glomerulocystic disease
   C. Autosomal recessive polycystic kidney disease (ARPKD)
   D. Autosomal dominant polycystic kidney disease (ADPKD)

107. Which of the following lesions is the most common primary benign tumor of the bowel in childhood?

    A. Polyp
    B. Lymphoma
    C. Hemangioma
    D. Duplication cyst

108. On ultrasound the normal spleen typically appears:

    A. Less echogenic than the adrenal gland
    B. More echogenic than the renal cortex
    C. More echogenic than the pancreas
    D. Less echogenic than the liver

109. Which sonographic finding helps differentiate between a neuroblastoma and a Wilms tumor?

    A. A solid mass
    B. Invasion or displacement of vessels
    C. A well-defined mass
    D. Lymphadenopathy

110. The phase of the endometrial cycle that occurs after ovulation is the:

    A. Secretory phase
    B. Luteal phase
    C. Menstrual phase
    D. Proliferative phase

111. What minimally invasive procedure is performed to diagnose disorders of the brain and spinal cord?

    A. Epidural
    B. Quad screen
    C. Laminotomy
    D. Lumbar puncture

112. The most common dorsal cutaneous stigma is a:

    A. Hemangioma
    B. Skin tag
    C. Sacral dimple
    D. Hair tuft

113. Name the sonographic characteristic that is associated primarily with acute renal failure:

    A. Large, edematous kidneys
    B. Decreased blood urea nitrogen (BUN) and creatinine (CR) levels
    C. Small, echogenic kidneys
    D. Thinned renal parenchyma

114. A penetrating injury or a femoral artery catheterization is commonly associated with which vascular complication?

    A. Nidus
    B. Arteriovenous malformation (AVM)
    C. Pseudoaneurysm
    D. Deep venous thrombosis (DVT)

115. Which pediatric malignancy of the spleen is most common in the presence of both non-Hodgkin and Hodgkin disease?

    A. Metastasis
    B. Leukemia
    C. Hamartoma
    D. Lymphoma

116. Which rare malignant liver tumor originates from the hepatic mesenchyme?

    A. Hepatoblastoma
    B. Hemangioendothelioma
    C. Hepatocellular carcinoma
    D. Undifferentiated embryonal sarcoma

117. What does an inflamed blind-ending, fluid-filled tubular structure arising from the ileum most likely indicate?

    A. Crohn disease
    B. Normal appendix
    C. Meckel diverticulum
    D. Appendicitis

118. What infection is the most common cause of meningitis in newborns?

    A. Group B streptococcus
    B. Haemophilus influenzae
    C. Cytomegalovirus (CMV)
    D. Enterococcus

119. An adolescent patient presents with symptoms of gradual acute scrotal pain and edema. What is the most likely diagnosis given this history and the findings in this image?

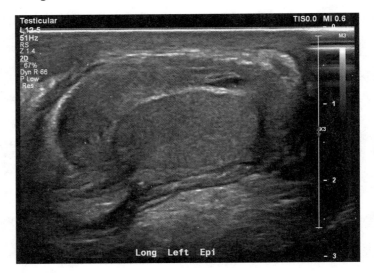

    A. Appendiceal torsion
    B. Epididymitis
    C. Testicular torsion
    D. Orchitis

120. Which of these procedures is performed by aspirating fluid from the chest?

    A. Paracentesis
    B. Pericardiocentesis
    C. Amniocentesis
    D. Thoracentesis

PART 21

Suggested Readings

Cohen HL, Sivit CJ: *Fetal and Pediatric Ultrasound: A Casebook Approach*. New York, McGraw-Hill, 2001.

de Bruyn R (ed): *Pediatric Ultrasound: How, Why and When*, 2nd edition (e-book). Philadelphia, Churchill Livingstone/Elsevier, 2010.

Deeg KH, Rupprecht T, Hofbeck M: *Doppler Sonography in Infancy and Childhood*. New York, Springer, 2015.

Hagen-Ansert SL (ed): *Textbook of Diagnostic Sonography*, 8th edition. St. Louis, Elsevier, 2018.

Husain AN, Stocker JT, Dehner LP (eds): *Pediatric Pathology*, 4th edition. Philadelphia, Wolters Kluwer, 2016.

Keough J: *Nursing Laboratory and Diagnostic Tests Demystified*, 2nd edition. New York, McGraw-Hill, 2017.

Kremkau FW: *Sonography: Principles and Instruments*, 9th edition. St. Louis, Elsevier, 2016.

Lazo DL: *Fundamentals of Sectional Anatomy: An Imaging Approach*, 2nd edition. Stamford, CT, Cengage Learning, 2015.

Riccabona M: *Pediatric Ultrasound: Requisites and Applications*. Berlin, Springer, 2014.

Rumack CM, Levine D (eds): *Diagnostic Ultrasound*, 5th edition. Philadelphia, Elsevier, 2018.

Scholz S, Jarboe MD (eds): *Diagnostic and Interventional Ultrasound in Pediatrics and Pediatric Surgery*. New York, Springer, 2016.

Siegel MJ (ed): *Pediatric Sonography*, 4th edition. Philadelphia, Lippincott Williams & Wilkins, 2011.

Stocker JT, Dehner LP, eds: *Pediatric Pathology*, 2nd edition, Philadelphia, Lippincott Williams & Wilkins, 2001.

PART 22

ARDMS Exam Content Outline Tasks Cross-Referenced to Mock Exam Questions

Publisher's note: *For your convenience, question numbers in this mock exam are arranged below under the task-related topics and subtopics of the latest ARDMS exam content outline for the Pediatric Sonography (PS) specialty exam. The questions and/or the explanations of the answers refer to the tasks for which they are listed. And if a question is relevant to more than one task, it is listed for every task to which it pertains. Why? To provide you with a framework for targeting study on specific clinical tasks.*

Remember that the ARDMS exam content outlines may be updated every few years. Always be sure to visit the ARDMS "Get Certified" page at www.ardms.org to view the latest exam content outlines.

Anatomy & Physiology—26%

Normal Anatomy

Evaluate anatomy of the neonatal brain and skull: *See questions* 1, 2, 3, 4, 6, 7, 8, 10, 11, 12, 13, 15, 16, 18, 23, 24, 30, 31, 34, 38, 39, 40, 41, 42, 46, 47, 48, 49, 51, 53, 54, 55, 56, 57, 58, 59, 60, 63, 65, 66, 67, 68, 69, 70, 71, 72, 73, 74, 75.

Evaluate anatomy of the neck and head (e.g., parotid glands, submandibular glands, thyroid): *See questions* 101, 102, 103, 104, 105, 106, 108, 109, 111, 112, 113, 114, 115, 119, 121, 122, 126, 127, 134, 135, 571.

Evaluate anatomy of the chest (e.g., pleural space, lung, thymus, diaphragm): *See questions* 136, 137, 138, 139, 140, 141, 142, 144, 147, 150, 153, 154, 417.

Evaluate anatomy of the gastrointestinal tract (e.g., esophagus, pylorus, stomach, bowel, appendix): *See questions* 161, 163, 165, 183, 417, 418, 419, 420, 421, 422, 424, 425, 426, 427, 428, 430, 437, 438, 439, 440, 446.

Evaluate anatomy of abdominal organs (e.g., liver, gallbladder, biliary tract, adrenal glands, pancreas, spleen): *See questions* 156, 157, 158, 159, 161, 162, 163, 165, 168, 169, 171, 174, 175, 176, 177, 178, 181, 184, 185, 187, 188, 190, 193, 194, 195, 198, 199, 200, 202, 204, 205, 207, 208, 209, 211, 212, 214, 215, 217, 222, 224, 230, 234, 236, 239, 243, 246, 256, 258, 259, 261, 264, 266, 267, 269, 270, 273, 274, 275, 277, 278, 279, 280, 282, 283, 284, 288, 289, 293, 301, 303, 305, 309, 391, 392, 393, 395, 396, 401, 402, 403, 406, 408, 409, 410, 411, 412, 413, 414, 415, 416.

Evaluate anatomy of genitourinary system (e.g., kidneys, bladder, uterus, ovaries, scrotum): *See questions* 162, 311, 312, 313, 316, 317, 318, 320, 322, 323, 324, 325, 327, 330, 338, 340, 342, 346, 347, 352, 353, 358, 359, 361, 366, 367, 369, 370, 371, 373, 376, 378, 381, 382, 383, 384, 385, 386, 389, 390, 479, 481, 482, 483, 484, 485, 486, 487, 488, 489, 490, 491, 492, 494, 495, 496, 497, 498, 499, 500, 501, 502, 503, 504, 505, 506, 507, 508, 509, 510, 511, 512, 513, 514, 515, 516, 517, 518, 519, 520, 521, 522, 523, 524, 526, 527, 528, 529, 530, 532, 533, 534, 535, 536, 537, 538, 539, 540, 541, 542, 543, 544, 545, 546, 547, 548, 549, 550, 551, 552, 553, 554, 555, 556, 557.

Evaluate musculoskeletal anatomy (e.g., hips, joints): *See questions* 58, 63, 106, 108, 147, 310, 447, 448, 450, 451, 452, 453, 455, 456, 457, 458, 459, 460, 461, 462, 463, 464, 465, 466, 467, 468, 469, 470, 471, 472, 473, 474, 475, 476, 477, 478, 559, 566, 569, 570, 572, 573, 576, 577.

Evaluate anatomy of superficial structures (e.g., breast, abdominal wall, soft tissue): *See questions* 310, 526, 537, 548, 566, 571, 573.

Evaluate anatomy of the neonatal spine: *See questions* 71, 76, 78, 80, 81, 82, 83, 88, 89, 90, 91, 93, 94, 95, 96, 97, 98, 99, 100.

Developmental Changes

Identify normal age-specific changes: *See questions* 34, 48, 53, 126, 136, 157, 163, 258, 311, 312, 313, 314, 321, 326, 330, 342, 348, 349, 352, 355, 357, 358, 369, 381, 385, 393, 395, 398, 401, 410, 416, 419, 422, 428, 436, 439, 442, 450, 462, 464, 473, 479, 480, 532, 536, 545.

Perfusion and Function

Evaluate peripheral vascular anatomy: *See questions* 111, 210, 467, 542, 578, 579, 580, 581, 582, 583, 584, 585, 586, 587, 588, 589, 590, 591, 592.

Evaluate abdominal vascular anatomy: *See questions* 157, 158, 163, 164, 165, 169, 170, 177, 180, 181, 183, 190, 191, 198, 201, 204, 208, 211, 214, 217, 259, 266, 275, 282, 293, 314, 320, 328, 329, 331, 340, 363, 389, 390, 396, 409, 427, 437, 443, 508, 514, 523, 534, 540, 542, 579, 588.

Evaluate intracranial vascular anatomy: *See questions* 2, 4, 12, 24, 40, 73, 75.

Evaluate transplants: *See questions* 186, 328, 334, 336, 337, 339.

Congenital Variants Pathology & Pathophysiology—45%

Neonatal Brain

Evaluate for congenital intracranial abnormalities (e.g., Dandy-Walker malformation, holoprosencephaly, callosal agenesis): *See questions* 2, 6, 10, 11, 13, 15, 19, 20, 24, 27, 30, 39, 42, 46, 59, 65, 69, 72, 87, 90.

Evaluate for neurocutaneous syndromes (e.g., tuberous sclerosis, Von Hippel-Lindau, Sturge-Weber): *See questions* 46, 189, 271, 319, 350, 368.

Evaluate for hydrocephalus/ventriculomegaly: *See questions* 2, 7, 13, 24, 47, 52, 64.

Evaluate for findings of hypoxic-ischemic insults in preterm and term infants: *See questions* 13, 17, 22, 45, 406.

Evaluate for intracranial hemorrhage, infection, and masses: *See questions* 5, 8, 9, 10, 14, 16, 21, 25, 26, 27, 29, 32, 35, 36, 37, 43, 44, 45, 47, 52, 61, 64.

Evaluate for findings related to sickle cell disease: *See questions* 242, 296, 298, 461.

Head and Neck

Evaluate for neck abnormalities (e.g., thyroglossal duct cyst, branchial cleft cyst, fibromatosis colli): *See questions* 101, 103, 106, 109, 110, 116, 118, 126, 128, 130, 131, 571.

Evaluate for thyroid abnormalities (e.g., goiter, nodules, masses, enlargement): *See questions* 107, 109, 117, 119, 120, 123, 124, 125, 129, 132, 133.

Chest

Evaluate for chest abnormalities (e.g., pleural effusion, sequestration, congenital pulmonary airway malformation, masses): *See questions* 136, 137, 141, 143, 145, 149, 150, 151, 152, 155.

Evaluate for congenital diaphragmatic hernia and diaphragmatic paralysis (M-mode): *See questions* 139, 144, 148, 595.

Gastrointestinal

Evaluate for gastrointestinal abnormalities (e.g., appendicitis, volvulus, pyloric stenosis, necrotizing enterocolitis, intussusception, masses): *See questions* 146, 161, 183, 325, 418, 419, 421, 422, 423, 424, 426, 427, 428, 429, 431, 432, 433, 434, 435, 437, 439, 440, 441, 442, 443, 444, 445.

Hepatobiliary

Evaluate for hepatobiliary disease (e.g., infection, obstruction, parenchymal liver disease, biliary atresia, hepatoblastoma): *See questions* 160, 163, 168, 170, 172, 176, 179, 180, 182, 183, 184, 185, 189, 190, 191, 193, 194, 195, 196,

197, 199, 200, 202, 203, 205, 207, 209, 210, 211, 212, 213, 216, 218, 219, 220, 223, 224, 225, 226, 227, 228, 229, 230, 231, 232, 233, 235, 237, 238, 240, 241, 242, 244, 247, 248, 249, 250, 251, 252, 253, 254, 255, 257, 369.

Adrenal Glands, Pancreas, and Retroperitoneum

Evaluate adrenal glands for abnormalities (e.g., neuroblastoma, hyperplasia, hemorrhage): *See questions* 393, 398, 399, 401, 405, 406, 407, 409, 410, 411, 412, 413, 414, 415, 416.

Evaluate for pancreatic abnormalities (e.g., pancreatitis, cystic fibrosis, congenital anomalies, fatty replacement): *See questions* 254, 260, 262, 264, 265, 267, 268, 271, 272, 276, 277, 279, 280, 281, 284, 285, 286, 287, 308.

Evaluate retroperitoneum for masses (e.g., lymphadenopathy): *See questions* 264, 268, 319, 330, 333, 352, 357, 385, 393, 401, 405, 409, 411, 412, 571.

Spleen and Peritoneal Cavity

Evaluate for splenic abnormalities (e.g., polysplenia, infection, masses): *See questions* 291, 292, 294, 295, 296, 297, 298, 300, 302, 303, 304, 305, 306, 307, 308, 461, 622.

Evaluate for peritoneal cavity abnormalities (e.g., ascites, abscess): *See questions* 149, 186, 209, 232, 291, 307, 429.

Genitourinary System

Evaluate for congenital renal abnormalities (e.g., horseshoe, duplication anomalies, cystic diseases): *See questions* 189, 311, 313, 314, 315, 319, 322, 324, 327, 329, 331, 332, 336, 337, 338, 341, 342, 349, 350, 355, 357, 360, 361, 363, 364, 365, 366, 367, 368, 369, 376, 377, 378.

Evaluate for acquired renal abnormalities (e.g., obstruction, infection, masses): *See questions* 311, 313, 314, 315, 319, 322, 324, 327, 329, 330, 331, 332, 333, 334, 335, 336, 337, 338, 341, 343, 344, 345, 348, 352, 353, 354, 355, 357, 360, 361, 363, 365, 369, 370, 376, 377, 381, 382, 383, 385, 386, 388, 390.

Evaluate for ureter and bladder abnormalities (e.g., infection, ureterocele, urachal anomalies, obstruction, vesicoureteral reflux, masses): *See questions* 311, 315, 323, 325, 326, 335, 338, 344, 346, 359, 360, 361, 362, 364, 365, 366, 370, 373, 379, 384, 387.

Evaluate female genital tract for abnormalities (e.g., hematometrocolpos, torsion, masses): *See questions* 325, 481, 484, 485, 487, 489, 491, 492, 493, 494, 496, 497, 498, 499, 500, 502, 503, 504, 505, 506, 507, 509, 511, 513, 515, 517, 518, 519, 520, 521, 522.

Evaluate male genital tract for abnormalities (e.g., infection, hydroceles, cryptorchidism, torsion): *See questions* 524, 527, 528, 529, 530, 531, 533, 534, 535, 536, 538, 539, 540, 541, 543, 546, 547, 550, 551, 552, 553, 554, 555, 556, 557.

Musculoskeletal, Superficial Structures, and Hernias

Evaluate the hip for developmental dysplasia: *See questions* 106, 447, 449, 451, 452, 455, 459, 462, 463, 468, 469, 471, 473, 474, 477.

Evaluate for joint effusion in hips or other joints: *See questions* 448, 454, 458, 461, 464.

Evaluate tendons and synovium for abnormalities (e.g., tenosynovitis, synovial hypertrophy): *See questions* 464, 558, 559, 563, 573, 577, 598.

Evaluate superficial structures for abnormalities (e.g., foreign bodies, infections, masses): *See questions* 79, 558, 561, 562, 563, 565, 567, 568, 574, 575, 576.

Evaluate glands and soft tissues for abnormalities (e.g., infection, lymph nodes, masses): *See questions* 106, 107, 109, 110, 116, 117, 118, 124, 125, 126, 129, 130, 132, 133, 145, 151, 200, 260, 264, 268, 271, 276, 281, 285, 286, 291, 393, 398, 401, 405, 406, 407, 410, 411, 412, 413, 414, 415, 416, 485, 487, 493, 496, 497, 498, 499, 502, 503, 504, 505, 506, 511, 513, 515, 517, 519, 520, 524, 527, 528, 530, 531, 533, 534, 535, 538, 539, 540, 541, 543, 547, 551, 552, 555, 556, 557, 558, 560, 561, 562, 563, 565, 567, 568, 571, 573, 574, 575, 576.

Evaluate for hernias (e.g., direct, indirect, inguinal): *See questions* 139, 144, 531, 553, 560.

Neonatal Spine

Evaluate for spinal malformations (e.g., tethered cord, myelomeningocele, caudal regression): *See questions* 11, 76, 77, 80, 81, 82, 85, 86, 87, 89, 90, 91, 93, 94, 96, 97, 98, 100.

Vascular and Transplants

Evaluate for peripheral vascular malformations: *See questions* 2, 4, 143, 205, 562, 580, 583.

Evaluate for abdominal vascular malformations: *See questions* 164, 165, 190, 205, 292, 580.

Evaluate for intracranial vascular malformations: *See questions* 2, 4, 12, 24, 40.

Evaluate vessels and intravascular lines for abnormalities (e.g., thrombosis, pseudoaneurysm, stenosis): *See questions* 164, 170, 180, 190, 210, 211, 308, 329, 331, 363, 579, 580, 581, 582, 583, 586, 587, 589, 619.

Evaluate transplant complications (e.g., thrombus, stenosis): *See questions* 186, 334, 336, 337, 339.

Data and Protocols—19%

Outside Data (clinical assessment, history and physical [H&P], lab values)

Verify appropriateness of the order and obtain pertinent clinical history from the patient and/ or medical records (including previous imaging): *See questions* 4, 21, 25, 27, 33, 35, 36, 59, 62, 80, 84, 89, 104, 114, 123, 136, 146, 153, 160, 193, 202, 207, 213, 240, 243, 262, 286, 296, 299, 304, 305, 330, 333, 341, 351, 375, 377, 417, 425, 427, 432, 436, 443, 462, 464, 473, 481, 568, 586, 600, 613.

Assess relevant patient signs and symptoms for examination being performed: *See questions* 5, 27, 28, 32, 33, 77, 79, 85, 88, 101, 106, 118, 125, 146, 182, 202, 229, 240, 250, 272, 296, 298, 307, 330, 332, 337, 341, 355, 356, 357, 365, 413, 418, 419, 422, 428, 429, 437, 439, 443, 445, 448, 449, 456, 460, 461, 467, 473, 497, 499, 509, 511, 517, 535, 552, 558, 563, 567, 574, 617.

Explain examination requirements to patient (positioning, gel application, transducer pressure): *See questions* 166, 220, 224, 229, 374, 623.

Clinical Standards and Guidelines

Communicate examination preparation requirements (e.g., fasting, bladder filling): *See questions* 166, 201, 220, 224, 229, 236, 262, 374, 462, 494, 623.

Modify imaging protocols based on clinical history and/
or sonographic findings (e.g., premature, critically ill,
uncooperative patients): *See questions* 23, 33, 41, 50,
62, 87, 356, 442, 449, 458, 462, 464, 494, 623.

Utilize multiple patient positions: *See questions* 78, 167, 215,
220, 231, 234, 242, 252, 316, 339, 345, 358, 425, 454,
457, 471, 540, 623.

Utilize appropriate acoustic windows and scanning planes:
See questions 23, 38, 40, 43, 49, 62, 84, 105, 122, 146,
167, 177, 204, 206, 234, 283, 339, 417, 425, 440, 454,
455, 458, 477, 494, 586.

Communicate ultrasound findings and relevant patient
information to interpreting healthcare provider: *See
questions* 201, 617, 622.

Measurement Techniques

Obtain appropriate measurements: *See questions* 7, 64, 83,
126, 163, 180, 181, 203, 224, 225, 258, 267, 273, 326,
349, 358, 415, 418, 422, 429, 433, 440, 441, 447, 451,
452, 455, 468, 469, 477, 479, 482, 489, 495, 497, 498,
511, 512, 515, 540, 545, 604, 610.

Obtain Doppler velocities and measurements: *See questions*
40, 180, 201, 203, 206, 314, 329, 331, 390, 443, 499,
581, 610.

Physics and Instrumentation—5%

Imaging Instruments

Select appropriate examination techniques (e.g., M-mode,
B-mode, Doppler, harmonic imaging): *See questions* 50,
61, 84, 136, 143, 148, 150, 206, 207, 220, 263, 340,
354, 356, 358, 372, 398, 415, 440, 454, 525, 564, 572,
594, 595, 596, 597, 602, 604, 607, 611, 612.

Adjust console settings to optimize images (e.g., depth
settings, artifact recognition, artifact correction when
appropriate): *See questions* 21, 35, 206, 215, 223, 231,
344, 354, 363, 441, 499, 525, 564, 593, 594, 596, 598,
599, 601, 602, 603, 605, 606, 607, 608, 609, 612.

Apply as low as reasonably achievable (ALARA) principle
(e.g., thermal index, mechanical index): *See questions*
600, 605.

Treatment and Emerging Technology—5%

Managing Medical Emergencies and Traumatic Injury

Recognize findings that require immediate attention: *See questions* 21, 25, 97, 182, 183, 192, 249, 286, 296, 332, 334, 337, 356, 365, 380, 422, 427, 428, 429, 436, 437, 439, 464, 499, 517, 524, 547, 552, 567, 613, 617, 622.

Evaluate for abnormalities due to traumatic events: *See questions* 13, 17, 21, 22, 25, 33, 35, 41, 44, 45, 97, 148, 192, 195, 249, 286, 300, 302, 304, 334, 339, 346, 356, 380, 398, 406, 547, 567, 574.

Interventional Procedures

Assist/support ultrasound guidance during interventional procedures: *See questions* 92, 131, 149, 197, 339, 343, 436, 568, 600, 622.

Evaluate for post-procedure changes: *See questions* 186, 337, 339, 356, 380, 467, 619, 622.

Disinfection

Maintain infection control (e.g., low-level disinfection techniques, high-level disinfection techniques, sterile techniques): *See questions* 87, 90, 92, 131, 149, 614, 615, 618, 620.

Emerging Technology

Recognize emerging technology applications (e.g., elastography, contrast): *See questions* 197, 203, 600, 604, 611, 616.